Designing Intelligent Healthcare Systems, Products, and Services Using Disruptive Technologies and Health Informatics

Disruptive technologies are gaining importance in healthcare systems and health informatics. By discussing computational intelligence, IoT, blockchain, cloud and big data analytics, this book provides support to researchers and other stakeholders involved in designing intelligent systems used in healthcare, its products and its services.

This book offers both theoretical and practical application-based chapters and presents novel technical studies on designing intelligent healthcare systems, products and services. It offers conceptual and visionary content comprising hypothetical and speculative scenarios and will also include recently developed disruptive holistic techniques in healthcare and the monitoring of physiological data. Metaheuristic computational intelligence-based algorithms for analysis, diagnosis and prevention of disease through disruptive technologies are also provided.

Designing Intelligent Healthcare Systems, Products, and Services Using Disruptive Technologies and Health Informatics is written for researchers, academicians and professionals to bring them up to speed on current research endeavours, as well as introduce hypothetical and speculative scenarios.

Artificial Intelligence in Smart Healthcare Systems

Series Editors:
Vishal Jain and Jyotir Moy Chatterjee

The progress of the healthcare sector is incremental as it learns from associations between data over time through the application of suitable big data and IoT frameworks and patterns. Many healthcare service providers are employing IoT-enabled devices for monitoring patient health care, but their diagnosis and prescriptions are instance-specific only. However, these IoT-enabled healthcare devices are generating volumes of data (Big-IoT Data), that can be analysed for more accurate diagnosis and prescriptions. A major challenge in the above realm is the effective and accurate learning of unstructured clinical data through the application of precise algorithms. Incorrect input data leading to erroneous outputs with false positives shall be intolerable in healthcare as patient's lives are at stake. This new book series addresses various aspects of how smart healthcare can be used to detect and analyse diseases, the underlying methodologies and related security concerns. Healthcare is a multidisciplinary field that involves a range of factors like the financial system, social factors, health technologies and organisational structures that affect the healthcare provided to individuals, families, institutions, organisations and populations. The goals of healthcare services include patient safety, timeliness, effectiveness, efficiency and equity. Smart healthcare consists of m-health, e-health, electronic resource management, smart and intelligent home services and medical devices. The Internet of Things (IoT) is a system comprising real-world things that interact and communicate with each other via networking technologies. The wide range of potential applications of IoT includes healthcare services. IoT-enabled healthcare technologies are suitable for remote health monitoring, including rehabilitation, assisted ambient living, etc. In turn, healthcare analytics can be applied to the data gathered from different areas to improve healthcare at a minimum expense.

This new book series is designed to be a first choice reference at university libraries, academic institutions, research and development centres, information technology centres and any institutions interested in using, design, modelling and analysing intelligent healthcare services. Successful application of deep learning frameworks to enable meaningful, cost-effective personalised healthcare services is the primary aim of the healthcare industry in the present scenario. However, realising this goal requires effective understanding, application and amalgamation of IoT, Big Data and several other computing technologies to deploy such systems in an effective manner. This series shall help clarify the understanding of certain key mechanisms and technologies helpful in realising such systems.

Designing Intelligent Healthcare Systems, Products, and Services Using Disruptive Technologies and Health Informatics
Teena Bagga, Kamal Upreti, Nishant Kumar, Amirul Hasan Ansari and Danish Nadeem

Designing Intelligent Healthcare Systems, Products, and Services Using Disruptive Technologies and Health Informatics

Edited by
Teena Bagga, Kamal Upreti, Nishant Kumar,
Amirul Hasan Ansari and Danish Nadeem

CRC Press
Taylor & Francis Group
Boca Raton London

CRC Press is an imprint of the
Taylor & Francis Group, an **informa** business

First edition published 2023
by CRC Press
6000 Broken Sound Parkway NW, Suite 300, Boca Raton, FL 33487–2742

and by CRC Press
4 Park Square, Milton Park, Abingdon, Oxon, OX14 4RN

CRC Press is an imprint of Taylor & Francis Group, LLC

© 2023 Taylor & Francis Group, LLC

ISBN: 978-1-032-10800-1 (hbk)
ISBN: 978-1-032-10801-8 (pbk)
ISBN: 978-1-003-21710-7 (ebk)

DOI: 10.1201/9781003217107

Typeset in Times
by Apex CoVantage, LLC

Contents

Editor Biographies

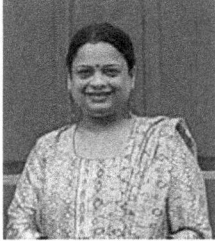

Teena Bagga is an instructor and researcher with over 20 years of experience. Since 2001 she has been a professor at Amity Business School, Amity University, Noida. Her areas of specialisation are information systems, business analytics and project management. She has published around 80 research papers in various national and international journals and has written case studies which are included in the Case Centre, UK. Her research interests are e-business, digital marketing, education quality, strategy, information systems, e-governance, smart applications and business analytics. She has organised several guest lectures, seminars and conferences and delivered keynote addresses at various platforms. In addition, she is an active editorial board member and reviewer of reputed national and international journals. She also has one copyright and one patent to her credit.

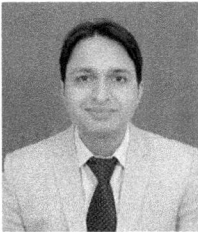

Kamal Upreti is currently working as Associate Professor in the Department of Computer Science and Engineering, Dr. Akhilesh Das Gupta Institute of Technology and Management affiliated to Guru Govind Singh Indraprastha University, Delhi, India. He previously worked with HCL, NECHCL, Hindustan Times, Dehradun Institute of Technology and Delhi Institute of Advanced Studies, gaining more than nine years of rich experience in research working in academia and the corporate environment. He also worked at NECHCL in Japan on the project 'Hydrastore' funded by a joint collaboration between HCL and NECHCL Company. Dr. Upreti has attended national and international conferences as a session chair and been a keynote speaker in various platforms. He was awarded best teacher, best researcher, extra academic performer and gold medalist in the M. Tech program. He has published patents, books, magazines and research papers in various national and international conferences and journals. His research area includes cyber security, data analytics, wireless networking, embedded system, neural networks and artificial intelligence.

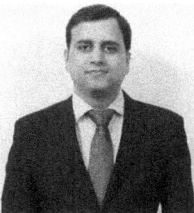

Nishant Kumar is currently working as an assistant professor in the Amity School of Business, Amity University, Noida (India). Previously to that he worked with Doon University, Delhi Institute of Advanced Studies, HCL Infosystems Ltd., gaining more than nine years of rich experience in academics, research and the corporate environment. Dr. Kumar has published patents, book chapters and research papers in journals with ABDC classification and is also a member and on the editorial review board of national and international journals. He has presented papers at various national and international conferences and has won an outstanding research paper award. His research interests include intelligent computation technologies, data analytics, customer relationship management techniques, e-commerce, multivariate statistical analysis, model development and validation using PLS-SEM and AMOS.

Amirul Hasan Ansari is the director of the Centre for Management Studies, Jamia Millia Islamia. He entered academia with national and international corporate experience, with an acclaimed career span of about 30+ years in teaching, research and consultancy. He has been invited to be a part of several prestigious national and international academic and professional bodies. His current research interest is focused on issues related to emotional intelligence, knowledge management, leadership, HR analytics and hospital administration. He has a good number of national and international publications to his credit and has published two books. Dr. Ansari has successfully completed several UGC-sponsored major projects and is a team leader who leads by example. He is respected for his humble demeanour and visionary administrative skills. During his distinguished career he has had many accomplishments and is hailed as an institution builder, a be loved teacher and a passionate researcher.

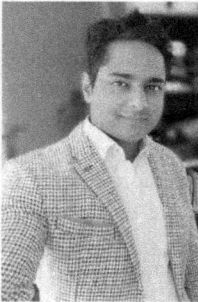

Danish Nadeem is a senior data scientist and technical consultant working in the Netherlands. Along with his education in computer science and artificial intelligence from Germany, he has over 18 years of industry and research experience in the applications of cutting-edge artificial intelligence (AI)–based and machine learning technologies while working within EU-funded framework and Horizon 2020 projects. Working in industries such as education, health, pharmaceuticals, media and entertainment, finance and logistics, he has also contributed to about 13 research publications in various international conferences and journals. He spent several years working in research and development at the German Research Centre for Artificial Intelligence before moving to the Netherlands to further develop his career by taking up leading roles advocating for innovative information and communication technologies.

Contributors

Chaitanya P. Agrawal
Makhanlal University
Bhopal, India

Meena Agrawal
Maulana Azad National Institute of
    Technology
Bhopal, Madhya Pradesh, India

Mohammad Rehan Ajmal
University of Tabuk
Saudi Arabia

Mohammad Shabbir Alam
Jazan University
Saudi Arabia

Ahmad Mohammad Ayaz
University of Tabuk
Saudi Arabia

Sushant Bhargava
Indian Institute of Management
Lucknow
Lucknow, India

Akshita S. Chanchlani
Sant Gadge Baba Amravati University
Amravati, India

Sangya Chattopadhyay
MCKV Institute of Engineering
India

Richi Chhabra
Deenbadhu Chotu Ram University of
Science and Technology
India

Elisandro Pires Frigo
Federal University of Paraná
Brazil

Ankit Garg
Institute of Management Studies
Ghaziabad, India

Vivek Garg
University of Greenwich
United Kingdom

Dhanashri H. Gawali
Sant Gadge Baba Amravati
University
Amravati, India

Anil Hiwale
MIT World Peace University
Pune, India

Rituraj Jain
Wollega University
Nekemte, Ethiopia

S. Kannadhasan
Cheran College of Engineering
India

Deepak Kumar
Amity Institute of Geoinformatics &
Remote Sensing
India

Ela Kumar
Indira Gandhi Delhi Technical
University for Women
India

Juli Kumari
Indira Gandhi Delhi Technical
University for Women
India

Soma Mitra
Brainware University
Kolkata, West Bengal, India

Venkatesh Krishna Murthy
Wharf Street Strategies Limited
London, United Kingdom

Syed Khalid Mustafa
University of Tabuk
Saudi Arabia

R. Nagarajan
Gnanamani College of
Technology
India

Mauparna Nandan
Brainware University
Kolkata, West Bengal, India

Mohammad Shahnawaz Nasir
Jazan University
Saudi Arabia

Kumud Ranjan Pal
Seharabazar C.K. Institution
India

Divya Pant
Institute of Management Studies
Ghaziabad, India

Antara Parai
Siliguri Institute of Technology (SIT)
Siliguri, West Bengal, India

Minakshee Patil
Sinhgad Academy of Engineering
Pune, India

Sourik Pyne
MCKV Institute of Engineering
India

Khalid Ali Qidwai
Jazan University
Saudi Arabia

Archana Ranade
Deenanath Mangeshkar Hospital and
Research Centre
Pune, India

Archisman Roy
Banaras Hindu University
India

Neha P. Sathe
MIT World Peace University
Pune, India

Saumya Satija
Indira Gandhi Delhi Technical
University for Women (IGDTUW)
India

Shampa Sengupta
MCKV Institute of Engineering
India

Umesh Kumar Singh
Vikram University
Ujjain, India

Mohd Tajuddin
Jeddah Regional Lab
Mahjar, Jeddah, Saudi Arabia

Charles Roberto Telles
Federal University of Paraná
Brazil

Vilas M. Thakare
Sant Gadge Baba Amravati University
Amravati, India

Anuj Tripathi
Affle (India) Limited
India

Binu Kuriakose Vargis
Inderprastha Engineering College
Ghaziabad, India

Naveen Virmani
Institute of Management Studies
Ghaziabad, India

Sushant Kumar Vishnoi
Institute of Management Studies
Ghaziabad, India

Vijay M. Wadhai
D.Y. Patil College of Engineering
Pune, India

1 Telemedicine (e-Health, m-Health)

Requirements, Challenges and Applications

Mauparna Nandan[1], Soma Mitra[1], Antara Parai[2], Rituraj Jain[3], Meena Agrawal[4] and Umesh Kumar Singh[5]

[1] Brainware University West Bengal, India
[2] Siliguri Institute of Technology (SIT), West Bengal, India
[3] Electrical and Computer Engineering, Wollega University, Ethiopia
[4] Maulana Azad National Institute of Technology, Bhopal, India
[5] Vikram University, Ujjain, India

CONTENTS

DOI: 10.1201/9781003217107-1

1

1.1   INTRODUCTION

The increase in population and the increase in life expectancy in populated countries creates a severe problem in terms of catering to the healthcare facilities in the remote corners of the country [1]. In the 21st century, with the invention of new information and communication technology (ICT) tools, telemedicine technology has emerged as a stepping stone to address some of the challenges in providing rapid accessibility, cost-effective and high-quality healthcare services, especially for the people residing in remote and underprivileged areas and is now heralding a new genre in the healthcare industry. Telemedicine primarily focuses on the use of ICT tools, namely the Internet, computers and cell phones, which have great potential in bringing innovative approaches and providing a sustainable solution to address the contemporary global health issues confronted by developing countries [2]. It is implemented by sending electronic information, thereby providing and supporting healthcare when it becomes impossible to cater to distant people. It has emerged as a revolutionary tool that aids in digitising patient information, providing online appointments with doctors, generating online reports and providing remote access to such medical imaging and online payment modes for patient empowerment [3].

The term telemedicine originated from the Greek word '*tele*', which means 'distance' and the Latin word '*mederi*', which means 'to heal'. It was coined in the 1970s and literally means 'healing at a distance'. Although at a rudimentary level, it is considered 'futuristic' and 'experimental', in the future, telemedicine is going to be the lifeline of millions of citizens in a country. It has an assortment of implementations in education, administration, research and patient care. Throughout the world people living in distant corners of the country strive to have good-quality specialty medical care in time. People in these areas could only find poor-quality access to healthcare, chiefly because specialist physicians are reluctant to relocate themselves in the sparsely populated areas instead of the areas of concentrated urban populations [4]. Telemedicine has emerged with the immense potentiality to bridge the gap between quality healthcare and these remote areas. To summarise, although telemedicine literally means 'medicine at a distance', in a broader sense, telemedicine is the usage of innovative telecommunication technologies to deliver healthcare services to persons who are separated by geographic, temporal, social or cultural barriers. From the technological point of view, telemedicine can be conceived as a confluence of medical informatics, healthcare services and telecommunications which incorporates hardware, software, medical equipment and fast and uninterrupted communication links for its implementation. In other words, telemedicine encompasses all aspects of healthcare from one location to another, including diagnosis, consultation, treatment, education, data transmission and all other facets of healthcare.

Thus, the significance of telemedicine lies in the optimisation of all possible existing healthcare systems and for the development of efficient, in-time, standard, patient-oriented healthcare worldwide. Telemedicine encompasses healthcare services like disease diagnosis, treatment and proper monitoring of patients, delivering expert advice to patients and enhancing the knowledge base of patients as shown in Figure 1.1. Apart from these, telemedicine also includes services like teleradiology or telepathology beyond the conventional medical facilities [5].

Telehealth, a broader aspect of telemedicine, specifically refers to providing both remote medical services like telemedicine as well as remote non-clinical services such as providing a training facility to medical staff, conducting administrative meetings and promoting medical education.

Telehealth is an agglomeration of numerous technologies to ensure a compact and total package of medication, medical treatment and continuous monitoring of the health data of the patient in a real-time format [5]. Clinical services are not always incorporated in telehealth. Videoconferencing, still picture transmission, remote vital sign monitoring, ongoing medical education and supportive call centres are all examples of telehealth. Telehealth encompasses the following concepts, as illustrated in Figure 1.2.

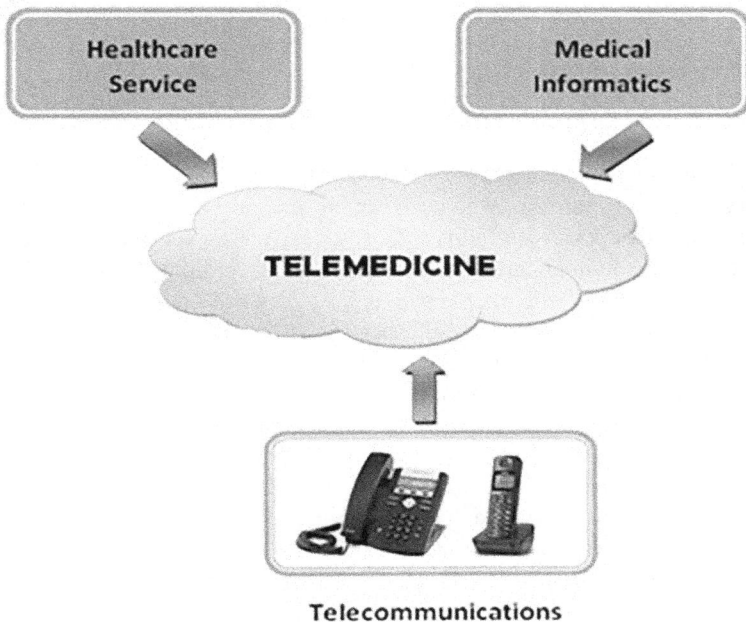

FIGURE 1.1   Telemedicine from a technological viewpoint.

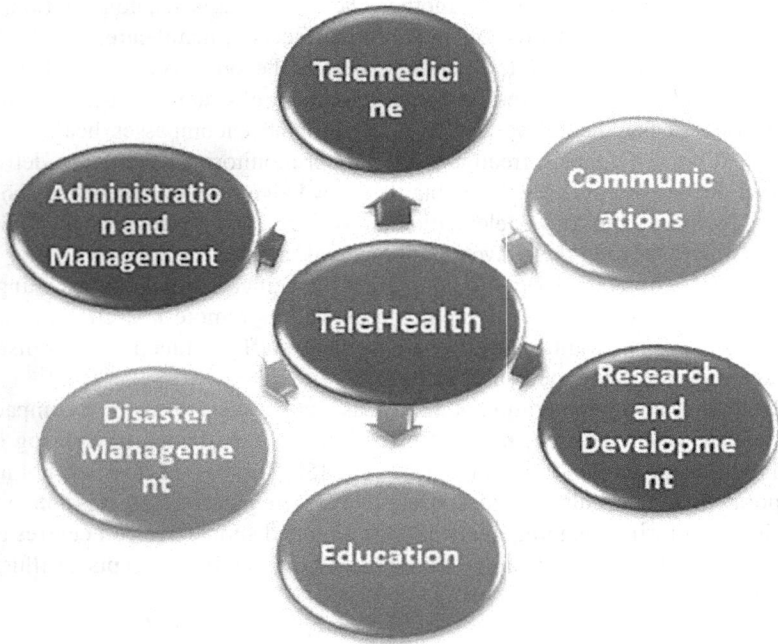

FIGURE 1.2   Relationship between telehealth and telemedicine.

1.2   ORIGINS AND HISTORY

The origins of current telemedicine applications were pioneered in 1905 by a Dutch physician, Willem Einthoven, who used remote-distance electrocardiogram (ECG) transmission. After reviewing numerous sources, it was verified that the earliest clinical telemedicine application was in the field of cardiology and not in radiology. In the early 1900s, patients onboard ships at sea and on distant islands used to receive radio consultations from health centres in Norway, Italy and France. Thus, telemedicine has a long history as per Table 3, when it first evolved in the mid-to-late 19th century when electricity and radio [6] were invented, and then in the early 20th century, when one of the earliest recorded examples of electrocardiograph data was transferred via telephone wires [7] with the advancement of television and the Internet. Telemedicine began to boom in the 1960s, where it was mainly implemented in the military and space technology industries [6, 8]. In early days, telemedicine was mainly used in the psychiatric institutes to arrange a face-to-face consultation between a patient and doctor, using a primitive technology, a television set [9], as well providing real-time medical advice from a nearby medical college to the airport medical centre [10–11].

1844	1875	1905	1927	1972	1990	2003	2015-
•Electric Telegraph invented by Samuel Morse	• Alexander Graham Bell invented Telephone	• William Einthoven invented the EKG machine	• Philo Taylor Farnsworth invented the world's first electronic television	• NASA developed STARPAHC project	• Tim Berners-Lee invented World Wide Web (WWW)	• Skype Video chat was introduced	• Healthcare mobile apps, Video Conferencing

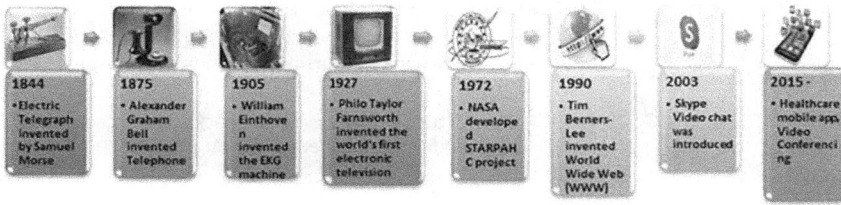

FIGURE 1.3 Evolution of telemedicine.

Telemedicine grew in popularity in rural areas, where people have very restricted access to healthcare but can now consult professionals from remote areas. The Public Health Service, National Aeronautics and Space Administration (NASA), the Department of Defense and the United States government all worked together in the 1960s and 1970s to develop new technologies. The Department of Health and Human Services (DHHS) has invested both time and money towards telemedicine research. The relationship between the Indian Health Services and NASA was one of the most successful and pioneering projects of government undertakings as shown in Figure 1.3.

Although today's telehealth gadgets resemble older telemedicine technology, they are smaller in size but possess a wider range of functionality. Mobile health gadgets that measure patients' critical data in real time include wearables like fitness wristbands and heart rate monitors. Physicians currently use smart glasses and smart watches, which relieves them of onerous paperwork. Augmedix is a digital health company that utilises Google Glass to automatically transcribe medical records while a patient is being examined. For the telemedicine sector, there still exist a lot of unexplored challenges that need to be addressed. And thus, the corporate and government-owned research companies are engaging themselves extensively in telemedicine, such that the technology advances at a breakneck pace and becomes the future in every human life. Broadly speaking, the healthcare market operates through these different segments which are illustrated in Figure 1.4.

1.3 LITERATURE REVIEW

A few decades back the healthcare system gave little priority to ICT tools because the Internet and web-based technologies were in a nascent stage then. In spite of this, the need for a hospital information system standard was necessary. The international Health Level Seven (HL7) standards [12] were first formed in 1987. In 1994, the organisation received accreditation from the American National Standards Institute (ANSI). The OSI Reference Model refers to the seventh layer as the application layer of the Open Systems Interconnection protocol. This international standardisation standard is currently used as a reference by ISO, publishing a number of frameworks and standards related to healthcare. As e-health took off at the beginning of the

Hospitals	• **Government Hospitals** - Healthcare centres, district hospitals • **Private Hospitals** - Nursing homes, private hospitals
Pharmaceutical	• Manufacturing, processing and packaging of chemical compounds used for medication purposes
Diagnostics	• Comprises of companies and labs that provide diagnostics or analytical services
Medical Equipments and Supplies	• Establishments primarily manufacturing medical equipment and supplies
Medical Insurance	• Incorporates both health insurance and medical services like reimbursement facility
Telemedicine	• Provides healthcare delivery to rural and remote areas

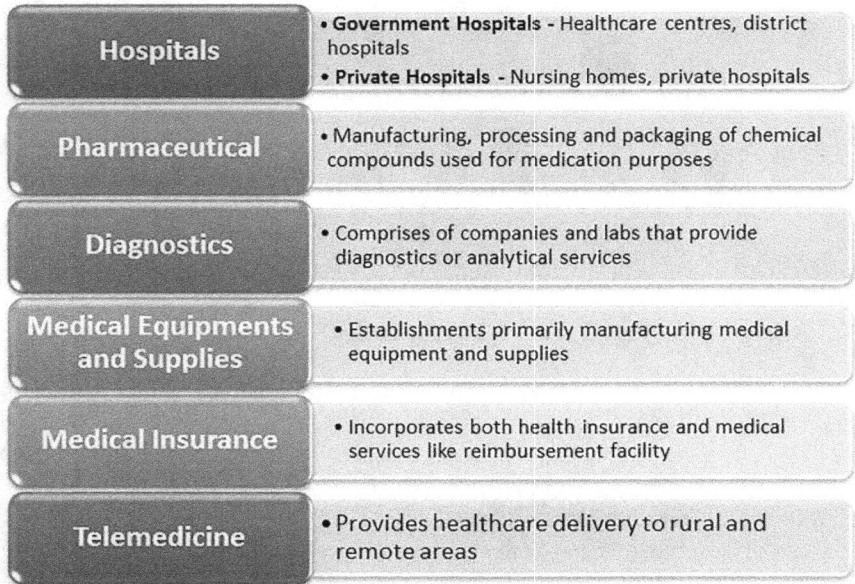

FIGURE 1.4 Healthcare segments.

new century, from 1999 to 2002, it grew rapidly. It paralleled the rapid development of ICT to ease the availability of the clinical data. Web 2.0 and Web 3.0 have provided unprecedented opportunities to access and analyse large amounts of clinical data for medical professionals [13]. Additionally, electronic health records (EHRs) and personal health records (PHRs) are key elements in healthcare systems. These days, patients are more likely to ask for access to their health information as well. It is possible to access medical records without having to ask a doctor directly [14]. EHR systems are basically computerised databases of health records for patients and consumers [15]. It is possible to leverage the advantages of public EHR systems to improve public healthcare systems. For example, they are cost-effective and more efficient to manage large amounts of patient data, and they facilitate the centralised management of records [16].

The Center for Medicare & Medicaid Services (CMS), which is part of the DHHS, endorsed incentive payment programs for the preliminary care that incorporates chronic care management (CCM) on 1 January 2015 [17]. A qualified professional, hospital and critical access hospital (CAH) may participate as long as they use and implement certified EHR technology. Certification by the National Coordinator for Health Information Technology is required for this technology [Office of the National Coordinator (ONC)] under the Office of the Secretary for DHHS [18].

Different communication technologies are widely used to deliver healthcare through telemedicine and e-Health systems. A compilation of up-and-coming health technologies, under research but already commercialised by the World Health

Organization (WHO), was released in 2011 [19]. A number of health technologies presented in this report may provide low-cost solutions for unmet medical needs. At present, these technologies use handheld healthcare devices for measuring pulse rate, percentage of haemoglobin and oxygen saturation level, among other things [20], and a communication is established between a doctor and a patient using the Internet and a mobile phone [19].

Using a mobile phone, a critical heart rate monitor [21] calculates the heart rate and analyses the fetal heartbeat using a beat-to-beat algorithm. Midwives can access the stored data by using a web browser to examine it on a server.

M-health for paediatric HIV [22]: A paediatric HIV knowledge database with a clinical decision-making system is used by the physicians to manage paediatric HIV by integrating clinical information.

Transmission of images using a mobile phone [23]: An embedded camera in a mobile phone is used as an image to acquire units, whereas the Internet is used as the image transferring medium. By using this system, remote areas can access medical image diagnostics facilities that provide more specialised healthcare. Mobile phones transmit the images as Multimedia Message System (MMS) files.

Embedded oximeter [24]: A mobile phone is endowed with a sensor which sends the information received from the finger sensor. It can be analysed and can aid physicians to detect the patient's condition and to take appropriate decisions.

Small telemedicine unit [25]: In addition to aiding physicians in detecting clinical events, it can help them make decisions. Through Code Division Multiple Access (CDMA), Global System for Mobile communication (GSM), the Internet and satellite, both the patient and the doctor can communicate with each other. In addition to its use in rural areas, the device can assist with teleconsultation and several other health services.

Hossain et al. [26] presented in 2012 continuous research and implementation of multimedia services and technologies in every sphere of medical healthcare. An innovative bio-patch and a low-power sensor system-on-chip (SoC) is presented by Yang et al. [27]. Hossain and Ahmed suggested an instantaneous helping system for the all-day caregivers of older people who constantly need assistance to survive [28]. Zhang et al. [29] tested a protocol to protect medical data over wireless networks in order to maintain integrity, privacy and security. A paper [29] presents a virtual reality–based surgical simulator on a CLOUD-based platform for the reduction of the mandibular angle. For surgeons operating instruments in a variety of surgical environments and situations, this simulator provides stimulus and sensations.

The use of mobile technologies and m-health services is growing every day, both for patients and providers. The healthcare industry has been impacted greatly by these services, and the way healthcare is delivered is being revolutionised [30].

1.4 LITERATURE GAP

Many papers gather information about the meteoric rise of telemedicine in terms of clinical diagnosis, but there is a lack of research papers regarding the sociocultural influence on the spread of the telemedicine. The influence of culture on telemedicine adoption must be addressed, as it shows a diversified growth in the different countries. How it spreads among the different cultures and how the cultural competence influences the efficacy of healthcare providers to deliver healthcare services that better suit the social, cultural and linguistic needs of patients need to be examined. Language barriers can be a major difficulty for healthcare providers, as we all know that language issues are more frequent in the mental health area – what patients face here are mostly internal. So, research works must be carried out on the sociocultural aspect in telemedicine that analyses its growth in different cultures and what cultural aspects are influencing the adoption of telemedicine in different countries.

1.5   e-HEALTH

e-Health is emerging as a giant source of good online, real-time clinical caregiving from anywhere in the world. It harnesses the power of the Internet in combination with web-based multimedia and network technologies. The growing Internet-based technologies gave birth to e-Health. It was born as a result of e-applications, which spurred development by implementing the idea of telemedicine [31]. Telemedicine and e-Health are now well-known terms, and now a variety of academic institutions, professional bodies and funding organisations are using them interchangeably. Nowadays, e-Health is taken as the 'use of information and communication technologies locally and at a distance' that interweaves health, information and network technologies. Telemedicine and e-Health are referred as the use of ICT embedded in software programs with speedy communication systems to timely deliver, manage and monitor healthcare services in the remote areas [32]. That's why it is termed 'e-Health', where 'e' stands for electronic, though 10 other factors are similarly responsible for shaping its characteristics. They are discussed in the following section.

1.6   THE 10 E'S IN 'e-HEALTH'

- *Efficiency* – Efficiency in healthcare is increased due to decreases in cost by avoiding repeated or unnecessary diagnostic interventions, as direct communication is possible between patients and the healthcare establishment though they are located far away from the patient.
- *Enhancing quality of care* – e-Health may enhance the quality of healthcare by providing enormous options to compare between different providers and select the best-quality providers among them.
- *Evidence based* – e-Health interventions should be based on evidence such that their efficacy and effectiveness should be verified through thorough scientific review rather than assumed.
- *Empowerment of consumers and patients* – It is possible that personal electronic records and patient-centred medicine can be made accessible to consumers over the Internet.
- *Encouragement* to build up a new relationship between the patient and health professional as constant sharing of decisions is possible using the Internet.

- *Education* of physicians as well as consumers through online sources. Patients can gather information regarding health services.
- *Enabling standardised information exchange and communication* between different healthcare organisations.
- *Extending* the scope of healthcare has no conventional boundaries. Consumers can choose health services online from global providers.
- *Ethics* – With the emergence of e-Health, new difficulties and risks to ethical concerns such as online professional practise, privacy and equity issues have emerged.
- *Equity* – Ensuring that e-Health can be accessed by all irrespective of gender, culture, age or financial status has become a major equity concern.

1.7 APPLICATIONS OF e-HEALTH

1.7.1 EMR AND EHR APPLICATIONS

The most important application of e-Health is the electronic medical record (EMR), as a patient's medical history is stored digitally in EMR applications. These records are known as EHRs. Since records may be quickly exchanged between healthcare professionals, specialists, hospitals and nursing homes, EHRs provide better stability of treatment; as a result, information sharing is not restricted to specific geographical areas. These records can store data of the patients during their treatment period as well as preserve registered data like laboratory results, medical instructions, imaging records and bio-signal records for future use as well. The leading EHR companies include Epic, Allscripts, CureMD, eClinicalWorks, GE Healthcare, Cerner, Practice Fusion and Athena Health [33].

1.7.2 COMPUTERISED PHYSICIAN ORDER ENTRY

Computerised physician order entry (CPOE) is used by medical professionals to enter medical data or instructions electronically. Healthcare providers can prescribe medicines, create orders for labs, radiology, etc., electronically.

1.7.3 CLINICAL DECISION SUPPORT

Clinical decision support (CDS) is specially designed to support healthcare professionals in the diagnosis and treatment of patients. Various tools like automated alerts for patients and doctors, clinical guidelines and diagnostic support are provided.

1.8 m-HEALTH

Mobile health (m-Health), another aspect of telemedicine, is a branch of e-Health broadly. It is the use of mobile in healthcare. As mobile phones are personal and are always used by people, they are becoming very popular in disease management nowadays. So constant monitoring of the patients is possible by the doctors and nurses through mobiles. During emergency or routine visits, patients can be efficiently managed through mobiles.

This has the potential to promote patient self-management in remote areas where the possibility of a doctor's intervention is very slim. It further encourages more participation in medical decision making. Recent research works unveil some interesting facts about the recent trends of gathering health information using mobile phones. Nowadays, smartphone owners tend to get health information through their phone, and this has spurred the production of health apps in recent years. For hypertensive patients, the most popular apps include tracking functions, including blood pressure tracking (BPT). Thus, e-Health and m-Health are progressively gaining an edge in the treatment of hypertensive patients, delivering quality healthcare to prevent cardiovascular consequences of high BP [34].

1.9 APPLICATIONS OF m-HEALTH

Areas and applications of m-Health can be considered from the perspective of users [35]. The major areas where m-Health is used can be broadly stated as follows:

- remote monitoring of the patient's environmental conditions
- remote monitoring of the development of disease in patients
- supporting the treatment process, like advising about medicine, etc., from remote locations
- communication between the healthcare worker and the patient or between the healthcare professionals can be also done using mobiles
- promotion of a healthy lifestyle
- combating addiction

Nowadays, m-Health applications are widely used in emergency response, disease surveillance and control of chronic diseases like malaria, HIV, etc., as well as self-management of diabetes, weight loss, support for physical activity, remote monitoring and patient care.

1.10 u-HEALTH (UBIQUITOUS HEALTHCARE)

u-Health, or ubiquitous healthcare, refers to providing healthcare to any person at any time and at any place by eliminating geographic, temporal and other barriers while enhancing coverage and quality of healthcare services. This is feasible due to the prominence of healthcare awareness and the boom of Internet and mobile wireless technologies. According to Lievens and Jordanova (2007), u-Health is described as 'the ability to give healthcare to individuals anywhere, at any time, through the use of internet and wireless mobile technologies' [36].

People can check their health without visiting the hospital in a ubiquitous healthcare system. Hospitals, on the other hand, can disburse effective medical services based on a computerised medical database and associated resources. A ubiquitous healthcare system typically comprises three components: a portable device to receive the patient's bio-signals, a smartphone device application to transmit the bio-signals received to a server with filtering and a server to monitor and analyse the patient's bio-signals with continuous data [37].

1.11   APPLICATIONS OF u-HEALTH

*   *Mobile medical system:* The mobile medical system provides emergency or quick medical assistance. Ambulance, patient monitoring and sensor networks, medical equipment, medical personnel and the remote hospital are all part of it. This method enables the patient to be treated while on the road to the hospital.
*   *Homecare medical system:* Wireless body sensors, portable medical devices and means of sending medical data to a hospital-based medical system for better diagnosis make up the homecare medical system. The mobile medical facility can make arrangements for the patient to be sent to the hospital for immediate or emergency treatment.
*   *Hospital-based medical system:* This system is housed in a hospital and incorporates the patient's entire database. When the patient is taken to the hospital, this system takes care of the treatment. Disease-diagnosis gadgets, monitoring systems and even healthcare information systems are examples of ubiquitous healthcare applications.

1.12   BROADER ASPECTS OF TELEMEDICINE

There is a slew of additional terminology linked with long-distance healthcare delivery, which are briefly defined as follows:

*   *Telediagnostics:* Telediagnostics is the application of information and communication technology to allow for patient diagnosis across geographically separated domains. It is usually a real-time, live conversation between the doctor and the patient at the remote location. Telediagnostics can also encompass a store-and-forward architecture, in which the patient's data is forwarded to a specialist for consultation [38].
*   *Teleconsultation:* Teleconsultation is the use of information and communication technology to connect individuals beyond geographic barriers, such as healthcare professionals and their patients, for clinical consultations. Diagnostic, treatment, mentoring and other clinical activities connected to the delivery of healthcare services performed by healthcare professionals [39].
*   *Telemonitoring:* Telemonitoring refers to the remote monitoring of vital signs and symptoms in patients. Patients with chronic diseases such as heart or respiratory disorders who live in their own homes and must be observed on a regular basis are the most prominent examples of telemonitoring. Telemonitoring systems notify practitioners to abnormal findings, allowing them to intervene quickly [40].

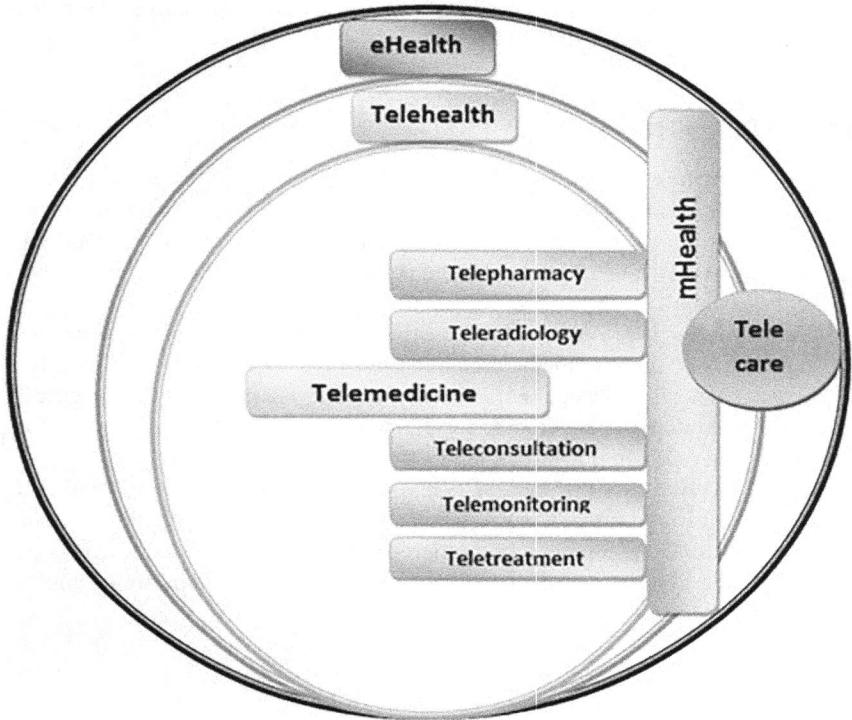

FIGURE 1.5   Review of telehealth service implementation framework.

- *Teletreatment:* Teletreatment is the use of telemedicine to deliver therapy to patients in inaccessible or remote locations. The specialist at the specialty centre could give advice to the doctor treating the patient on the best course of treatment.
- *Telecare:* Telecare is defined as the provision of support and help to persons in need across a long distance using ICT. It is the use of sensors to provide continuous, automatic and remote monitoring of elderly and fragile people, allowing them to remain in their own homes. Personal alarms with remote support, monitoring of environmental alarms (e.g. smoke and gas detectors) and automatic falls detection technology are all examples of telecare applications.

The relationship between these various aspects of healthcare services over a distance is depicted in Figure 1.5.

1.13   APPLICATIONS OF TELEMEDICINE

Throughout the entire world, the applications of telemedicine in various fields of healthcare are numerous [41]:

- *Teleradiology*: It helps to send a patient's x-rays and records securely to a radiologist located in other areas.
- *Telepsychiatry*: Telepsychiatry allow psychiatrists to provide treatment to remote patients. As psychiatry does not require physical examination of patients and there is a shortage of psychiatrists in several areas, this makes telepsychiatry very popular.
- *Teledermatology*: Teledermatology solutions allow remote diagnosis of skin diseases using photos of rashes, moles, etc., sent by the patient.
- *Teleophthalmology*: Using teleophthalmology solutions, ophthalmologists can treat eye diseases by examining patients' eyes from remote locations.
- *Telenephrology*: Telenephrology solutions are used to consult a nephrologist for kidney disease.
- *Teleobstetrics*: Teleobstetrics allow parents to consult with a obstetrician in an emergency.
- *Teleoncology*: Cancer patients can be treated from remote areas using tele-oncology solutions. This field has become very popular to attend the cancer patients in their last stages.
- *Telepathology*: With the help of telepathology solutions, pathologists can share pathology for diagnosis, research and education from remote locations.
- *Telerehabilitation*: Rehab services are provided by telerehabilitation remotely.
- *Telemedicine in surgery*: In the post-surgery period a doctor may check the healing wounds for further clinical advice.
- *Telemedicine in gynaecological disease*: Live telemedicine solutions might be provided for birth control counselling.
- *Telemedicine in endocrinology*: A live chat may happen between a doctor and patient depending on the criticality of the situation.
- **Support for cardiovascular disease prevention**: A typical blood pressure telemonitoring (BPT) application is a telemedicine application for cardiovascular disease treatment that allows for remote transmission of blood pressure and other health data from patients' homes to neighbouring hospitals or designated doctor's chambers. Several randomised studies have shown that regular BPT lowers blood pressure significantly compared to normal care, particularly in high-risk hysterectomy patients. They can avail themselves of additional benefit when this treatment comes with a group of supervision teams of doctors grouped with community pharmacists.
- **Support for diabetic prevention**: Younger groups, such as teenagers from low-income, urban and minority backgrounds, may find telemedicine and m-Health (mobile health) interventions particularly appealing due to their familiarity with, and everyday use of, technology such as mobile phones, the internet and smartphone applications (apps). For patients suffering from chronic diseases, technology can be used to communicate knowledge about self-management practices and provide psychosocial support.
- **Interactive health communication and disease prevention**: Adoption of healthy lifestyles utilising information technology and telemedicine is becoming popular day by day.

- *Epidemiological surveillance*: In epidemic situations, it has proved to be a handy technology in protecting both medical practitioners and patients, as well as to restrict patients' social mobility, thereby reducing the chances of the spreading disease. The researcher uses current literature to explain how telemedicine and e-Health can be used as an imperative measure to enhance clinical care. This study's recent findings highlight the importance of telemedicine and contemporary applications used during the epidemic. More importantly, the data shows how telemedicine and e-Health can be used in clinical services. In the COVID-19 situation telemedicine and e-Health can deliver timely information in health emergencies, as a convenient, secure, scalable and efficient method of providing clinical care [42].
- *Interactive health communication and disease prevention*: Individuals and population organisations may well be aware, educated and inspired about healthcare, health-related issues and the adoption of healthy lifestyles utilising information technology and telemedicine. Central, secondary and tertiary health promotion and disease prevention agendas will all gain from the various approaches and applications of telemedicine.

From this discussion it is evident that throughout the underdeveloped countries good clinical facilities are meagre. The progress of medical technologies are restricted to the developed and low-population-density countries. In recent decades, all over the world, the life expectancy of people is increasing, which triggers changes in demographic patterns with increasing numbers of elderly people. A continuous demand of attending to chronic diseases is shooting high. So, with increasing elderly populations, telemedicine could be an answer to cater to the online real-time clinical advice and assistance these people need.

1.14 TELEMEDICINE ARCHITECTURE AND ITS FUNCTIONALITY

In general, telemedicine systems possess a hierarchical three-tiered architecture that comprises the following:

Level 1 – Local/remote telemedicine centre: Rudimentary healthcare units are located at the remote villages.

Level 2 – City/district hospital: In the next level, the nearby major city is connected with the level 1 rudimentary or primary level 1 units.

Level 3 – Specialty centre: For disease-specific help and assistance, the city hospital is linked with the specialty centres.

Figure 1.6 depicts the architecture of the telemedicine where a patient first gets his basic medical services from a local health professional. The third unit may contain teleconsultation gadgets that are connected to the city hospital via PC sand the Internet. This unit collects the physiological data of the patient and communicates the information to the remote city hospital. After receiving the records, the remote medical practitioner reviews them thoroughly before engaging in a live patient interaction.

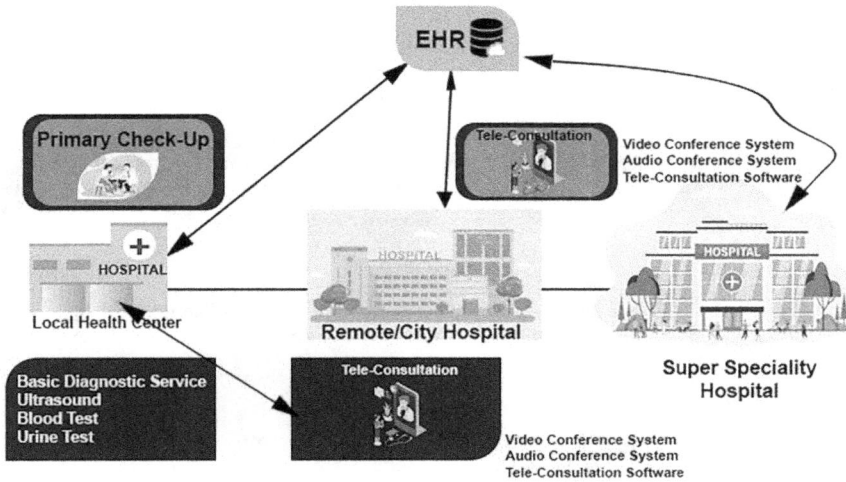

FIGURE 1.6   Telemedicine architecture.

A live interaction may happen between the patient and the specialist depending on the criticality of the situation. These remote hospitals are linked to a centralised database that stores all of the patient's data, as well as other information and even the audio/video contact between the doctor and the patient. Mobile apps or a web-based interface can be used to access the saved data [43].

1.15   PLATFORMS AND TOOLS USED FOR m-HEALTH

The advent and popularisation of the internet and its widespread adoption has expedited the speed of information communication technology tools (ICT) using the web-based platform and multimedia related technologies. m-Health primarily functions through the implementation of various types of ICT tools and applications. KineQuantum, for example, is a French ICT whose goal is to project physiotherapy patients in 3D and virtual-reality games, which could monitor their muscle movements in order to track and visualise their improvement. There are innumerable m-Health applications that are specially designed for mobile devices and can be generalised into the following technical types (Figure 1.7).

1.16   GROWTH OF TELEMEDICINE IN THE LAST DECADE

Telemedicine and e-Health are registering a steady growth in the world market (Figure 1.8). It is forecasted that in 2025, it could reach near 657 billion U.S. dollars [44].

North America is projected to be the dominant telemedicine market in the world. Due to technological advancements and the peoples' lifestyle, they are keen to use

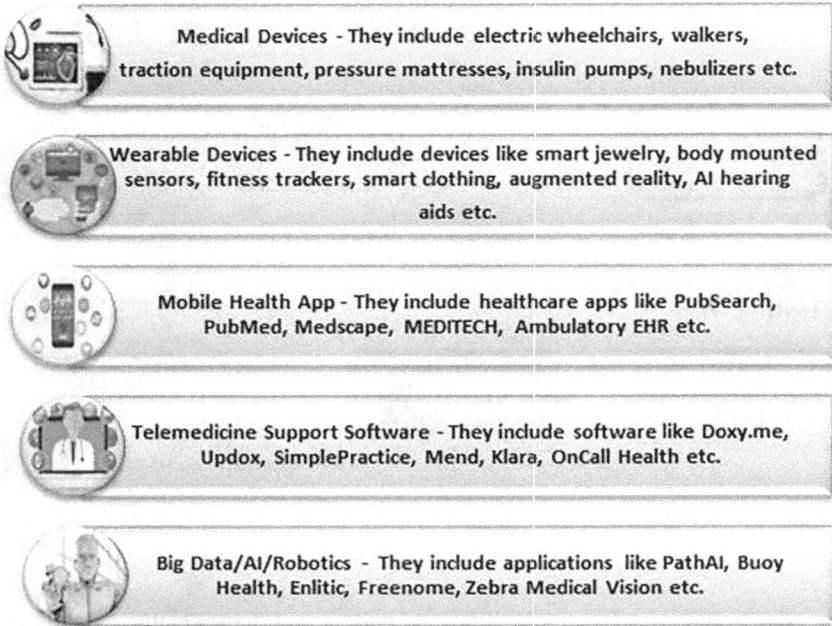

Medical Devices - They include electric wheelchairs, walkers, traction equipment, pressure mattresses, insulin pumps, nebulizers etc.

Wearable Devices - They include devices like smart jewelry, body mounted sensors, fitness trackers, smart clothing, augmented reality, AI hearing aids etc.

Mobile Health App - They include healthcare apps like PubSearch, PubMed, Medscape, MEDITECH, Ambulatory EHR etc.

Telemedicine Support Software - They include software like Doxy.me, Updox, SimplePractice, Mend, Klara, OnCall Health etc.

Big Data/AI/Robotics - They include applications like PathAI, Buoy Health, Enlitic, Freenome, Zebra Medical Vision etc.

FIGURE 1.7   Applications and tools used in telemedicine.

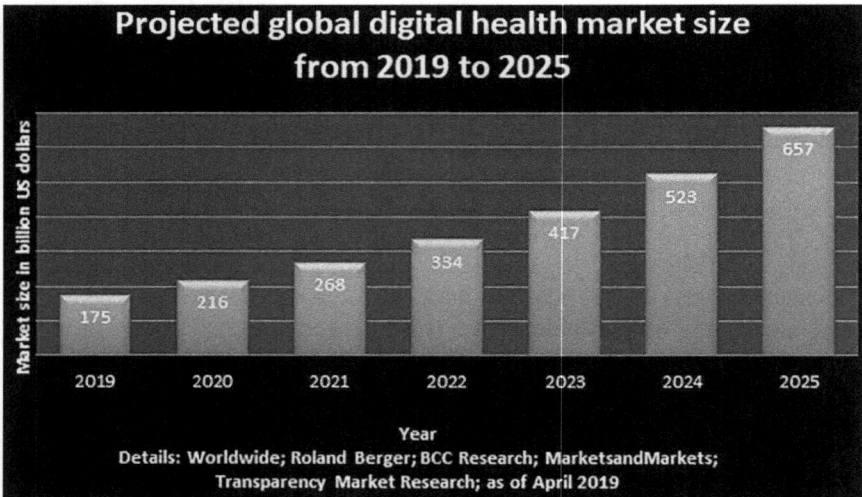

FIGURE 1.8   Global digital health market survey results.

technology to get the e-health information soon. Because of increasing health awareness grouped with cloud-based technology and handheld interconnected devices, a
new era of the telemedicine growth is apparent. According to the Amwell Physician
and Consumer's survey in 2020, in the United States, 59% of patients are attended
to through video calls. The use of tele-Health registered in 2015 was 57%, with an
encouraging growth in 2019 of 69%. It fuelled the telemedicine market with a huge
worldwide funding (Figure 1.9) [45].

In the digital health market, there are various categories like social health network, wellness, telemedicine, etc. Among these, telemedicine has got top priority
and the highest funding throughout the world (Figure 1.10). We can get a hint of

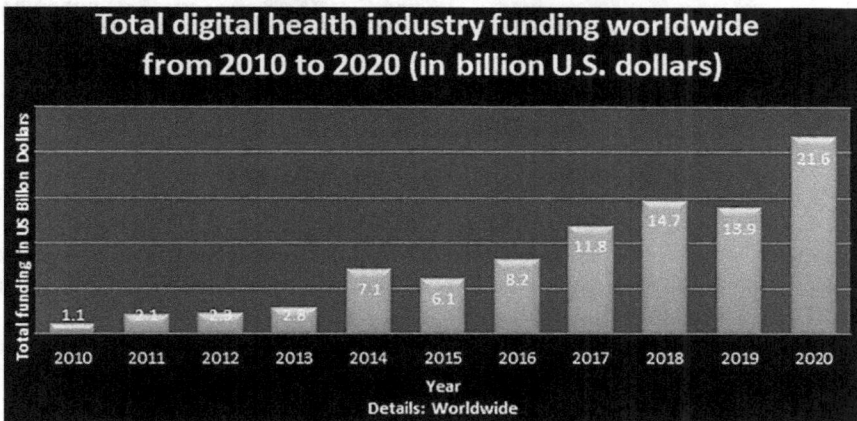

FIGURE 1.9   Digital health industry funds worldwide.

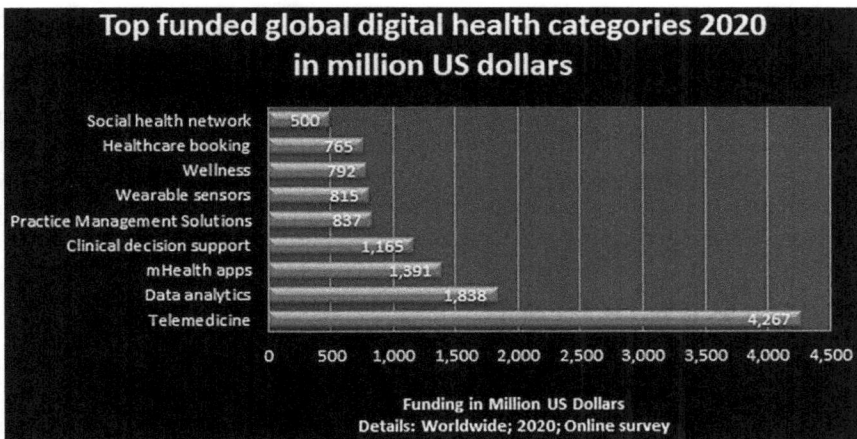

FIGURE 1.10   Top funding global digital health categories.

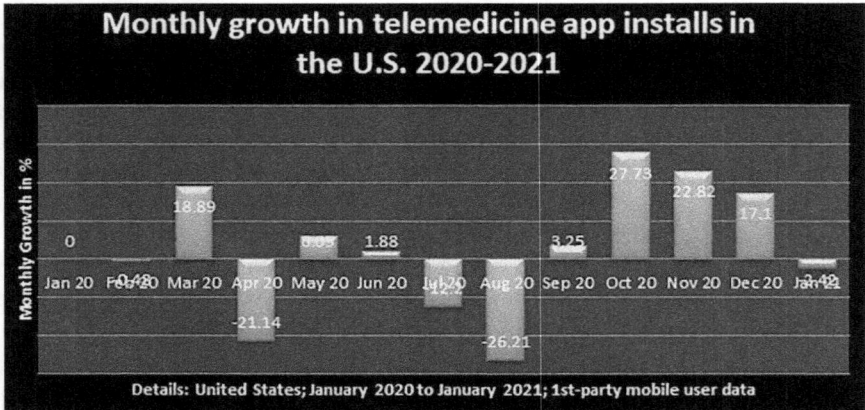

Monthly growth in telemedicine app installs in the U.S. 2020-2021

Details: United States; January 2020 to January 2021; 1st-party mobile user data

FIGURE 1.11 Growth of telemedicine apps in the United States.

this by analysing the data of monthly growth of telemedicine app installation in the United States during the COVID-19 time (2020–2021) (Figure 1.11). In Figure 1.12, a dramatic growth is registered in telemedicine response during the COVID-19 period, but according to the forecast it will likely to maintain this uptrend during the post–COVID-19 period [46].

In the COVID-19 time due to lockdowns and social distancing, the availability of instant healthcare was out of reach in remote places as well as in the urban areas. Telemedicine removes the barrier between the healthcare providers and the patients. In Figure 1.11 an overall 65% increase in medical app download is registered all over the world. Asian countries like India and South Korea show a staggering growth of app downloading: 90% and 135%, respectively [47].

Compared to the United States, Europe has the second largest share of the telemedicine market, as the government's guidelines for using digital health have improved and chronic disease prevalence has risen. Among the millions of deaths worldwide due to dietary issues, around 16% were related to diet, according to the report published by the National Institutes of Health. The death rate from tobacco consumption was estimated at 14.4%. The contribution of alcohol consumption to deaths is about 4% and that of low physical activity is about 3%. Due to this, 20 of the Italian regions had adopted telemedicine guidelines. The service thus facilitates a greater demand for telemedicine in the region as it facilitates greater use of the service.

1.17 OVERVIEW OF TELEMEDICINE INDUSTRY IN INDIA

The COVID-19 outbreak posed a number of obstacles on physical healthcare systems, as citizens have been unable to physically consult with doctors. By 2025, the telemedicine business is estimated to generate a market worth more than $5.4 billion and country wise telemedicine application download is detailed in Figure 1.13. Some of the telemedicine apps that give the best telemedicine service in India include Practo

Past, present and future use of telemedicine in response to COVID-19 U.S. April 2020

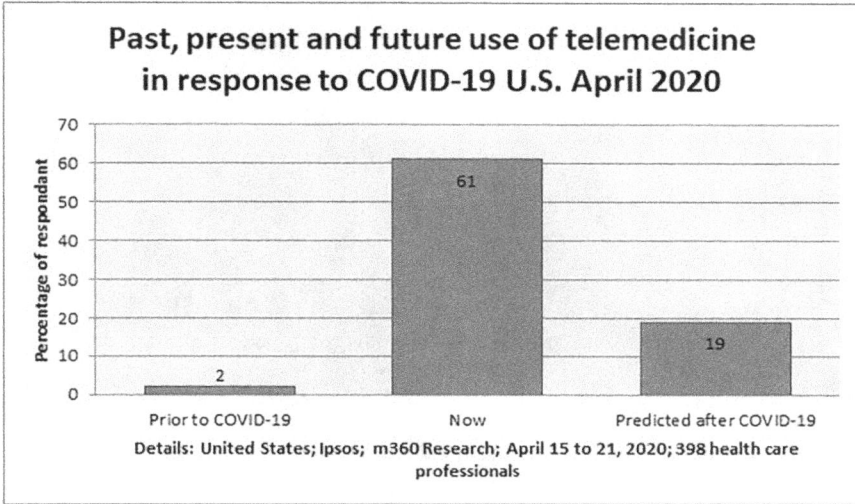

Details: United States; Ipsos; m360 Research; April 15 to 21, 2020; 398 health care professionals

FIGURE 1.12   Application of telemedicine with respect to COVID-19 in the United States.

Increase in medical app downloads during peak of COVID-19 crisis by country 2020 (In %)

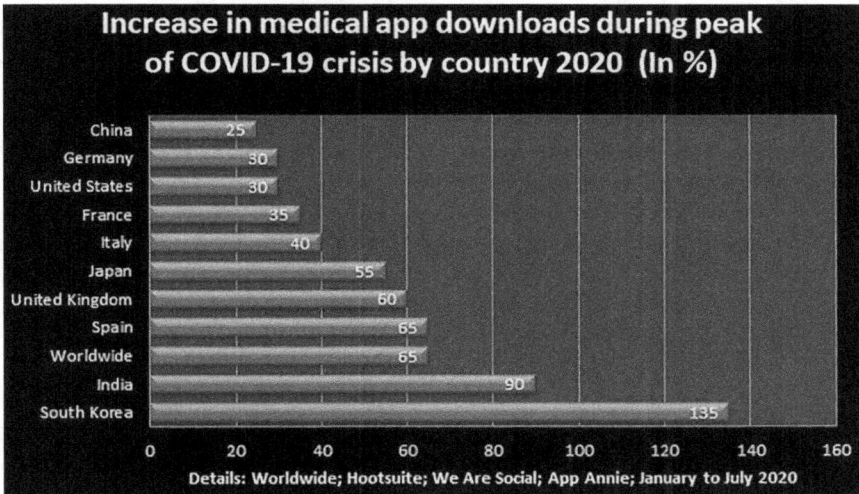

Details: Worldwide; Hootsuite; We Are Social; App Annie; January to July 2020

FIGURE 1.13   Mobile app downloads during COVID-19.

and DocPrime, mFine, CallHealth and Lybrate. As a consequence, the government has reformed its rules on remote healthcare delivery, allowing telemedicine by video, voice or text. Not only will telemedicine assist these firms in combating the spread of the coronavirus, but it will also enhance the access to healthcare in remote areas. Through real-time consultations with doctors via smartphones, tablets, laptops or PCs, innovative technologies are consenting health organisations to enhance access

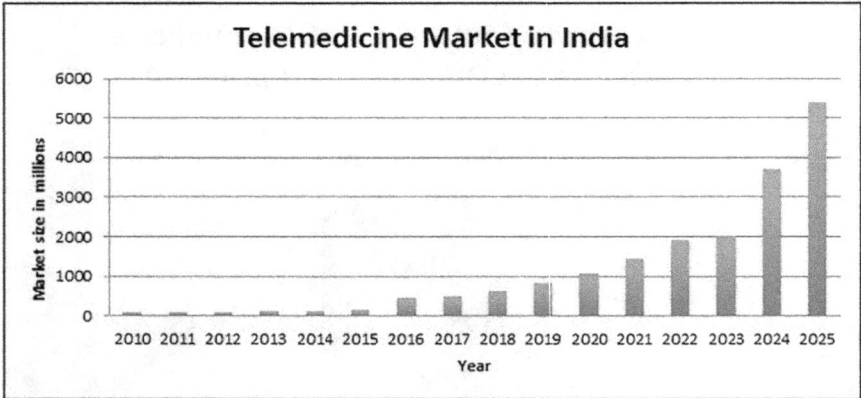

FIGURE 1.14   The telemedicine market in India.

and in order to minimise the burden on hospitals. With a compound annual growth rate (CAGR) of 31%, India's telemedicine market is expected to reach $5.4 billion by 2025 [48]. It will curtail the consultation time and enhance the clinical expertise in terms of accessibility in remote areas as shown in Figure 1.14. According to Statista, the business is expected to reach $280 billion by the end of 2021.

The doctor-to-population ratio as recommended by the World Health Organization (WHO) should be 1:1000, however, India currently holds a doctor-to-population ratio of 0.62:1000 [49].

This hinders the spreading of telemedicine in India because the online consultation takes more time to complete. The Ministry of Health and Family Welfare and the Department of Information Technology have joint efforts to promote the telemedicine market. The National Telemedicine Portal, a division of the Ministry of Health and Family Welfare, is working on a greenfield project in e-health, establishing a National Medical College Network (NMCN) [50] to connect medical colleges across the country for e-education and a national rural telemedicine network for e-healthcare delivery. Another project is ISRO's Village Resource Centre (VRC), which provides the online real-time information about agriculture, ground water management, tele-medicine, real-time weather information, etc.

1.18   CHALLENGES OF TELEMEDICINE

- **Doctors' perspectives**: Doctors are not fully equipped with the knowledge about e-medicine and are unfamiliar with it.
- **Patients' concern and deficit of confidence**: Patients suffer from the lack of faith regarding the outcome of e-medicine.
- **Financial crisis**: Telemedicine is sometimes financially impracticable due to high technology and communication costs.

- *Absence of fundamental amenities*: In countries like India, most of the people (40%) belong to the below poverty level where the fundamental necessities of life are not fulfilled. Here, accessing the newly developed technologies are beyond the reach of the people.
- *Literacy rate and language diversity*: The world is full of diverse languages. There are a lot more countries in the world where the literacy rate barely reaches 2% with a handful of people familiar with the English language.
- *Technical restrictions*: E-medicine technologically is still in its nascent stage with yet to be developed highly sensible biomedical sensors and high bandwidth network.
- *Aspect of quality*: While 'quality is of the essence' and everyone desires it, it can occasionally cause problems. In the case of healthcare, there is no competent regulatory authority to set rules and drive organisations to follow them – it is entirely up to the organisations to decide how they will handle it.
- *Government assistance*: Both the government and private businesses organisations possess restrictions. Any technology in its early stages necessitates attention and support. Only the government has the resources and authority to assist it in survival and expansion. But the government has taken no such initiative for its development [51].

1.19 THEORETICAL IMPLICATION AND DISCUSSION

No doubt, the world is experiencing a boom in telemedicine which bridges the physical distance between the medical professional and the patients. Surely, it will cater a lot to serve the high-quality medical services at the distant corners of each country of the world in the near future. But still its growth is restricted by the internet services and the technical infrastructure available in the country. Mainly the developed countries are reaping its good harvest due their technical advancement and country-wide high-speed internet services. Long-term development of telemedicine in a country depends on the use of a national agency, national strategy, scientific development and evaluation. The post-COVID period is seeing the world experience a surge in the telemedicine field which can be preserved in the long run by employing a proper infrastructure and national policies backed by technical advancement.

1.20 CONCLUSION AND FUTURE PROSPECTS

Nowadays, each country in the world is striving to develop an infrastructure for e-Health, m-Health and telemedicine to promote a real-time healthcare system for the remote population. This infrastructure will eventually bring advanced medical care and technology closer together, but also generate awareness among the stakeholders and the community. Various government agencies and private agencies must come together to create the necessary plans to implement the system. Over the past few years, digitisation has gained importance in medical practice. A large part of the people is not sufficiently aware of the advantages of the telemedicine, e-Health and m-health in spite of the tremendous growth of the mobile and embedded technologies. The new generation is tech-savvy but the elder generations are reluctant to operate on mobile technologies. We may hope that wider acceptance of telemedicine and its attendant technologies will give a renewed impetus to the exponential growth of the telemedicine in the forthcoming decades.

It is believed that the primary responsibility of m-Health/e-Health care promoter groups in 2021 will be to spread knowledge about electronic health technologies and to provide recommendations for their implementation in accordance with 'good practices' for using such technologies. In m-Health and e-Health investigation and implementation, we need to discuss the possibilities and difficulties of new methodologies that could be implemented.

1.21   REFERENCES

[1] D. Lupton and S. Maslen, "Telemedicine and the senses: A review," *Sociology of Health and Illness*; vol. 39(8), pp. 1557–1571, 2017.

[2] B. Cabieses, G. Faba, M. Espinoza and G. Santorelli, "The link between information and communication technologies and global public health: pushing forward," *Telemedicine and e-Health*, vol. 19, pp. 879–887, 2013. [Online] Available at: https://doi.org/10.1089/tmj.2012.0232

[3] B. Rao and A. Lombardi II, "Telemedicine: Current status in developed and developing countries," *Journal of Drugs in Dermatology*, vol. 8(4), pp. 371–375, 2009.

[4] P.J. Heinzelmann, N.E. Lugn and J.C. Kvedar, "Telemedicine in the future," *Journal of Telemedicine and Telecare*, vol. 11(8), pp. 384–390, 2005.

[5] R. Bashshur, G. Shannon, E. Krupinski and J. Grigsby, "The taxonomy of telemedicine," *Telemedicine Journal and e-Health*, vol. 17(6), pp. 484–494, 2011.

[6] J. Craig and V. Patterson, "Introduction to the practice of telemedicine," *Journal of Telemedicine and Telecare*, vol. 11(1), pp. 3–9, Jan. 2005.

[7] W. Einthoven and Le télécardiogramme, "The telecardiogram," *Archives Internationales de Physiologie*, vol. 4, pp. 132–164, 1906.

[8] R. Currell et al., "Telemedicine versus face to face patient care: Effects on professional practice and health care outcomes," *Cochrane Database of Systematic Reviews*, 2000, Issue 2. Art. No.: CD002098.

[9] R.A. Benschoter, M.T. Eaton and P. Smith, "Use of videotape to provide individual instruction in techniques of psychotherapy," *Academic Medicine*, vol. 40(12), pp. 1159–1161, 1965.

[10] T.F. Dwyer, "Telepsychiatry: Psychiatric consultation by interactive television," *American Journal of Psychiatry*, vol. 130, pp. 865–869, 1973.

[11] R. Wootton, L.S. Jebamani and S.A. Dow, "E-health and the Universitas 21 organization: 2. Telemedicine and underserved populations," *Journal of Telemedicine and Telecare*, vol. 11(5), pp. 221–224, 2005.

[12] R.H. Dolin, B. Rogers and C. Jaffe, "Health level seven interoperability strategy: Big data, incrementally structured," *Methods of Information in Medicine*, vol. 54(01), pp. 75–82, 2015.

[13] S. Subramoniam and A. Saifullah Sadi, "Healthcare 2.0," *IT Professional*, vol. 12(6), pp. 46–51, 2010. [Online] Available at: http://dx.doi.org/10.1109/MITP.2010.66.

[14] J. Li, L.P.W. Land, P. Ray and S. Chattopadhyaya, "E-health readiness framework from electronic health records perspective," *International Journal of Internet and Enterprise Management*, vol. 6(4), pp. 326–348, 2010. [Online] Available at: http://dblp.unitrier.de/db/journals/ijiem/ijiem6.html#LiLRC10

[15] M. Eichelberg, T. Aden, J. Riesmeier, A. Dogac and G.B. Laleci, "A survey and analysis of electronic healthcare record standards," *ACM Computing Surveys*, vol.37(4), pp. 277–315, 2005. [Online] Available at: http://dx.doi.org/10.1145/1118890.1118891.

[16] B. Martínez-Pérez, I. de la Torre-Díez, M. López-Coronado and J. Herreros-González, "Mobile apps in cardiology: Review," *JMIR M-health U-health*, vol. 1(2), 2013. [Online] Available at: http://dx.doi.org/10.2196/mhealth.2737. <http://mhealth.jmir.org/2013/2/e15/>.

[17] R.L. Gardner, R. Youssef, B. Morphis, A. DaCunha, K. Pelland and E. Cooper, "Use of chronic care management codes for Medicare beneficiaries: A missed opportunity?" *Journal of General Internal Medicine*, vol. 33(11), pp. 1892–1898, 2018.

[18] B.M. Silva, J.J. Rodrigues, I. de la Torre Díez, M. López-Coronado and K. Saleem, "Mobile-health: A review of current state in 2015," *Journal of Biomedical Informatics*, vol. 56, pp. 265–272, 2015.

[19] WHO, "Compendium of new and emerging technologies," pp. 7–30, 2011. [Online] Available at: www.who.int/medical_devices/innovation/new_emerging_techs/en/.

[20] C. Imison, S. Castle-Clarke, R. Watson and N. Edwards, *Delivering the benefits of digital health care*, pp. 5–6, London: Nuffield Trust.

[21] C.S. Lee, M. Masek, C.P. Lam and K.T. Tan, "Advances in fetal heart rate monitoring using smart phones," in: *Proceedings of the 9th international conference on Communications and information technologies*, ISCIT'09, IEEE Press, Piscataway, NJ, USA, 2009, pp. 735–740. [Online] Available at: http://dl.acm.org/citation.cfm?id=1789954.1790134.

[22] S. Paul, S. Bhattacharya, A. Sudar, D. Patra, A. Majumdar, J. Mukhopadhyay and B. Majumdar, "A web-based electronic health care system for the treatment of pediatric HIV," *11th International Conference on e-Health Networking, Applications and Services*, 2009. Healthcom 2009, pp. 175–180, 2009. [Online] Available at: http://dx.doi. org/10.1109/HEALTH.2009.5406192.

[23] L. Bellina and E. Missoni, "M-learning: Mobile phones' appropriateness and potential for the training of laboratory technicians in limited-resource settings," *Health and Technology*, vol. 1(2–4), pp. 93–97, 2011. [Online] Available at: http://dx.doi.org/10.1007/s12553–011–0008-x.

[24] D. Dunsmuir, C. Petersen, W. Karlen, J. Lim, G.A. Dumont and J.M. Ansermino, "The phone oximeter for mobile spot-check," *Anesthesia and Analgesia*, pp. 18–21, Jan. 2012.

[25] E. Sutjiredjeki, S. Soegijoko, T.L.R. Mengko and S. Tjondronegoro, "Development of mobile telemedicine system with multi communication links to reduce maternal mortality rate," *Proceedings of the Sixth IASTED International Conference on Biomedical Engineering*, BioMED'08, ACTA Press, Anaheim, CA, USA, pp. 402–407, 2008. [Online] Available at: http://dl.acm.org/citation.cfm?id=1713360.1713444.

[26] G. Yang, L. Xie, M. Mäntysalo, J. Chen, H. Tenhunen and L.-R. Zheng, "Bio-patch design and implementation based on a low-power system-on-chip and paper-based inkjet printing technology," *IEEE Transactions on Information Technology in Biomedicine: A Publication of the IEEE Engineering in Medicine and Biology Societ*, vol. 16, pp. 1043–1050, 2012. [Online] Available at: http://dblp.uni-trier.de/db/journals/titb/titb16. html#YangXMCTZ12.

[27] M. Hossain and D. Ahmed, "Virtual caregiver: An ambient-aware elderly monitoring system," *IEEE Transactions on Information Technology in Biomedicine: A Publication of the IEEE Engineering in Medicine and Biology Societ*, vol. 16(6), pp. 1024–1031, 2012. [Online] Available at: http://dx.doi.org/10.1109/TITB.2012.2203313

[28] Q. Wang, H. Chen, W. Wu, H.-Y. Jin and P.-A. Heng, "Real-time mandibular angle reduction surgical simulation with haptic rendering," *IEEE Transactions on Information Technology in Biomedicine: A Publication of the IEEE Engineering in Medicine and Biology Society*, vol. 16(6), pp. 1105–1114, 2012. [Online] Available at: http://dx.doi. org/10.1109/ TITB.2012.2218114.

[29] C. Free, G. Phillips, L. Watson, L. Galli, L. Felix, P. Edwards, V. Patel and A. Haines, "The effectiveness of mobile-health technologies to improve health care service delivery processes: A systematic review and meta-analysis," *PLoS Medicine*, vol. 10(1), e1001363, 2013. [Online] Available at: http://dx.doi.org/10.1371/journal. pmed.1001363.

[30] D. Nicolini, "The work to make telemedicine work: A social and Articulative view," *Social Science & Medicine*, vol. 12, 2005.

[31] H. Oh, C. Rizo, M. Enkin and A. Jadad, "What is e-Health (3): A systematic review of published definitions," *Journal of Medical Internet Research*, vol. 7(1), e1, 2005.

[32] G. Eysenbach, "What is e-health?" *Journal of Medical Internet Research*, vol. 3(2), e20, 2005.

[33] World Health Organization Regional Office for Europe, "E-health," www.euro.who.int/en/health-topics/Health systems/e-health.

[34] R.S. Istepanian, E. Jovanov and Y.T. Zhang, "Guest editorial introduction to the special section on m-health: Beyond seamless mobility and global wireless health-care connectivity," *IEEE Transactions on Information Technology in Biomedicine*, vol. 8(4), pp. 405–414, 2004.

[35] S. Tachakra, X. Wang, R.S. Istepanian and Y. Song, "Mobile e-health: The unwired evolution of telemedicine," *Telemedicine Journal and e-Health*, vol. 9(3), pp. 247–257, 2003.

[36] N. Agoulmine, M.J. Deen, J. Lee and M. Meyyappan, "U-Health smart home," *IEEE Nanotechnology Magazine*, vol. 5(3), pp. 6–11, Sept. 2011. [Online] Available at: http://doi.org/10.1109/MNANO.2011.941951.

[37] O. -y. Kwon, S. -h. Shin, S. -j. Shin and W. -s. Kim, "Design of U-Health system with the use of smart phone and sensor network," *2010 Proceedings of the 5th International Conference on Ubiquitous Information Technologies and Applications*, pp. 1–6, 2010. [Online] Available at: http://doi.org/10.1109/ICUT.2010.5677830.

[38] P. Stamford, T. Bickford, H. Hsiao and W. Mattern, "The significance of telemedicine in a rural emergency department," *IEEE Engineering in Medicine and Biology Magazine*, vol. 18(4), pp. 45–52, July–Aug. 1999. [Online] Available at: http://doi.org/10.1109/51.775488.

[39] T.C. Chang, J.D. Lee and S.J. Wu, "The Telemedicine and Teleconsultation System Application in Clinical Medicine," *The 26th Annual International Conference of the IEEE Engineering in Medicine and Biology Society*, 2004, pp. 3392–3395. [Online] Available at: http://doi.org/10.1109/IEMBS.2004.1403953.

[40] P. Mendoza, P. Gonzalez, B. Villanueva, E. Haltiwanger and H. Nazeran, "A web-based vital sign telemonitor and recorder for telemedicine applications," *The 26th Annual International Conference of the IEEE Engineering in Medicine and Biology Society*, pp. 2196–2199, 2004. [Online] Available at: http://doi.org/10.1109/IEMBS.2004.1403641.

[41] N.F. Güler and E.D. Übeyli, "Theory and applications of telemedicine," *Journal of Medical Systems*, vol. 26, pp. 199–220, 2002. [Online] Available at: https://doi.org/10.1023/A:1015010316958.

[42] S.B. Thacker, R.G. Parrish and F.L. Trowbridge, "A method for evaluating systems of epidemiological surveillance," *World Health Statistics Quarterly*, vol. 41(1), pp. 11–18, 1988. Erratum in: *World Health Stat Q.*, vol. 42(2), 1989: preceding 58. PMID: 3269210.

[43] A.K. Maji et al., "Security analysis and implementation of web-based telemedicine services with a four-tier architecture," *2008 Second International Conference on Pervasive Computing Technologies for Healthcare*, 2008, pp. 46–54. [Online] Available at: http://doi.org/10.1109/PCTHEALTH.2008.4571024.

[44] Statista, "Global digital health market forecast 2025," Statista, 2021. [Online] Available at: www.statista.com/statistics/1092869/global-digital-health-market-size-forecast/.

[45] A. Williams, U. Bhatti, H. Alam and V. Nikolian, "The role of telemedicine in postoperative care," 2021. [Online] Available at: http://doi.org/10.21037/mhealth.2018.04.03, May 2 2018.

[46] Statista, "Telehealth visits before and during COVID-19 in the U.S. 2020," Statista, 2021. [Online] Available at: www.statista.com/statistics/1256789/telehealth-visits-before-and-during-covid-19-in-the-us/

[47] Statista, "COVID-19 growth in medical app downloads by country 2020," Statista, 2021. [Online] Available at: www.statista.com/statistics/1181413/medical-app-downloads-growth-during-covid-pandemic-by-country/

[48] The Financial Express, "Technology is on the verge of reshaping Indian Healthcare," Deepak Tuli, Co-founder, COO, Eka Care. 2021. [Online] Available at: www.finan cialexpress.com/healthcare/healthtech/technology-is-on-the-verge-of-reshaping-indian-healthcare-deepak-tuli-co-founder-coo-eka-care/2382757/

[49] P. India, "India's doctor-patient ratio still behind WHO-prescribed 1:1,000: Govt," *Business-standard.com*, 2021. [Online] Available at: www.business-standard.com/article/pti-stories/doctor-patient-ratio-in-india-less-than-who-prescribed-norm-of-1–1000-govt-119111901421_1.html

[50] Main.mohfw.gov.in. 2021. [Online] Available at: https://main.mohfw.gov.in/sites/default/files/20Chapter.pdf

[51] S. Dash, R. Aarthy and V. Mohan, "Telemedicine during COVID-19 in India – a new policy and its challenges," *Journal of Public Health Policy*, vol. 42, pp. 501–509, 2021. [Online] Available at: https://doi.org/10.1057/s41271-021-00287-w

2 Future Risk Analysis of the Health Public Sector During COVID-19 Period (2020 to March 2021)

Charles Roberto Telles[1], Ahmad Mohammad Ayaz[2],
Syed Khalid Mustafa[2], Archisman Roy[3],
Mohammad Rehan Ajmal[2] and Elisandro Pires Frigo[1]
[1] Federal University of Parana, Brazil
[2] University of Tabuk, Saudi Arabia
[3] Banaras Hindu University, India

CONTENTS

2.1   INTRODUCTION

The COVID-19 pandemic period exposed abnormal manufacturing and logistical conditions for the consumption and demand of products/services in health units worldwide [1–5]. Initially, in the absence of knowledge about the disease, new items and techniques emerged, creating a stressful condition in terms of fulfilling healthcare

DOI: 10.1201/9781003217107-2

units in logistics, planning, investment and operational demands [6–10]. In addition to these problems discussed in recent research [1–10], this chapter addresses the background of this scenario, that is, if the public sector could respond promptly and resiliently to an increased demand of administrative work, that is ultimately the necessary asset to deliver help for populations in terms of robustness and reliable actions.

Political reasons generally keep this type of information apart from populations, configuring for the democratic process little information and lack of transparency [11–12]. Aiming to know about how public administrations worldwide can fail internally to process information in terms of the role of actions of new public policies to be implemented to tackle COVID-19 is not something science can solve easily since data is commonly restricted. This problem faces a conflictual analysis on how science must also be closely linked to the political structure of governments and why their internal productivity processes must be transparent and very well structured [13–14].

A case analysis was evidenced in an institution of the public administration in Brazil, which was already precarious under normal conditions before COVID-19 and which under this new stress had a collapse in the first semester of 2021 [15–17].

At the beginning of the pandemic, the state public institution in question demanded new biddings of products like masks, respirators, alcohol 70%, protective equipment and face shields for healthcare workers, needles, syringes, intubation kits and sedatives to be purchased at a large scale. In Brazil, during this period, it was up to public institutions themselves to seek their quantitative parameters of items to endure COVID-19, and it was observed that stressful conditions in the public administrative work were found both for federal and state administration, which culminated in an inadequate health-related products/services supply chain for the population [15–17].

Focusing on how the public sector deals with information processing in the daily administrative work of collaborators and how it influences the final outcomes for the population, the case study is going to be presented based on the bidding data collected at Portal da Transparência (www.transparencia.pr.gov.br/) and a methodology developed for future risk analysis in which it is possible to evaluate how an institution responded to abnormal conditions in the perspective of the workforce and data processing available during COVID-19.

The results of this research present an algorithm and graph analysis that can mainly analyse the load of political and administrative projects in the institution, considering for it the parameters such as time, failure and the active projects in a given time (sample of analysis) set as two possible optimal performances: stability or stress of production. It takes into consideration the aspect of resilience for disrupting events as the need of an adaptive management where the interconnectedness of social, economic, environmental [18] and other systems is existent, and therefore, risk mitigation and monitoring aspects need to be evaluated with more complex forms [19]. Then, approximating to this scenario of analysis, the method of this research resulted in a predictive and monitoring tool, where the algorithm is able to identify a surface integral in order to plot nonlinear data at the graph with the given desired solutions of the problem. By performing this task, it is possible to observe the collective phenomena (swarm intelligence) in terms of 'future behaviour' by using horizontal visibility graphs [20–21].

2.2 PAST STUDIES/LITERATURE REVIEW

Administrative workflows of every type with massive loads of information, human resources procedures, geographic distance, intersectorial work and other features are complicated environments where productivity can be hard to achieve regarding precision and time reliability [22–23]. On the democracy basis of analysis, the problem is to achieve a common solution in a world full of strong emergencies where the organisation of all events can't be always defined linearly. Since many administrative workflows are mainly hybrid (composed of human processing skills and machines), it is sometimes impossible to have predefined control over productivity due to the human cognitive performance that might differ in time and intensity for each collaborator, and therefore, new approaches are needed to address this basis of production for every society [24–25].

Unexpected behaviour, uncertainty and information processing are something natural to the human cognitive processes [26]. For this, although unpredictable, any probability distribution of the cognitive performance for multiple tasks in a given work activity might appear, and establishing a way to measure it can be useful for the prediction of how the complexity and nonlinearity on this type of events work as a whole (collective phenomena). The method presented in this research allows us to evaluate how a given sample of analysis will have its standards of productivity for a future time (future risk analysis). Also, other implications are found to enhance productivity performance and the relation between humans and machines.

Considering that work demands on the public sector have grown exponentially during COVID-19 [27–28], the role of human resources and computing is to generate a linear probability where all demands are executed in a certain period of time and the efficiency/effectiveness needs to be 100% or as close as possible. If the productivity is inefficient and imprecise, so will be the democratic process and its achievements [29–31]. This happens because the volume of information raised within a system also raises uncertainty and complexity of how work should be executed, aiming for efficiency and efficacy to populations and especially during disrupting events [32–33]. This point is very connected with the need for parameterisation and standardisation of how to perform a given work activity in a public or private system known as KPI (key productivity indicators). For governments, this main objective, which is to design and execute public policies, is limited insofar as the administrative work base is outdated in terms of data treatment, performance indicators and risk mitigation.

In this sense, hybrid organisations need to be supported by a real-life closed loop control system, and outputs derived from it can be reached towards the micro dimension of information processing (cognitive level) to the global dimension of performance expected (public sector productivity level) [22–26]. This method makes it possible for decision makers to carry out strategic planning, assets relocation, money allocation, time prediction and control over productivity.

2.3 METHODOLOGY

This research sought to identify in a sample of bidding procedures in the state administrative unit of Paraná, Brazil, from 2020 to March 2021, the factors that promoted ineffectiveness in budget execution and of public policies during the COVID-19 period. To carry out this bidding analysis, descriptive statistics were used to collect parametric data on the terms of reference and instruction of 26 bidding protocols, correlating the variables time (to deliver goods/services to population) and notes (procedural failures observed by the state attorney general Pacific gas and energy company [PGE] and the state comptroller general Computable general equilibrium [CGE]) in bidding procedures, including bidding waivers that occurred during the pandemic period.

The legal action adopted in Brazil to provide support during the pandemic, Federal Law No. 13,979, of 6 February 2020 [34], seeks to find measures that may be adopted to face the public health emergency of international importance resulting from the coronavirus – COVID-19 – with the objective of verifying the guarantee of the principles and norms that guide the public administration, in particular the legality, impersonality, economy, publicity and administrative morality, aiming at the protection of probity and the federal/state treasury. The considerations regarding this legal action were based on the new hypothesis of waiver of bidding modality of auctions (basic provider), created specifically to tackle the public health emergency. The notes performed by the PGE and CGE were carried out in accordance with the auditing and control standards of the Brazilian Technical Standards on Auditing, the International Standards of Supreme Audit Institutions (INTOSAI), the standards and guidelines of the Institute of Internal Auditors (IIA) and the internal and external control institutions that are referenced in the country.

Bidding procedures in the modality of basic providesr are processes occurring in public administration that allow the functioning of the public system with a view to providing essential services to the democratic role of the government regime adopted by Brazil. The provision of these procedures can occur through the acquisition of products or services according to the management of each government for a period of four years.

For a bidding procedure to be carried out effectively and efficiently, it is necessary that the administrative basis of the public sector, which starts with the responsible sectors, human resources, workflows, information systems and relevant legislation, can be optimally functioning in terms of the processing of information, aiming at a precision about the work to be performed [22–24]. Considering that this information processing initially results from human work factors, there is necessarily the possibility that failures are made during the work activity in such a way as to delay or make the completion of this administrative routine work impossible [25]. Likewise, in addition to the human workforce, there is the non-human work structure defined by the information systems, workflow of the institution and the legislation of a certain government units. In this sense, there is a hybrid work system in which the variables of information source are of natural origin (human resources) and artificial in work environments (systems and information organisation).

As a point of analysis, two sectors that integrate the main input and output nodes of information on bidding projects from the institution were verified: the Permanent Bidding Commission (CPL) and the Purchasing and Agreements sector (CCC). These sectors, the analytical base, together with the other internal and external sectors, were evaluated in its work performance in terms of time and failures.

About 300 PGE and CGE notes in the 26 protocols were analysed (17 bidding waivers and 9 normal biddings), and they, through the proposed analysis methodology, present critical points regarding the future risk of implementing new administrative and mainly political projects of the current administration, as well as to address the society's needs during COVID-19.

2.3.1 HUMAN RESOURCES

Considering that an analysis of how human information processing can occur always with 100% precision is uncertain, given the nature of the object of investigation, it is only possible to identify whether there are failures in this event when the final result of the activities to be performed can be observed by its efficiency and effectiveness in achieving the objectives.

For the analysis of these variables of a subjective order in the execution but objective in the completion of a proposed objective, an on-site interview and a questionnaire were conducted to understand how bidding sectors (CPL and CCC and other requesting sectors that require bidding procedures) were composed. The questionnaire (Supplementary Data 1) was sent in March and April 2021. As for the questionnaire, it was verified that there are human resources with academic training and professional experience adequate to the execution of the work role that is part of the workflow for the execution of a bidding procedure. However, regarding the investigated sectors, there is a diversity in the academic backgrounds and time of experience with this type of work, generating instabilities as to the knowledge required to the execution of bidding procedures.

2.3.2 DATASET: TIME AND NOTES FROM PGE AND CGE

The time estimated by the CPL for a normal bidding procedure to be completed was listed as 30, 90 and 180 days, while for layoffs during the time of COVID-19, they needed the shortest time possible, on smaller time scales than for a normal bidding. Regarding the processing time of the protocols, the average time for the bidding waiver protocols (reduced time modality that should end in 90 days) was 4.64 months, while the normal bidding protocols were 8.77 months. And the types of projects in the sample were divided between political projects and administrative infrastructure projects (Table 2.1), which, the latter is of vital importance to structure the

---

TABLE 2.1

Types of Objects of Bidding Procedures

Types of Objects	Political	Administrative Structure
Normal bidding	3	6
Bidding waiver	17	0

Source: transparencia.pr.gov.br compiled by Telles, C. R.

TABLE 2.2

Notes Made by the Control Institutions of the State of Paraná

	μ	n	p
Number of notes per normal bidding	15,66	141	9
Number of notes due to bidding waiver	9,35	159	17

* μ = average of notes per protocol, n = number of notes and p = number of protocols.
Source: transparencia.pr.gov.br compiled by Telles, C. R.

political projects that are dependent on the public administrative base in its strength of the work in order to achieve high efficiency and effectiveness.

Regarding the notes made by the PGE and CGE, a total of 300 notes were listed in the 26 samples analysed (Table 2.2) along its frequency (Figure 2.1).

2.4   RESULTS/FINDINGS

2.4.1   PARAMETERISATION

Some parameters were listed on the bidding procedures which served as a basis for analysis to verify in which criteria the notes given by the CGE and PGE are more frequent, as shown in Supplementary Data 2.

Based on the items of Supplementary Data 2, the notes can be seen as shown in Figures 2.2 and 2.3. In Figure 2.2, items 2.5 and 2.7 were not pointed out. And the number of notes in the term of reference were 104 and in the protocol instruction, 37.

In Figure 2.3, items 2.1 and 2.4 were not pointed out. And the number of notes in the term of reference were 93 and in the protocol instruction, 66.

2.4.2   CORRELATION BETWEEN PROTOCOL FREQUENCY
AND VARIABLES TIME AND FAILURE

According to Figure 2.1, with the increase in the frequency of execution of new bidding protocols, between the months of April and June, there was also an increase in the time needed to complete these protocols, especially for the period of April to August 2020. Likewise, there was a higher incidence of notes in the protocols for the months of June to July, as can be seen in Figures 2.4 and 2.5.

The month of February was not considered because there was only one sample and it was not possible to obtain an average from protocols in this month. For the other months, the time and failures values were obtained by the arithmetic mean of the samples. In Figure 2.5, the month of December had no samples. Roughly speaking, it is possible to verify that, as there was an increase in the number of protocols in the analysed sectors; there was also an increase in the incidence of failures and time.

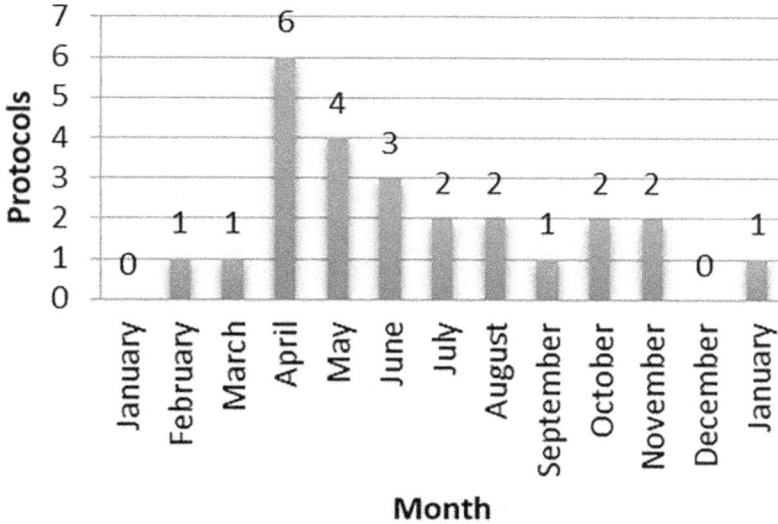

FIGURE 2.1 Frequency of biddings during 2020 and March 2021. Note that no bidding was created during February and March 2021.

Source: transparencia.pr.gov.br compiled by Telles, C. R.

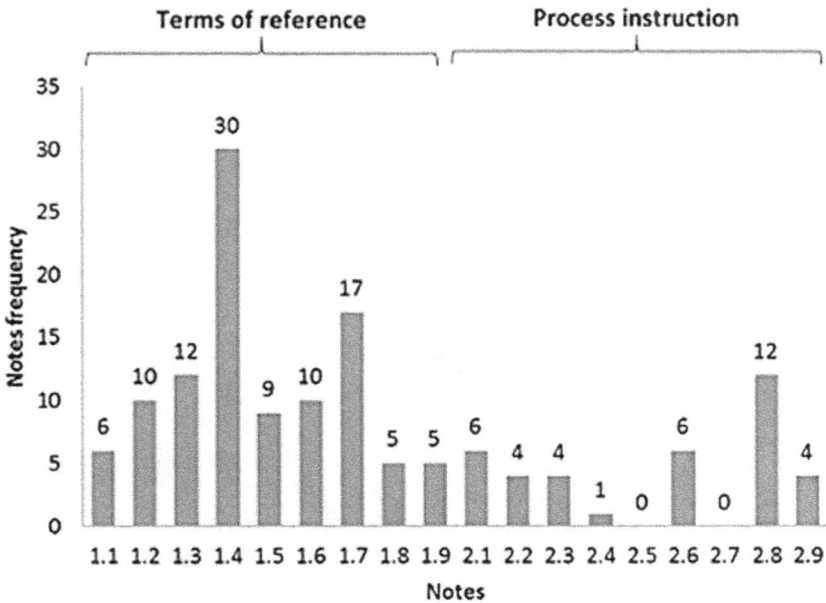

FIGURE 2.2 PGE's notes on bids.

Source: transparencia.pr.gov.br compiled by Telles, C. R.

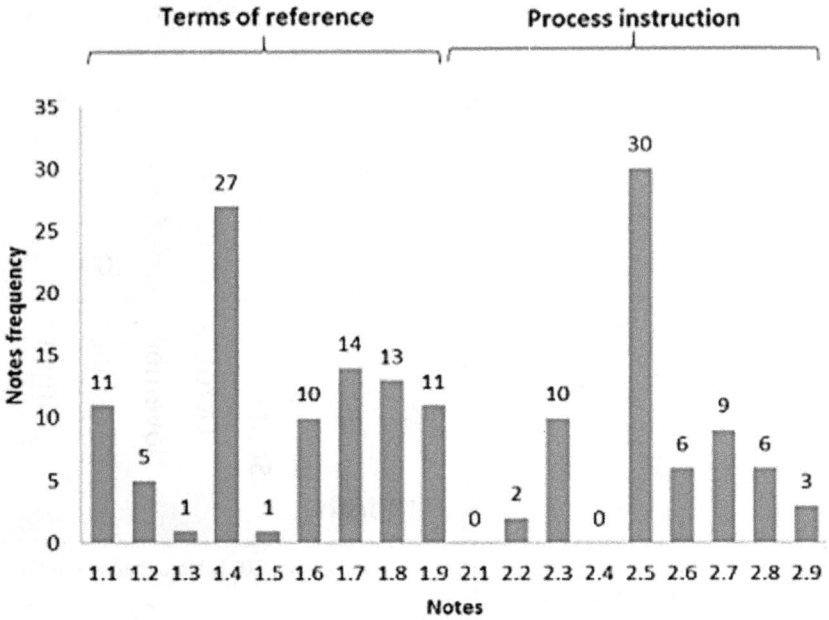

FIGURE 2.3   PGE and CGE's notes on bidding waivers.

Source: transparencia.pr.gov.br compiled by Telles, C. R.

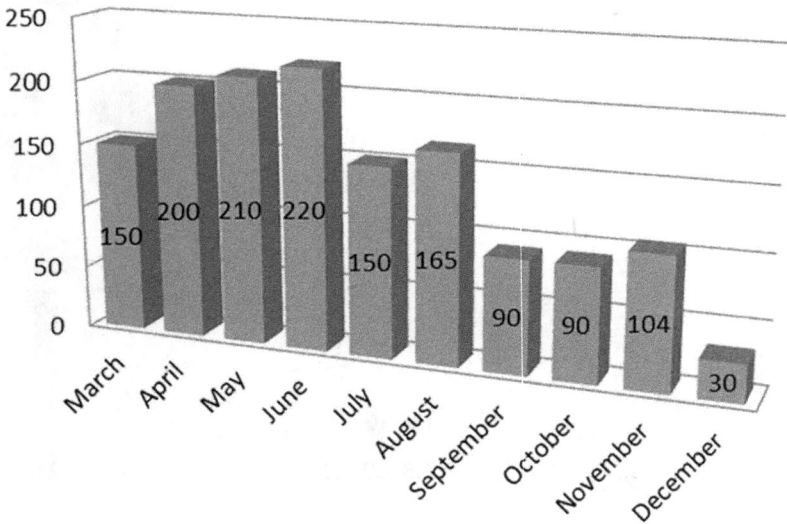

FIGURE 2.4   Incidence of time for the processing of bidding procedures during 2020.

Source: transparencia.pr.gov.br compiled by Telles, C. R.

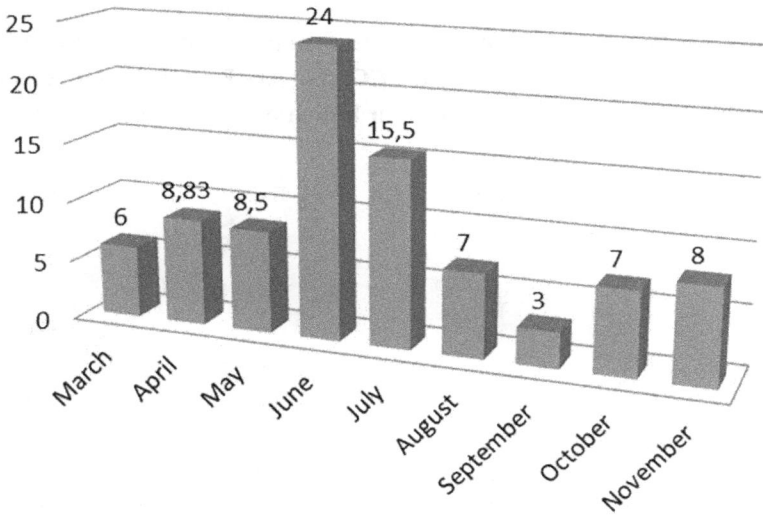

FIGURE 2.5   Incidence of notes (failures) in bidding procedures during 2020.

Source: transparencia.pr.gov.br compiled by Telles, C. R.

2.4.3   FUTURE RISKS ANALYSIS AND GRAPH REPRESENTATION

An analysis of the performances of the sectors that work with bidding procedures on stress was carried out, identifying, based on the history of the year 2020, how these sectors would respond to a future work demand.

Table 2.3 was prepared to compose Figure 2.6. In it, a sample of the period of 2020 between the months of April and July, a period of great stress in the sector, provided the proportion between the number of bidding projects in the period, the number of failures and time (period mean value) required to complete these projects. The analysis was also performed for a normality of the period (N), in which the execution of activities was stable, considering for failures and time (mean value), the period from March and August to November.

Now considering the grey marked months from Table 2.3, stressful condition values were extracted as parameters of productivity in the public sector sample for future risk analysis. In Table 2.4, P/A presents the growing ratio of political and administrative projects, notes and time as the mean of the given month and object ID calculated as input to Figure 2.6 data with the equation for future risk predictive

analysis $f\,dF,t = \dfrac{P}{A}\sqrt{\dfrac{\dfrac{1}{n}\sum_{i=1}^{n\to\infty} t_i}{\dfrac{1}{n}\sum_{i=1}^{n\to\infty} F_i}} = \dfrac{dF,t}{dt}$, where t_i refers to the time and F_i refers to

failures (notes). This equation was designed to obtain the numerical value of bidding

TABLE 2.3
Database for Analysis of the Period of Stress and Stability of the Execution of Activities in the Sectors (CPL and CCC) that Are Part of the Analysis Base of the Bidding Procedures. Grey Colour Indicates a Period of Analysis of the Sector under Stress.

Month	Failures	Time	P/A*
February	13	390	1/2
March	6	150	1/3
April	8,83	200	6/3
May	8,5	210	9/4
June	24	220	11/5
July	15,5	150	13/5
August	7	165	14/6
September	3	90	15/6
October	7	90	17/6
November	8	104	19/6
December	0	30	20/6

*P/A: Political (P) and administrative (A) projects of the period. Note: In the months of February and December there was no average to calculate, as there was only one current political project.

Source: transparencia.pr.gov.br compiled by Telles, C. R.

TABLE 2.4
Database for Viewing Future Risk

Month	April	May	June	July	N
P/A	5	9	12	14	N
Notes	8,83	8,67	13,78	14,21	6,2
Time	200	205	210	195	119,8
Object ID	1.6161	1.6267	1.5203	1.4961	1.5770

Source: transparencia.pr.gov.br compiled by Telles, C. R.

procedures and failures over time, considering for it every political and administrative project in the given period as $\iiint f\,dF, t = \oint_1^9 f\left(P\left(y'_{45}\left|y''_{90}\right|y'''_{180}\right)\right)dt'$. Since the graph representation is built with specific formula where nonlinearity prevails to plot the samples, there is no linear information (variables with possible and direct discrete numerical value) tracked in the time series in which connected points (nodes) could be overwhelmed in the visibility graph nodes intersections. This approach does not look to nodes or points that are displayed linearly among the graph axis in terms of values in discrete form. Conversely, the graph axis is shaped by time and by the risk analysis formula where each sample's continuous value obtained is linear to each other numerically, but not empirically in discrete form. That's why nodes connected do not break the visibility graph rules [21].

In addition, the measuring of local states of the real-life event can be representative in order to extract information about its behaviour along time. For this, the comparison of node states can be visualised as a series of discrete observable values showing increasing, unchanged and decreasing behaviour. With this technique, non-stationary time series, which is the one that is the subject of this research, can be evaluated by its output performances (time-dependent) [20].

In Figure 2.6, bidding waivers and the normal bidding protocols were analysed within the institution. It was found that to fulfill the political desire to provide supplies for healthcare units during the COVID-19 crisis in 2020, 26 bidding procedures (black dots) took more time and failed to achieve its completion than expected (grey dots), resulting in the whole year of 2020 with a low response of government to tackle the problems. It is possible to see in the graph grey dots that represent the appropriate time for a bidding waiver or normal bidding, that is 45, 90 and 180 days and black dots indicating how those projects were completed, having from 120 to 210 days as the mean value, and having some protocols with a superior time of 300 days. And concerning failures in the protocols (that is grammar, logical reasoning of the project, legal aspects and inconsistencies of every sort), they were found in more

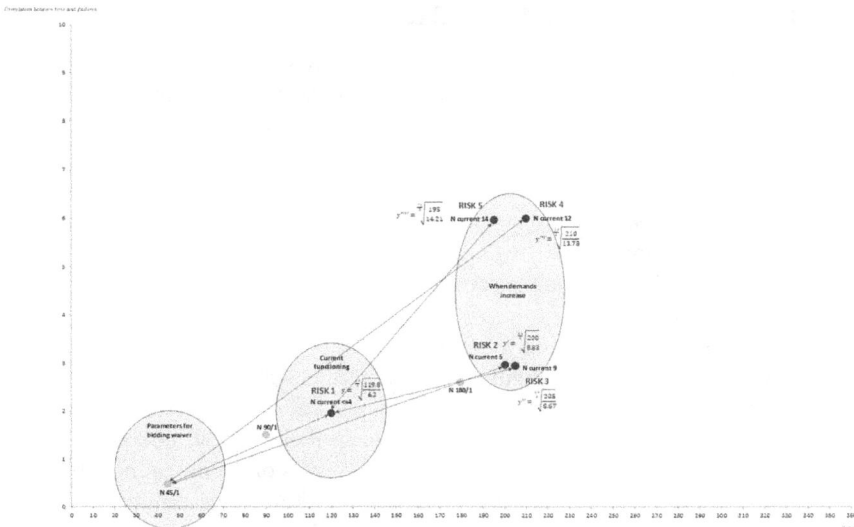

FIGURE 2.6   Future risk for biddings.

Source: transparencia.pr.gov.br compiled by Telles, C. R.

than 300 notes and the mean failure rate went from 8 to 14 per protocol, having some specific protocols with more than 40 failures.

Thus, although the object of this research is to verify the productivity performance of the work carried out by the CPL and CCC under stress (third sphere) or normal conditions (second sphere) and to produce the future risk analysis, it is not understood as a cause of the addition of time and precision factors, the way these sectors work. It is recommended for this approach to use SWOT analysis. Based on Figure 2.6, it is possible to make the following risk identifications:

Risk 1: Bidding waiver protocols that should take 45 days to complete or a maximum 90 days are far from the required period in normal conditions of work in the institution, considering the current normality of productivity (second sphere);

Risk 2: Under stress conditions, where productivity started to fail (third sphere = grey colour of Table 2.4), a bidding waiver has a high risk of taking on times and failures that are totally out of tolerance for this type of bidding modality;

Risk 3: As the institution assumes more bids, it assumes more time and failures beyond the 180-day margin;

Risks 4 and 5: Under stress, with 12 more projects being executed in the period, the sectors present for a bidding waiver have an intolerable margin of time and failures (risk 5) and for normal bidding an intolerable margin of failures and time relatively similar to the other performances under stress.

2.5 DISCUSSION AND IMPLICATIONS

It is not uncommon that public administration finds some limitations in addressing citizens' needs for the best performances for public services or really supportive infrastructure [29–31]. Also, it's not uncommon that the public sector comes up with a totally poor quality of information, services or political planning available to citizens, considering the vertical degree of organisation that we know as top-down approaches, even for democratic governments [11–12]. And concerning the method used and future risk analysis during COVID-19, it was verified that am agent's performance of work influenced public sector promptness and efficiency to provide solutions for democratic tasks.

When these precarious political system scenarios come up, the information used to execute a work tends to be individualised and also under subjectivity scales, or in other words, the discretisation of information and knowledge necessary to execute a task is not well performed, leaving individuals to create their own ad hoc methods [24]. The main task of the future risk analysis method consists of, from the input of data of administrative workflows, a performance-based algorithm, a graph analysis of how multiple tasks are performed in terms of precision and time, resulting in a monitoring and predictive tool. Continuous variables such as the human processing of information are hard to put in a standard in administrative workflows with traditional methods such as Lean, SWOT, Kanban and so on. Therefore, to avoid biases and unknown nature of the investigation, specific parameters were used to compose the equation for future risk analysis, and these parameters can assume as numerical outputs the subjective scale as performances under normal and stressful conditions of work.

The future risk analysis takes into consideration that if policy making is controversial or not issues that need to be achieved, certainly a control of the input-output of the administrative data and agent's work performance need to be used, because, if basic administrative tasks fail, they also fail to achieve policies, resulting in turn, in a failure of democratic process in the society along the years.

Also, specifically in the subject of this research, it reported some consequences for the delayed response of the public sector to the health system during COVID-19 in Brazil and in the state investigated:

• Deaths;
• Lack of equipment or drugs;
• Stress condition is forwarded to the next agents in the workflow that is hospitals, clinics and so on;
• Lack of confidence to government and democratic stability;
• Delayed response to new technologies or drugs;
• Wrong choices by buying wrong items – no testing performances, but an attempt to give a final hit;
• Increase in demand for hospitals and other services by time;
• Chaotic pattern formation to generate new policies and expected indicators performances;
• Uncertainty in the actions taken and results expected;
• Corruption increase.

2.6 LIMITATIONS OF THE STUDY AND SCOPE FOR FURTHER RESEARCH

One limitation of this study refers to the confounding scenario where COVID-19 took place worldwide. It has implications towards which factors influenced most the instability of countries' governments in terms of policies to be adopted and science itself being in a phase of discussion mostly. For this reason, the study tried to have as a scope a specific scenario of analysis where democratic achievements and public administration have its role.

And concerning the scope for future researches, it's possible to consider that in many cases of democratic divergences, solutions to the problems are the least observed issue, but that really should concern us all [35]. Following this path, not even governors worry about finding solutions to divergences, and top-down or popular approaches are considered as the first tool of governing. More experienced and organised societies expend more money to find solutions in a given modern problem than struggling with each one's opinions/subjectivity. That can be considered the true value of a control system in complex and massive hybrid organisations or societies where computerisation, discretisation of information and working skills are mandatory concepts.

2.7 CONCLUSION

The confrontation with COVID-19 today is something that required and is still demanding that countries have their infrastructure in good condition in order to respond in an immediate and well-designed way to avoid the virus spreading. Therefore, the use of resilient risk analysis can be helpful for public institutions to mitigate their own and natural limitations imposed by disruptive events.

From the 26 examples on bidding procedures of the Paraná State administrative unit analysed during the COVID-19 period, a risk analysis of the samples indicated that work performance to endure COVID-19 is very disqualified and does not achieve the proper standards of efficiency and effectiveness that this pandemic time required. This study showed new governments come with new management systems. For each new administration, new political projects are devised, which, when they start to come out of the paper, strongly collide with the inefficiency and inefficiency of implementation, given that the base that supports the entire system does not allow for it. Democratically, the lack of fulfillment of goals for the population makes the political system itself seriously falliable, as well as the role of institutions, leading to believe that the failures to fulfill constant goals accumulate and affect the existence of the democratic regime over the years.

Funding: This research received no external funding.

Conflicts of Interest: The authors declare no conflict of interest.

Data availability: all the data used in the tables and figures were compiled by the author Charles Roberto Telles and they are available upon request or they can be found as raw information from the webpage transparencia. pr.gov.br: www.transparencia.pr.gov.br/pte/home;jsessionid=Ir8m0viFb-7fY0pNZ0Jt-fKMw09weQUle3x4KtDdE.ssecs75004?windowId=748, also for biddings waivers, www.transparencia.pr.gov.br/pte/compras/dispensasInexigibilidade?windowId=992 and normal biddings at www.transparencia.pr.gov.br/pte/compras/licitacoes/inicio?windowId=483.

2.8 REFERENCES

[1] S. Turale et al., "Challenging times: Ethics, nursing and the COVID-19 pandemic." *International Nursing Review* vol. 67 no. 2, pp. 164–167, 2020. https://doi.org/10.1111/inr.12598.

[2] A. Kumar, S. Luthra, S. Kumar Mangla, and Y. Kazançoğlu, "COVID-19 impact on sustainable production and operations management." *Sustainable Operations and Computers* vol. 1, pp. 1–7, 2020. https://doi.org/10.1016/j.susoc.2020.06.001.

[3] D. Ivanov, "Predicting the impacts of epidemic outbreaks on global supply chains: A simulation-based analysis on the coronavirus outbreak (COVID-19/SARS-CoV-2) case." *Transportation Research Part E: Logistics and Transportation Review*, vol. 136, 101922, 2020. https://doi.org/10.1016/j.tre.2020.101922.

[4] J. L. Hick, D. Hanfling, M. K. Wynia, and A. T. Pavia, "Duty to plan: Health care, crisis standards of care, and novel coronavirus SARS-CoV-2." *Nam Perspectives*, 2020. https://doi.org/10.31478/202003b.

[5] C. Bryce, P. Ring, S. Ashby, and J. K. Wardman, "Resilience in the face of uncertainty: Early lessons from the COVID-19 pandemic." *Journal of Risk Research* vol. 23, no. 7–8, pp. 880–887, 2020. https://doi.org/10.1080/13669877.2020.1756379.

[6] M. Alkahtani, M. Omair, Q. S. Khalid, G. Hussain, I. Ahmad, and C. Pruncu, "A covid-19 supply chain management strategy based on variable production under uncertain environment conditions." *International Journal of Environmental Research and Public Health* vol. 18, no. 4, pp. 1662, 2021. https://doi.org/10.3390/ijerph18041662.

[7] M. S. Golan, B. D. Trump, J. C. Cegan, and I. Linkov, "Supply chain resilience for vaccines: review of modeling approaches in the context of the COVID-19 pandemic." *Industrial Management & Data Systems*, 2021. https://doi.org/10.1108/IMDS-01-2021-0022.

[8] C. L. Atkinson, C. McCue, E. Prier, and A. M. Atkinson, "Supply chain manipulation, misrepresentation, and magical thinking during the COVID-19 pandemic." *The American Review of Public Administration* vol. 50, no. 6–7, pp. 628–634, 2020. https://doi.org/10.1177/0275074020942055.

[9] Jr. Ketchen, J. David, and C. W. Craighead, "Research at the intersection of entrepreneurship, supply chain management, and strategic management: Opportunities highlighted by COVID-19." *Journal of Management* vol. 46, no. 8, pp. 1330–1341, 2020. https://doi.org/10.1177/0149206320945028.

[10] A. S. Sangeetha, S. Shunmugan, and G. Murugan, "Blockchain for IoT enabled supply chain management-a systematic review." In *2020 Fourth International Conference on I-SMAC (IoT in Social, Mobile, Analytics and Cloud)(I-SMAC)*, pp. 48–52. IEEE, 2020. https://doi.org/10.1109/I-SMAC49090.2020.9243371.

[11] T. Dai, M. H. Zaman, W. Padula, and P. M. Davidson, "Supply chain failures amid Covid-19 signal a new pillar for global health preparedness." *Journal of Clinical Nursing*, 2020. https://doi.org/10.1111/jocn.15400.

[12] G. Gereffi, "What does the COVID-19 pandemic teach us about global value chains? The case of medical supplies." *Journal of International Business Policy* vol. 3, no. 3, pp. 287–301, 2020. https://doi.org/10.1057/s42214-020-00062-w.

[13] P. Aubrecht, J. Essink, M. Kovac, and Ann-Sophie Vandenberghe, "Centralized and decentralized responses to COVID-19 in federal systems: US and EU comparisons." Available at *Social Science Research Network (SSRN)* 3584182, 2020. http://dx.doi.org/10.2139/ssrn.3584182

[14] D. Ivanov and A. Dolgui, "OR-methods for coping with the ripple effect in supply chains during COVID-19 pandemic: Managerial insights and research implications." *International Journal of Production Economics* vol. 232, 107921, 2021. https://doi.org/10.1016/j.ijpe.2020.107921.

[15] R. Barifouse, "Covid-19: Por que a pandemia saiu do controle no Paraná." *BBC News Brasil*, December 06, 2020. [Online]. Available: www.bbc.com/portuguese/brasil-55201873. [Accessed July 25, 2021].

[16] G1PR, "Curitiba completa 10 dias com superlotação de UTIs para adultos com Covid-19." G1 PR, June 4, 2021. [Online]. Available: https://g1.globo.com/pr/parana/noticia/2021/06/04/curitiba-completa-10-dias-com-superlotacao-de-utis-para-adultos-com-covid-19.ghtml. [Accessed July 25, 2021].

[17] *Redação Paraná*, "Colapso: Curitiba registra 104% de ocupação de leitos de UTI, com fila de espera.". Redação Paraná, June 2, 2021. [Online]. Available: www.brasildefato.com.br/2021/06/02/colapso-curitiba-registra-104-de-ocupacao-de-leitos-de-uti-com-fila-de-espera. [Accessed July 25, 2021].

[18] E. B. Connelly, C. R. Allen, K. Hatfield, J. M. Palma-Oliveira, D. D. Woods, and I. Linkov, "Features of resilience." *Environment Systems and Decisions* vol. 37, no. 1, pp. 46–50, 2017. https://doi.org/10.1007/s10669-017-9634-9.

[19] M. S. Golan, L. H. Jernegan, and I. Linkov, "Trends and applications of resilience analytics in supply chain modeling: Systematic literature review in the context of the COVID-19 pandemic." *Environment Systems and Decisions* vol. 40, pp. 222–243, 2020. https://doi.org/10.1007/s10669-020-09777-w.

[20] M. Stephen, C. Gu, and H. Yang, "Visibility graph based time series analysis." *PloS One* vol. 10, no. 11, e0143015, 2015. https://doi.org/10.1371/journal.pone.0143015.

[21] A. M. Núñez, L. Lacasa and B. Luque, "Mapping dynamics into graphs. The visibility algorithm." Ph.D. dissertation, Universidad Politécnica de Madrid, 2014.

[22] B. T. Pentland and M. S. Feldman, "Organizational routines as a unit of analysis." *Industrial and Corporate Change* vol. 14, no. 5, pp. 793–815, 2005. https://doi.org/10.1093/icc/dth070.

[23] S. Ranson, B. Hinings, and R. Greenwood, "The structuring of organizational structures," *Administrative Science Quarterly* vol. 25, no. 1, pp. 1–7, 1980. www.jstor.org/stable/i341306.

[24] B. T. Pentland, T. Haerem, and D. W. Hillison, "4. Using workflow data to explore the structure of an organizational routine." *Organizational Routines: Advancing Empirical Research* vol. 47, 2009. https://doi.org/10.4337/9781848447240.00010.

[25] J. Birkinshaw, R. Nobel, and J. Ridderstråle, "Knowledge as a contingency variable: Do the characteristics of knowledge predict organization structure?" *Organization Science* vol. 13, no. 3, pp. 274–289, 2002. www.jstor.org/stable/3086021.

[26] J. Cardoso, "Approaches to compute workflow complexity." In *Dagstuhl Seminar Proceedings*. Schloss Dagstuhl-Leibniz-Zentrum für Informatik, 2006.

[27] K. Garber, M. M. Ajiko, S. M. Gualtero-Trujillo, S. Martinez-Vernaza, and A. Chichom-Mefire, "Structural inequities in the global supply of personal protective equipment." 2020. *British Medical Journal*. https://doi.org/10.1136/bmj.m2727.

[28] L. Young, "Our economic systems have failed. Will Covid-19 shock us into sense?" *Varsity Publications Ltd*. University of Cambridge Newspaper, March 2, 2021. [Online]. Available: www.varsity.co.uk/opinion/20789. [Accessed March 14, 2021].

[29] R. E. Glover and N. Maani, "Have we reached 'peak neoliberalism' in the UK's covid-19 response?" *British Medical Journal*, January 27, 2021. [Online]. Available: https://blogs.bmj.com/bmj/2021/01/27/have-we-reached-peak-neoliberalism-in-the-uks-covid-19-response/. [Accessed March 20, 2021].

[30] N. Chomsky and V. Prashad, "Why neoliberal leaders who failed to protect their countries from COVID-19 must be investigated." *Alice News: Centro de Estudos Sociais*, January 1, 2021. [Online]. Available: https://alicenews.ces.uc.pt/index.php?lang=1&id=32471. [Accessed May 2, 2021].

[31] M. Šumonja, "Neoliberalism is not dead – On political implications of Covid-19." *Capital & Class* 0309816820982381, 2020. https://doi.org/10.1177/0309816820982381.

[32] L. Jones, and S. Hameiri, "COVID-19 and the failure of the neoliberal regulatory state." *Review of International Political Economy* pp. 1–25, 2021. https://doi.org/10.1080/09692290.2021.1892798.

[33] N. P. Isaković, "Covid-19: What has Covid-19 taught us about neoliberalism?" WILPF International. 2020. [Online]. Available: www.wilpf.org/covid-19-what-has-covid-19-taught-us-about-neoliberalism/. [Accessed March 20, 2021].

[34] J. Bolsonaro, S. Moro, and L. H. Mandetta, *DOU-Federal Oficial Diary Newspaper*. "Lei n° 13.979, de 6 de fevereiro de 2020." 2020. Brazil.

[35] M. H. Moore, "Creating public value: The core idea of strategic management in government." *International Journal of Professional Business Review* vol. 6, no. 1, pp. 219, 2021. https://doi.org/10.26668/businessreview/2021.v6i1.219.

2.9   SUPPLEMENTARY DATA 1

Questionnaire sent to the CPL and CCC sector to verify the work performed based on the availability and characteristics of the sector's human resources.

Questionnaire	CPL	CCC
1. How many employees currently work in your sector?	4	8
2. What would be the ideal number in case you understand that there is still a lack of collaborators?	6	9
3. All employees have what level of education?	4 undergraduate	6 undergraduate /2 high school
4. Does each employee have working time (experience) with their role in the sector?	4[a]	1: 1 year 3: 2 years 4: 3 years
5. Is your sector's workflow well defined? (Or there are work assignments that you feel should not be in the sector, or there is a lack of organisation in stages prior to yours, describe the situation if necessary)	Yes	Yes
6. If you could highlight the main problem (between sectors or other) that there is for the work to be carried out efficiently and effectively, what would you point out?	The workflow and procedures must be set up in a clear, objective manner and in accordance with current legislation.	The planning of service contracts/ material acquisitions must be done within a minimum period of 6 months, as the bidding protocols last an average of 3 months, from the preparation of the Terms of Reference for the signing of the contract, and then start the period of contract execution. Other than that, the sectors should have the ability to prepare the Terms of Reference, as it is the main document of the protocols, which guides everything else.
7. In relation to information systems: e-protocol, or other systems that you use to be able to register, work with data, control input and output of information from your sector: Is there a good control of information in your sector by each employee and the existing systems work well, or would you have suggestions for the implementation of new systems?	They work.	Yes, requests arrive via e-protocol and are logged for tracking purposes.

[a] Where 1 means a lot of experience and 3 an average of since 6 protocols each since 2019. *Source*: Telles, C. R.

2.10   SUPPLEMENTARY DATA 2

Parameters used to check frequency of CGE and PGE notes.

1. Terms of reference

ID*	Parameters
1.1	Object description
1.2	Price quotation
1.3	Draft notification
1.4	Technical detail of the object and the intended solution (project instruction, legislation and/or the protocol itself/execution/nature of the object)
1.5	Indication of micro and small businesses (ME) and small businesses (EPP)
1.6	Content organisation (trivial errors regarding numbering, grammar, sequence and missing items)
1.7	Legislation
1.8	Authorisation and/or approval of responsible person
1.9	Statements signed by the contractor (18 years old, nepotism, sustainability)

2. Protocol instruction

ID*	Parameters
2.1	Indication of budget resources for the expenditure
2.2	Authorisation from the expense organiser
2.3	Materials and Services Management System: consults the price registration minutes and other system records.
2.4	Price justification
2.5	Technical opinion on the normal or the COVID-19 bidding waiver and issues related to the virus
2.6	Technical qualification documents and economic-financial qualification documents, when applicable.
2.7	Tax and labor regularity
2.8	Contract execution
2.9	Monitoring, inspection and management of the contract

*ID: object identification for analysis purposes. *Source*: transparencia.pr.gov.br compiled by Telles, C. R.

3 Role of Advanced Technologies in Gait Analysis and Its Importance in Healthcare

Neha P. Sathe[1], Anil Hiwale[1] and Archana Ranade[2]
[1] MIT World Peace University, Pune, India
[2] Deenanath Mangeshkar Hospital and
Research Centre, Pune, India

CONTENTS

DOI: 10.1201/9781003217107-3

3.1 INTRODUCTION

The study of locomotion or mobility of humans is called gait, and analysis of each phase of ambulation is defined as gait analysis. A systematic study of human movement done through the observer with eyes and brain in terms of qualitative method or through instrumental assistance quantitative methods are clinically accepted to infer the deviation in the human gait pattern. Even though considering subjectivity, gait analysis has contributed from decades in support of rehabilitation process, but changes in lifestyle and its replications in terms of lifestyle diseases are at the forefront and need to be take upon as a priority as pre-habilitation. As an illustration, the factsheet of the World Health Organization (WHO) regarding diabetes specifies that a healthy diet and regular physical exercise help to prevent or delay type 2 diabetic [1]. The WHO promotes the adaption of digital health for accelerating well-being [2]. Understanding our health, daily activity monitoring, nature of work, variation in eating habits and a lot more are contributing directly in maintaining the fitness graph of an individual. Awareness about preventive care is increasing day by day to tackle lifestyle disease, and for the masses, adaption to walking exercise is a common place to begin. The simplest way of exerting for fitness is to walk. Due to the availability of technological support with fitness bands and activity monitoring applications, people have started to speak about their daily step count target, calory chart, sleep time record, etc. To comprehend the role of balance, symmetry, stability, movement control and weight transfer on both legs

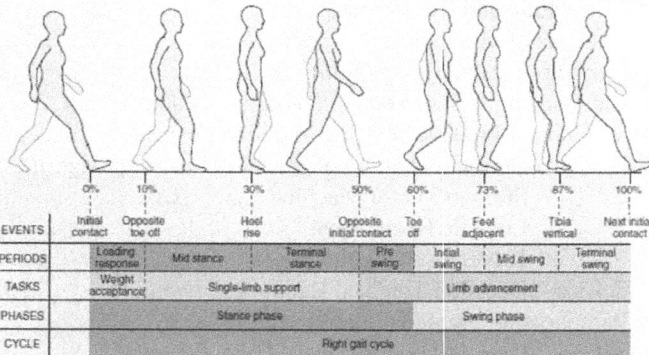

FIGURE 3.1 Gait cycle phases.

Source: Di Gregorio et al. Biomimetics 6.2 (2021): 22[3].

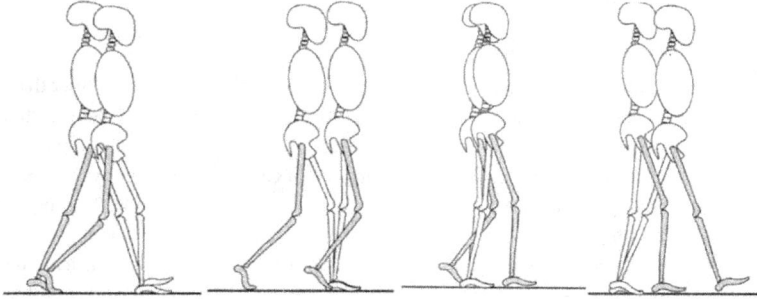

FIGURE 3.2   Swing phases (pre, initial, mid and terminal).

Source: Jacquelin Perry, New Jersey: SLACK (2010) [4].

and walking speed during walking, it is essential to analyse and differentiate a normal gait with any deviations within it. Thus, gait analysis will provide the insight.

3.2   GAIT PATTERN

The human gait comprises of number of repetitive events in association with musculoskeletal support used to move the body in a forward direction. Both legs follow the small event in a cyclic pattern to move the body. In an alternate manner both legs touch the ground, a preform swinging action in the air will take care of load balancing by managing the weight transfer. Such repetitive gait cycles constitute the gait pattern of the human. Figure 3.1 [3] shows the typical stages of the gait cycle (GC).

Each GC is divided in two stages: stance and swing. The stance phase resembles to all the event where the foot remains in contact with the ground. In the swing phase the foot is in the air for mobility. In the case of a normal person, the GC starts with a heel strike, first floor contact for movement termed initial contact. Stance phase covers three different steps: in the beginning and at the end of stance both legs contact with the ground (double stance or double limb support) and in middle of the stance only one foot contacts the ground (single limb support). In the start of GC, the double stance performs the weight acceptance and balancing. During the single support time or single limb support, the complete load is on one foot while other is in the swing phase. The longer single support holding duration specifies the stability of that leg. Double stance at the end of GC (terminal double stance) starts with the floor contact of the foot contralateral to initial contact and continues until the original stance foot is lifted for the swing phase.

Swing is subdivided in four stages: pre-swing, initial swing, mid swing and terminal swing as shown in Figure 3.2 [4]. The pre-swing phase is followed after the terminal stance which is a double stance phase, thus shifting from double support to single and preparation of the transfer of body weight from double to single foot initiates through the pre-swing phase for movement in a forward direction. In the initial swing phase advancement of the foot from its latest position is started by lifting the foot, covering the mid swing andtTerminal swing completes the advancement of the foot opposite to the foot in stance phase.

Altogether, considering each sub-phase of GC, the contribution of each one and critical functionalities performed over the time are listed in Table 3.1 [4].

TABLE 3.1

Gait Cycle Phases and Intervals

Sr No.	Name of the Phase	Interval in Terms of %	Objective
1.	Initial Contact - Foot touches the floor and perform weight transfer.	0% to 2% GC	Start of stance with heel rocker position
2.	Loading Response – Initial double stance followed after initial contact with ground	2% to 12% of GC	Performs weight bearing and shock absorption Start preparation for progression
3.	Mid Stance – beginning of single limb support	12% to 31% of GC	Assure limb and trunk stability and start progression with stationary foot
4.	Terminal stance – complete the single limb support phase and begin heel rise and other foot will strike the ground	31% to 50% of GC	Progression of body beyond the mid-stance phase with supporting foot
5.	Pre-Swing –– Initial terminal stance with double stance interval and initiate in initial contact of other foot with toe off.	50% to 62% of GC	Release of weight from prior foot and transfer to other and accelerate progression
6.	Initial Swing – starts with lifting the foot from the ground contact	62% to 75% of GC	Assures the foot clearance from the ground Initiate movement of foot from its trailing position
7.	Mid-Swing- swinging limb is moved forward	75% to 87% of GC	Advancement of the foot
8.	Terminal Swing – swinging foot touches the ground	87% to 100% GC	Complete the advancement phase and prepare the foot for next cycle of stance

Source: Jacquelin Perry et al. New Jersey: SLACK (2010) [4].

3.2.1   DEFINITIONS OF SPATIOTEMPORAL PARAMETERS

To monitor the gait pattern, the movement of the person observed across the surface provides the details regarding the distance covered and number of instances covered during the period in association with the time taken to complete all the minor activities. To elaborate, spatial (space) and temporal (time) parameters are taken into consideration. The typical spatiotemporal parameters used in gait analysis are:

- **Step length and stride length**

  When person starts walking with the initial position of both feet together and takes a first step: left or right foot for advancement and place it on the ground then the distance between right foot heel strike to left foot heel strike is specified as step length (cm), replicated graphically in Figure 3.3.

  The stride length is the distance between two consecutive advancements of the foot which will cover one advancement of the left and right foot

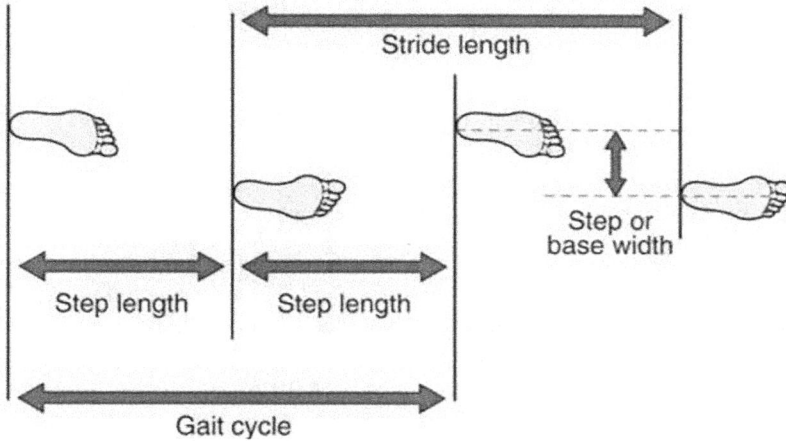

FIGURE 3.3   Step length and stride length.

covering two steps. If we start with a right foot step then that would be followed by a left foot step and the distance between heel strike of the right foot until the next heel strike of the right foot (cm), replicated graphically in Figure 3.3.

- **Step time and stride time**

  In line with the step length and stride length the step time is the duration elapsed in the foot advancement of one foot. The heel strike of the right leg to heel strike of the left leg is the one step time (sec), and the time elapsed in executing a stride or two steps is specified as the stride time covering the advancement of two feet or two steps. Calculated as time elapsed in heel strike of the right foot and next consecutive heel strike of the right foot (sec).

- **Cadence and velocity**

  Cadence specifies the number of steps taken per minute or steps covered per unit time by the person. Velocity specifies the distance covered by the person in unit time, measured in m/s, considering variation in instantaneous velocity, average velocity is calculated (m/min) by multiplying step length by cadence.

- **Stance % of cycle and swing % of cycle**

  The duration occupied by the stance and swing phase across the complete gait cycle in terms of percentage is specified. Out of 100% cycle time, the approximate division of 60% of stance and 40% of swing along with approximate standard deviation are considered.

- **Single support and double support time**

  Durations are taken into consideration providing the details about time duration in (sec), elaborate additional details if details regarding double support loading and unloading durations are considered. These parameters are used in a deeper level of analysis along with other parameters.

Thus, a combination of parameters describing distance covered and time taken for the same contribute a lot of information in gait analysis. Along with the listed parameters detailing through toe in/out angle, heel on/off time are also used. Based on the technique used to record the gait parameter, the feasibility of getting details changes and remains technology dependent definitely, with an increased set of parameters, detailed analysis becomes possible.

3.2.2 METHODS OF CAPTURING THE GAIT PATTERN

The way of capturing and analysing the gait pattern has had enormous developments across decades. Starting with the manual observer, use of image and video, marker infrared reflectors, electronic walkway, embedded sensor technology and a lot more with mobile and fitness band related application options have emerged. The validity of the measurement of gait parameters depends on the measuring instrument used.

3.2.2.1 Visual Gait Analysis

Performed by the physiotherapist to investigate the problem with a patient without any instrument aid. Becomes subjective and person dependent. Inference and decision remain subjective to the person, it would be difficult to recognise high-speed actions, details in term of quantity of any parameter is not possible, so it will provide superficial information. Repeated actions from the patient are advisable to get a thorough analysis. Maintaining a record manually becomes a tedious job with increasing number. Reliability completely depends on the personal skill of the observer. Typical abnormalities and best suitable angle for visual observation are specified as to a lateral, anterior or posterior trunk bending side view is appropriate, while the front view becomes helpful in identifying an abnormal walk [5].

3.2.2.2 Recorded Video Content

Various techniques like video cassette recording, recording through a specialised camera or mobile-based application are used to record the walk of the person and for analysis. If such a technique is provided for visual analysis, it will reduce the efforts of the patient for frequent or repetition of walking, and aminating will be easy. Playing the recorded content in slow motion may help to grab the details. The next advancement in recorded video content is using computerised assistance in extracting the features from the video and with the use of appropriate software getting additional inputs to complement the visual analysis. A specialised clinic would have setup of motion capture systems. With the use of reflective markers placed on the body, and recording done through infrared cameras capturing body motion with high sampling rate, detailed analysis is possible. Recording becomes environment dependent and a costly affair, and marker setup may disturb the comfort of the person when walking [6].

3.2.2.3 Force Plates and Electromyography

A force plate works on the princip;e of ground reaction force. The force plates are embedded in a rigid platform and analog to digital converted signals are recorded on a computer. Placement of a force plate beneath the walking area matters a lot. While recording the walk position of both legs on the force plate is essential for accurate data recovery, inappropriate placement of force plates may lead to collection of unsuitable data. To overcome the limitation of the motion capturing method, force plated or electromyography techniques are used. A combination of force plate technique and kinematic information retrieved through an optical motion capture system may provide kinetic information using inverse dynamics. Electromyography (EMG) is used to record the electrical activity generated by muscles and to study it. With development of a wireless EMG system, the involvement of EMG signal along with other sensors are providing complete system setup for gait recording.

3.2.2.4   Sensor-Based Techniques

Recent technological developments in body-worn sensors and availability of miniature sensors have put forwarded the easy technique of gait recording. With the use of an accelerometer, gyroscope, EMG sensor, pressure sensor, etc., the portable, low-cost modules are available. Embedded and miniature technology and inclusion of sensors in handheld devices like mobile phone or fitness bands has emerged with various solutions for daily activity monitoring. Extraction of features from data provided by sensors and further computerised analysis is common practice.

3.2.3   Review of Gait Analysis in Patient Monitoring

There are various clinical applications where gait analysis can be used. Table 3.2 provides the details about available sensor setup and its clinical application [6].

TABLE 3.2
Use of Various Gait-Related Sensors and Its Clinical Applications

Type of Sensors	Feature Extracted	Clinical Application
3D accelerometer mounted on thigh and shank	Range of motion of ankle and knee	For ankle fractures
3D accelerometer mounted on lower back	Local dynamic stability	Faller and non-faller group's stability
3D accelerometer and gyroscope embedded in shoe	Statistical feature extraction	Parkinson's for stability test
3D accelerometer and gyroscope mounted on waist	Total transition time, jerk, rotational speed	Geriatric rehabilitation
Sensors mounted on back – 3D accelerometer, gyroscope and magnetometer	Spatiotemporal parameters	Hemiplegic gait
Sensors placed in shoe – 3D accelerometer, gyroscope and magnetometer	Walk speed, spatiotemporal parameters	Hemiplegic gait
Sensors placed on wrist 3D – accelerometer and gyroscope	Symmetry index	Detecting asymmetry in early Parkinson's stage
Insole pressure sensors	Features extracted from centre of pressure data	Identifying gait deviation in children and cerebral palsy

Source: Chen, Shanshan, et al. IEEE journal of biomedical and health informatics 20.6 (2016): 1521–1537 [6].

Irrespective of the technology to be used for analysing the gait parameters, use of such technological advancement and improving the visibility of results are essential considerations in the latest developments. Use of gait parameters in normal patients, its applicability in rehabilitation or for achieving fitness will be of foremost importance when represented and described with an exact scope and by defining the applicability of it. Such a role of technological assistance used in research as a pathway is described in term of case studies.

3.2.3.1 Case Study of Cerebral Palsy

To decide the line of treatment in the case of cerebral palsy, the gait analysis has been used for decades in healthcare. Definitely after analysing each patient, the separate line of treatment must be decided, but the assistive use of a tool of gait parameters remains common. To specify the involvement of such technical assistance, some references are mentioned.

- *Journal of Pediatric Orthopaedics* published a research article in 2003 regarding altering decision making in cerebral palsy with assistance of gait analysis [7]. The decision regarding need for surgery in a few subjects was altered after gait analysis was combined with clinical examination. Good agreement of decision in case of bone surgery was observed, while poor agreement was observed in case of soft tissue operations. As mentioned in the paper, gait analysis alters 40% of the decisions in operative procedure, which is remarkable and must be considered.
- *The American Congress of Rehabilitation Medicine* and *the American Academy of Physical Medicine and Rehabilitation* published a research paper in 1992 which highlighted the use of gait analysis along with clinical examination for decision on surgery in treating patients with cerebral palsy. The author also covers the significance of postoperative development to know the fruitfulness of the combined strategy. The cases where surgery was recommended are also included to consider and improve the role of decision making by using gait analysis along with clinical examination [8].
- *Clinical Orthopaedics and Related Research* published a research article specifying the role of gait analysis in cerebral palsy treatment [9]. It mentioned the importance of stance phase stability, foot preposition in terminal swing, swing phase clearance, adequate step length and utilisation of energy as parameters to identify normal gait and comment that many or few of these are missing in the patient with cerebral palsy. Various methods are described to help out with decision making.

These case studies are added with the intention to specify the prolonged use of recommended assistive support of gait analysis along with clinical examination.

3.2.3.2 Case Study of Geriatric Care

Considering geriatric care, the serious concern is fall risk, as per the WHO falls are the second leading cause of unintentional injury and death and efforts need to be taken for gait training, balance and functional training to avoid the risk of falling. To describe the involvement of technological help in this category, a few test cases are described.

- The study carried out for understanding the effect of mild cognitive impairment in older people done through dual tasking – talking while walking on the electronic treadmill provides important findings. The test was carried out on 11 elderly people with mild cognitive impairment in two sessions and six gait parameters. Research work concluded with the outcome that in older people with mild cognitive impairment, temporal gait parameters are increased with dual tasking suggesting cognitive control [10].
- The study carried out for knowing the reliability of mobile instrumented gait analysis in older people who are facing mobility restriction. More than 100 patients were considered in the trial. Shoe-embedded inertial sensors are used, and they are asked to pass on an instrumented walkway used for recording of gait without gait support or as per needed required gait support. The obtained result highlights that use of wheeled walker in gait assessment can be quantified objectively by an instrumented method [11].

Thus, with the use of gait analysis in older people, a number of parameters can be evaluated to provide comfort to them.

3.3 STATISTICAL ANALYSIS OF GAIT FEATURES

Gait analysis will provide additional information by making perfect groupings of various spatial or temporal parameters. Knowing the relation among all parameters provides the insight towards linkages among them. Understanding the dependency or anti-dependency within these parameters helps out in related analysis. Whenever a scenario is necessary to deal with quantitative measure and analysis, it is essential to know the distribution, relation, ranges, variation, deviation, etc., associated with it. The statistical analysis tools provide the foundation to establish such all relations in an available quantitative dataset. Regarding statistical analysis of gait parameters, a few points are described which are commonly adopted and followed to take up research or to conclude certain findings. Based on statistical tests, comparative analysis and inferences are written and this helps to strengthen the clinical evidence.

3.3.1 DESCRIPTIVE STATISTICS REFERENCES

Use of descriptive statistics helps researchers to understand the exact information from the collected data. The collected data is represented in a different way with descriptive statistics to increase the visualisation and understanding of it. It will be better to begin with a selection of appropriate statistical reference tests to be used and formation of hypotheses as an indicator. Relating the work to be carried out, a required statistical tool is a crucial point of decision at different levels of work. Central tendency and dispersion are used as measures of descriptive statistics. Central tendency will provide details regarding mean, mode and median, while dispersion will provide details regarding variance and standard deviation. Table 3.3 gives the overview of commonly used descriptive statistic tools in clinical analysis [12].

3.3.1.1 Shape and Normality

Shape describes the pattern or distribution of the data available in the dataset. The data included within a dataset may be distributed symmetrically or asymmetrically specified as normal distribution and skewed distribution, respectively. In the case of the normal distribution of the dataset, the plotted histogram will follow a bell shape as shown in Figure 3.4.

Symmetry is measured with the skewness, which precisely checks for a lack of symmetry. If a distribution looks similar to the left and right sides of the centre point, then the dataset distribution is symmetric.

TABLE 3.3
Descriptive Statistics Tools in Clinical Analysis

Common Descriptive Statistic Tools Used

Central Tendency	Shape	Variation
Mode	Symmetry	Range
Median	Kurtosis	Variance
Mean		Standard Deviation

Source: Rodrigues et al., Revista brasileira de anestesiologia 67 (2017): 619–625 [12].

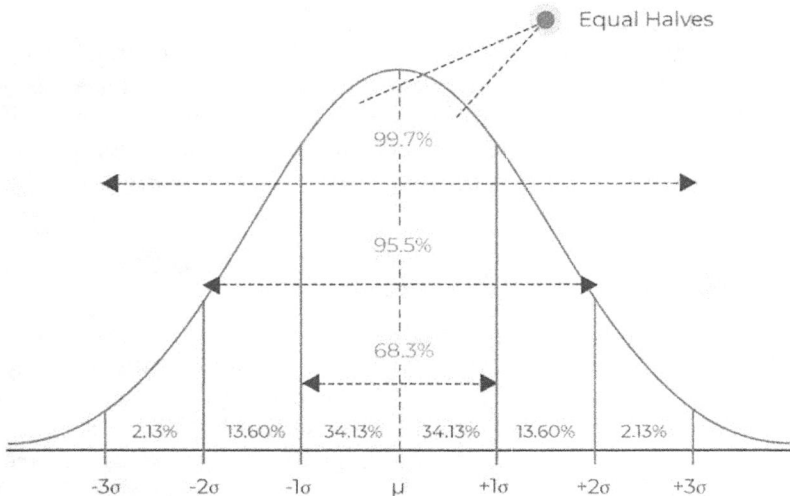

FIGURE 3.4 Bell curve: normal distribution.

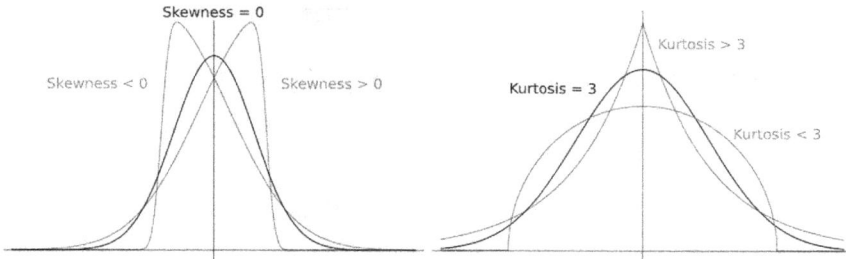

FIGURE 3.5 Skewness and kurtosis curve.

To understand the heavy-tailed or light-tailed distribution of data, kurtosis is used. The heavy tails with outliers are seen in high kurtosis, and light tails with lack of outliers shows low kurtosis value. A uniform distribution would be the extreme case. Figure 3.5 indicates the typical graph for skewness and kurtosis [13].

- Mean: it is an important measure, commonly referred as arithmetic mean, the sum of all the N contributors is divided by number of contributors (N) to get the mean of it. The mean value is useful to understand the overall trend of the dataset.
- Median: it is the middle value in distribution when the values are arranged in ascending order or descending order. This median is sometimes used to identify outliers. While calculating median, if the number of contributors is odd, then median is the middle number with equal count above and below it. If the number of contributors in the dataset is even, the middle pair must be added together and divided by 2 to identify the median value.
- Mode: it is defined as the value that has a higher frequency in a given set of values. It is the value that appears the most number of times. A set of data may have one mode, more than one mode or no mode at all.
- Variance: is the measure of variability; it specifies the spread between numbers in a dataset. If a dataset is spread then it will give a larger variance, which means numbers are far from each other.
- Standard deviation: spread of data around the mean is given by standard deviation. Wider spreading of data from the mean value indicates high standard deviation. A low standard deviation indicates data alignment with the mean. In a portfolio of data analysis methods, the standard deviation is useful for quickly determining the dispersion of data points.
- Range: range of a variable is the distance between the highest and lowest value available in the dataset. It will be calculated by identifying highest and lowest available value and subtracting it. But it never specifies anything about distribution.
- Interquartile range: indicates the position of the median. Quartiles represent the 25% and 75% positions in the scale: 25% shows the first quartile value and 75% indicates third quartile distribution. [12–14]

TABLE 3.4

Descriptive Statistical Sample Data

Parameters	Classification Based on Gender							
	Men				Women			
	Minimum	Maximum	Mean	SD	Minimum	Maximum	Mean	SD
Age	69	80	72.6	2.26	69	80	72.8	2.35
Stride length	0.836	1.902	1.471	0.159	0.745	1.721	1.325	0.142
Velocity	0.69	1.95	1.32	0.202	0.54	1.9	1.27	0.216
Body Height	1.44	1.94	1.78	0.059	1.48	1.80	1.645	0.052
Cadence	75.5	141.2	107.4	8.33	78.9	144.6	114.4	10.77

Source: Moe-Nilssen, et al. Gait & Posture 82 (2020): 220–226 [15].

Table 3.4 provides brief statistical information to decide the next step of implementation or to give a thought about further requirements [15].

These parameters are treated as a baseline to start evaluation of the dataset. To work upon any retrieved or derived information, it is essential to understand the distribution of the dataset, the skewness of it. Variations observed in mean, median, etc., values definitely provide a baseline to start, as well as help out to identify outliners which need to be treated separately. Once reference values are available, comparative analysis provided guidelines for the initial path. Comparative analysis covers glimpses of demographic involvement and its influence on possible variation. Independently knowing certain ranges and minimum or maximum values in reference to the available dataset is fundamental information. At the next level it becomes important to know the existence of any relation amid multiple entities available in terms of parameters.

3.3.2 CORRELATION AND COVARIANCE

Correlation coefficients are used to identify the existence of any relation within data. It gets replicated in terms of different result conditions as existence of positive relation, no relation or negative relation. There are various available formulae available to calculate the correlation coefficient, but the most commonly used is Pearson's correlation coefficient which checks the possibility of linear relationships within parameters. The formula to calculate Pearson's correlation coefficient is given in equation 3.1.

$$r = n\left(\sum xy\right) - \left(\sum x\right)\left(\sum y\right) \Big/ \sqrt{\left[n\sum x^2 - \left(\sum x\right)^2\right]\left[n\sum y^2 - \left(\sum y\right)^2\right]} \qquad (3.1)$$

The linear relation is reflected within the range of +1 to -1. The +1 result specifies positive relation, 0 is used for no relation and -1 represents negative relation. When parameters show a positive relation then the increment observed in one must reflect the likely increment in the other, while a negative relation shows a reciprocal result. No relation does not reflect any linkage within parameters. Figure 3.6 shows the range of correlation coefficients and their meaning.

Table 3.5 indicates the stride length with spatiotemporal parameters, and Table 3.6 indicates it with walking velocity [16].

Covariance provides the information about how the two random variables vary together. It is reflected in terms of positive, negative and zero covariance. Movement of variables in the same direction shows positive covariance, while movement of variables in the opposite direction shows negative covariance.

$$cov(X,Y) = \Sigma(X_i - \bar{X})(Y_j - \bar{Y})/n - 1 \qquad (2)$$

Table 3.6 indicates statistical information regarding correlation coefficient and coefficient of variation collected for young and older subjects. Such statistical information helps in further analysis, as well as remains a reference for comparative study across the globe [17].

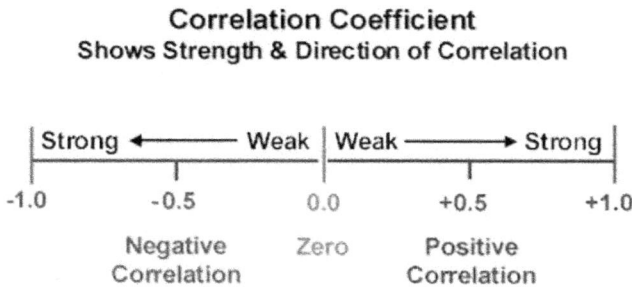

Correlation Coefficient
Shows Strength & Direction of Correlation

FIGURE 3.6   Correlation coefficient range and meaning.

TABLE 3.5
Sample Data for Correlation in Gait Parameters

Correlation	Correlation Coefficient	Regression
Cadence and stride length	0.81	0.0088 cad + 0.58
Candence and velocity	0.95	0.021 cad − 0.79
Stride length and cadence	0.81	75.6 str − 7.0
Stride length and velocity	0.95	1.89 str − 1.46
Velocity and cadence	0.95	44.1 vel + 45.4
Velocity and stride length	0.95	0.47 vel + 0.85

Source: Kirtley, et al. *Journal of Biomedical Engineering* 7.4 (1985): 282–288 [16].

TABLE 3.6
Statistical Details of Young and Older Subjects

Parameter	Younger Participants			Older Participants		
	Inter Class Correlation	Coefficient of Variation	Mean	Inter Class Correlation	Coefficient of Variation	Mean
Walking Speed	0.88 (0.77–0.94)	1.8	1.44 (1.31–1.55)	0.91(0.83–0.96)	3.5	1.17(1–1.33)
Cadence	0.83(0.67–0.91)	1.9	111.48 (102.34–117.77)	0.82(0.66–0.91)	3.1	107.89 (95.32–120.37)
Step Length Right	0.91(0.81–0.95)	1.4	77.30 (73.02–82.81)	0.89(0.78–0.94)	3.5	64.89 (55.65–71.77)
Step Length Left	0.92(0.84–0.96	1.4	77.12 (70–19–79.67)	0.88(0.77–0.94)	3.1	63.56 (55.67–71.17)

Source: Menz, Hylton B., et al. Gait & posture 20.1 (2004): 20–25 [17].

3.3.3 ANALYSIS OF VARIANCE

Analysis of variance (ANOVA) is used as an analysis tool. It is used to separate the observed variance data into two components as a systematic and random. To know the dependency of an independent variable on dependent variable, ANOVA analysis is used. Based on the expected outcome the type of test to be selected, one-way ANOVA test is used to compare more than two means from two independent groups. Two-way ANOVA considers an independent variable affecting the dependent variable. Along with these tests, calculating the standard deviation, confidence interval or prediction interval provides the path to process the data in clinical applications [18].

3.3.4 COMPARATIVE ANALYSIS WITHIN A DATASET

The typical statistical tool is mentioned to understand the applicability of the same few references' calculation are shown. A technical note published in the *Journal of Rehabilitation Research and Development* – Basic Gait Parameters: reference data for normal subjects 10–79 years of age [19] provides statistical references for the normal person within the age group of 10–79 years. Some references are shown in Table 3.7 specifying observed variations in gait speed at different paces in male and female groups with details of mean, standard deviation, confidence interval and prediction interval based on a dataset of 233 members.

On a similar line, calculated reference values are used for analysing the gait pattern. These statistical values are able to provide various guidelines to work on the basis of gait pattern like identifying abnormalities, early detection of unexpected variations, gender classification, verification of correlation within dependent parameters, etc.

3.3.5 CATEGORISATION BASED ON DEMOGRAPHIC FEATURES

Statistical data provides a lot of markers for further analysis, but inclusion of demographic consideration is very important to enhance the analysis level and understand the exact applicability. Based on the geographical regions the height, weight, walking style parameters show changes. That's why to select any statistical available reference to include in a study, it is essential to understand the demographical differences. For example, if the selected dataset has a record of subjects with average height of 5.4 feet and average age of 45+ years, then the observed step, stride and associated parameters cannot be used directly as a reference for a dataset an with average height of 5 feet and age group of 25+ years. In a similar way, gender makes difference in values retrieved as a reference. The values recorded for male and female groups must have markable variation in the range based on height, weight, etc. Thus, while selecting or during preparing the gait dataset, inclusion of demographic information is essential. Such practices are followed by researchers in domains; typical demographic characteristics used include height, weight and body mass index (Table 3.8) [20].

The role and influence of demographic features in gait analysis are of crucial importance. The standard to be referred to for a particular region needs to be compared with appropriate statistical figures; only then will appropriate analysis be feasible. To understand the role of various machine learning techniques and its application

TABLE 3.7
Normative Statistical Reference for Age Groups Based on Speed and Gender

Slow Gait Performance	Gender	Age	Mean	SD	CV	95% CI	95% PI
	Men	10–14	88.7	12	0.14	81.1–96.3	62.3–115.1
		30–39	88.3	18.9	0.21	78.1–98.5	48.6–128.0
		70–79	79.5	13.7	0.17	71.8–87.2	50.7–108.3
	Women	10–14	70.1	12.8	0.18	62.0–78.2	41.9–98.3
		30–39	86.7	15.7	0.18	78.2–95.2	53.7–119.7
		70–79	73.5	10.1	0.14	68.0–79.0	52.3–94.7
Normal Gait Performance	Men	10–14	108.6	11.2	0.10	101.5–115.7	84.0–133.2
		30–39	128.5	19.1	0.15	118.1–138.9	88.4–168.6
		70–79	111.3	12.5	0.11	104.5–118.1	85.1–137.6
	Women	10–14	132.3	19.6	0.15	119.9–144.7	89.2–175.4
		30–39	131.6	15.0	0.11	123.5–139.7	100.1–163.1
		70–79	118.2	15.4	0.13	109.8–126.6	85.9–150.5

Source: Öberg, et al. *Journal of Rehabilitation Research and Development* 30 (1993): 210–210 [19].

TABLE 3.8

Statistical Information on Demographic and Spatiotemporal Parameters

Parameters	Age 65–74		Age 75–84	
	Female	Male	Female	Male
BMI	25.6 ± 4.4	26.2 ± 3.2	26.2 ± 4.7	27.0 ± 3.4
Stride Time (Mean)	1081.5 ± 104.3	1147.3 ± 127.5	1124.3 ± 109.4	1140.7 ± 123.7
Walking Speed	126.1 ± 21.7	124.9 ± 21.6	109.7 ± 21.3	118.0 ± 24.9
Stride velocity (Mean)	123.6 ± 21.2	122.3 ± 21.0	111.1 ± 22.7	118.5 ± 22.5

Source: Beauchet et al. *Frontiers in Human Neuroscience* 11 (2017): 353 [21].

in gait analysis, few cases studies are added, considering a machine learning algorithm in the next section.

3.4 REVIEW OF CLINICAL PREDICTION USING MACHINE LEARNING

The expanded horizon of digitisation, advancement in data gathering techniques, numerous developments in body-worn sensors, evolution of internet of medical things along with machine learning, artificial intelligence and augmented reality are providing support in healthcare systems in different ways. These include technologies at various levels as in disease identification and diagnosis, data retrieving from records, data analysis, imaging techniques, personalised medication maintenance, etc. To know the role of machine learning algorithms in gait analysis prior implementation results are described in the following section.

3.4.1 REVIEW OF IMPLEMENTATION OF MACHINE LEARNING ALGORITHMS

Machine learning: The best suitable technology to learn from the past to perform prediction. The techniques which would help in early diagnosis or might provide some pathway with the prediction and classification technique. The mixed-model approach would become a great benefit by collaboration of technological help along with clinical analysis as a supporting tool. Based on the labelled dataset available, the classification techniques work suitably to provide quantitative data in support of clinical inference. The deployment of such machine learning algorithms to understand the gait characteristic or to identify any variation in spatiotemporal parameters, classifying the person within a diseased group, are described with few supervised machine learning approaches.

3.4.1.1 Support Vector Machine

Support vector machine (SVM) are supervised learning techniques used in the classification and regression prediction process. It is used to increase the maximum accuracy in prediction.

It defines the linear function in high dimensional feature space. SVM has been identified as useful in pattern classification [22].

- Source: Khera et al. [23] provided the detail review of various machine learning techniques used in gait analysis in depth in a research paper. Considering the performance of SVM in the diagnosis of gait disorder, the review results are shown in Table 3.9 [23].
- Source- Zheng et al.: Uses three models of SVM to perform classification: SVM based with all features (ABS), F-test based SVM (FBS), recursive feature elimination based SVM (RBS), the accuracy of classification of Parkinson's disease and healthy group in an imbalance class is shown in Table 3.10 [24].
- Source: Wang, Lei, et al. provides the details regarding classification of three neurological diseases using an inertial measurement unit. The intended classification groups are healthy control (HC), peripheral neuropathy (PC), post-stroke (PS) and Parkinson's disease (PD), which is done by performing daily activity monitoring of spatiotemporal gait parameters.

TABLE 3.9
Gait Disorder Statistical Data for SVM

Sr. No	Parameters	Accuracy of Classification %
1	Ground reaction force	85.19
2	GRF and kinematics	74.07
3	Kinematics and feature selection algorithm	95.2
4	Kinematics with no feature selection	90.5
5	Foot pressure data	94.36

Source: Khera et al. *Journal of Medical Engineering & Technology* 44.8 (2020): 441–467 [23].

TABLE 3.10
SVM Performance for Different Methods

Method	Accuracy %	Recall %
ABS	90	92.06
FBS	92.22	93.65
RBS	95.56	96.83

Performance of class imbalance case

Source: Zheng et al. (ISMICT). IEEE, 2021 [24].

The sensitivity and specificity of the implementation are mentioned in Tables 3.11 and 3.16 [25].

3.4.1.2 Logistic Regression

The logistic regression analyses the association within categorical dependent variables and independent variables. The output is binary: Yes or No. Logistic regression is versatile and a better option for modelling than discriminant analysis, as it does not assume that the independent variables are normally distributed as discriminant analysis does. It provides the confidence interval base on predicted values and provides cut-off points for classification [26].

- Source: Schniepp, Roman, et al. perform prediction of fall risk estimation within patients with gait impairment due to neurological disorders are addressed in the paper with 300+ patients and 60+ healthy person data received through an inertial sensor based daily monitoring system. Multivariate regression analysis was performed for predicting a Faller and Non-Faller Category, prediction of falling frequency and severity. Instrumented gait measure provides unique information for prediction [27]. Three different models tested are able to provide a correct prediction range from 0.78 to 0.92.
- Source: Gillani et al. Considers gait as an important biometric trait; the inertial sensor based dataset was used for age estimation and gender

TABLE 3.11

Sensitivity and Specificity of SVM in Four Classes

Performance of SVM	Sensitivity	Specificity
HC vs. Non-HC Group	0.900	0.886
PN vs. Non-PN Group	0.788	0.844
PD vs. Non-PS Group	0.933	0.903

Source: Wang, Lei, et al. *IEEE Robotics and Automation Letters* 5.2 (2020): 1970–1976 [25].

TABLE 3.12

Gender Classification Results [28]

Classifier	Recall in Male Category %	Recall in Female Category %	Accuracy %
Logistic Regression	72.2	63.9	68.2
Support Vector Machine	83.5	28.7	57
Random Forest	57.4	63.9	60.5

Source: Gillani et al. (ICETST). IEEE, 2020.

classification. The performance of a separate set of walking sequence used for gender classification is shown in Table 3.12 for various classifiers. [28]

The performance of logistic regression was superior in gender classification, while SVM gives better result in age estimation.

3.4.1.3 K-Nearest Neighbour

K- nearest neighbour is used in both classification and regression base problems. KNN assumes that similar things exist in close proximity. To perform the classification requires a record, distance metric and the value of k. To decide the appropriate value of k, an algorithm needs to be executed a number of times to decide the value of k giving minimal error.

- Source: Nam Nguyen et al. Considers the influence of neurodegenerative diseases on gait abnormalities. The classification model was developed using multiscale sample entropy and machine learning. Performance of support vector machine and K-nearest neighbour was tested to compare different groups and categories. Groups for comparative analysis and classification are healthy control (HC), Parkinson's disease (PD), Huntington's disease (HD) and amyotrophic lateral sclerosis (ALS). The performance in classification accuracy of both the classifiers ranges from 94 to 99.7% based on the selected features. The variation in the classification accuracy over the time period are observed in both KNN and SVM, but overall classification accuracy is on the higher side to discriminate groups [29].
- Source: Henderson et al. to detect the autism spectrum disorder (ASD) along with behavioural analysis, the focus on using gait analysis is increasing. The experiment was done on the recorded data through a motion tracking system and four machine learning classifiers: support vector machine, K-nearest neighbour, random forest and decision trees are tested for accuracy. The results are shown in Table 3.13 [30].

3.4.1.4 Decision Tree and Random Forest

The decision tree algorithm is used in classification and regression. For predicting in the decision tree, we need to start from the root node and split the dataset as per

TABLE 3.13
Classification Metric of Four Classifiers

Classifier	Accuracy	Precision
SVM	63.75	85.71
KNN	78.05	57.14
DT	76.47	69.64

Source: Henderson et al. (ISSC). IEEE, 2020 [30].

features. Expanding the tress through decision node, parent/child node, sub-tree and terminal node, the decision is made.

A random forest is a collaborative execution of a large number of decision trees. Each tree in the random forest splits into class prediction and based on the number of opinions, proceeds ahead.

- Source: Charbuty et al. reviewed 80+ references working on various datasets collected through different options and machine learning classifiers tested for accuracy. Through the reviewed literature, the accuracy of 99.9% was observed with decision tree and KNN [31].

3.4.2 PARAPHRASING PREVIOUS FINDINGS

Gait analysis has been used as a clinically adapted tool for a long time, and advancements in machine learning, deep learning and artificial intelligence are the extending technological role in the healthcare system. But the relevance of performance of gait analysis in certain diseases using available technologies of that time had proven its importance. Some test cases are paraphrased to clarify strong relation amid the need of gait analysis in healthcare. Definitely these are just a few test cases; use of it is not limited to this extent only.

- Source: Wren, Tishya AL, et al. The author does a thorough review to check the efficacy of gait analysis in the case of cerebral palsy patients. Efficacy was checked with various levels
  - Level 1 Technical accuracy
  - Level 2 Diagnostic accuracy
  - Level 3 and 4 Diagnostic thinking and treatment efficacy
  - Level 5 Patient outcome efficacy
  - Level 6 Societal efficacy

A reported 1528 references were identified and as a outcome specify that the gait analysis for the level 1 to 4, the gait analysis efficacy have evidence, but for higher-level evidences are not available. This systematic review provides the guideline to points to be emphasised in further studies.

3.4.2.1 Case Study of Cerebral Palsy Patients

Cerebral palsy affects the ability of person to move or in maintaining balance and posture. it results in uncontrolled movement, muscle stiffness or lack of coordination within movement. There are different levels and types but early detection definitely helps out.

- Source: Damiano et al., Specify that gait performance is representation of overall motor skills. In the case of cerebral palsy not only walking but other fine and gross motor skills also get affected. The Gross Motor Function Measure was done with five sets of activities in children with four cameras and then computerised motion analysis as done. The obtained ANOVA results are shown in Table 3.14 [32].

TABLE 3.14

Mean of Parameters as per Ambulatory Values in Children with Cerebral Palsy

Typical Parameters Selected	Performacne of Group 1	Performacne of Group 2
Age	7.25	12.1
Normalised Velocity	1.53	1.18
Cadence	141	120
Normalised Stride Length	1.28	1.18

Source: Damiano et al. *Developmental Medicine & Child Neurology* 38.5 (1996): 389–396 [32].

TABLE 3.15

Performance Analysis among Groups

	No. Surgical Procedures Recommended	Performance of Controlled Group			Performance of Experimental Group		
		Negative	No Change	Positive	Negative	No Change	Positive
Average	5	22.29%	51.88%	25.83%	23.13%	32.94%	43.96%
Standard Deviation	1.94	27.71%	29.54%	30.04%	17.69%	18.99%	22.57%

Source: Chang et al. *Journal of Paediatric Orthopaedics* 26.5 (2006): 612–616 [33].

Provides the conclusion that the clinical gait analysis and the Gross Motor Function Measure are valid indicators in testing of cerebral palsy.

- *Source* – Chang et al. covers different groups: experimental group and recommendation match control group for analysis. Groups are divided on the basis of adapting surgical treatment after initial gait analysis and group going with a non-surgical way. Table 3.15 shows the summary of change/no change/negative change in both groups [33].

Use of instrumented gait analysis and logistic regression observes a significantly higher outcome in the group who had adopted a surgical line of action after gait analysis.

3.4.2.2   Case Study of Parkinson's Patients

Parkinson's is the progressive nervous system disorder affecting the movement of the person. it leads to shaking of hands, short steps, each activity becomes time consuming, muscle stiffness, impaired posture and balance. The role of gait analysis is described in the following case studies.

- Source: Wren et al. analysed and identifies the fall risk in patients suffering from Parkinson's using wearable sensors. Compared with a health group, the gait variability in Parkinson's patients increases excessively. Table 3.16 provides the comparative analysis within faller and non-faller groups after six-month trials with a few selected parameters [34].

The observation through the study mentions two important points to think upon. Gait variability does exist in healthy persons, but those are considered to be beneficial and necessary with aging. An abnormal variability leading to loss of rhythm leads to fall risk in the case of Parkinson's disease [34].

- Source: Roiz et al. perform comparative analysis of healthy older and Parkinson's patients on spatiotemporal parameters and gait kinematics using a reflective marker method. Table 3.17 shows the performance indicator for 12 Parkinson and 15 healthy older patients [35].

In statistical analysis of spatiotemporal parameters, a significant difference in stride length and stride velocity was observed in both groups.

- Source: Pistacchi et al. performed the comparison of spatiotemporal and kinematic parameters of Parkinson's disease patients with a healthy group to

TABLE 3.16
Comparison of Gait Parameters in Non-Faller and Faller Group

Selected Parameters	No Fall Risk	Fall Risk
Stride Length	68.53 ± 12.27	65.34
Gait Cycle Time	1.04 (098–1.16)	1.00 (0.94–1.10)
Swing %	40 (37.58–42.06)	41 (38.12–42.19)

Source: Wren et al. *Gait & Posture* 34.2 (2011): 149–153 [34].

TABLE 3.17
Spatiotemporal Variables of Parkinson's and Healthy Older Persons Group

Parameters	Parkinson's Group	Older Persons Group
Stride Length	1.03±0.13	0.79±0.22
Cadence	89.87±6.86	87.97±16.75
Velocity	0.77±0.14	0.59±0.20

Source: Roiz et al. *Arquivos de neuro-psiquiatria* 68 (2010): 81–86 [35].

identify the possibility of early detection of gait abnormality in Parkinson's. Recording is done with the help of position markers, infrared camera and dynamometric platform. Table 3.18 shows the obtained statistical analysis of both groups [36].

This concluded with observations such as abnormal posture and ambulation and resting tremor may be early stages of Parkinson's and associated with reduced step length. But early gait variation may have different characteristics with Parkinson's disease. The study does specify various factors as its correlation to find out its use in therapeutic purpose [36].

3.4.2.3   Case Study of Geriatric Care

The biggest task considering the applicability of technological help in geriatric care needs to be explored. The awareness of technological enhancement, its use in home care or distant monitoring which would provide an independent safety environment for elderly, are key aspects while thinking about any technical engagement in healthcare [37].

- Source: Werner et al. Within the process of rehabilitation use of a body fixed sensor was tried for gait parameter measurement in older persons using rollator support. The objective of the study was to examine physical activity and mobility of acute hospitalised older persons. The test-retest and sensitivity to change are tested with a single body fixed sensor over a multisensor system. The efficiency and test-retest reliability were obtained. Typical results obtained are shown in Table 3.19 [38].

The result specifies that the sensor used is sensitive to recognise the variation in gait performance and helpful in early rehabilitation treatment. A single sensor as a cost-effective solution was tested for recording spatial and temporal parameters in geriatric care for the patients with rollator support.

TABLE 3.18
Statistical Analysis of Spatial-Temporal Parameters

Parameter	Right Limb Patients	Right Limb Controlled Subjects	Left Limb Patients	Left Limb Controlled Subjects
Step Length	0.48±0.13	0.619±0.04	0.49±0.13	0.74±0.19
Stride length	0.98±0.27	1.40±0.74	0.95±0.28	1.40±0.62
Velocity	0.84±0.28	1.33±0.06	0.83±0.28	1.33±0.06
Cadence	102.4±13.17	113.84±4.30	102.4±13.17	113.84±4.30

Source: Pistacchi et al. *Functional Neurology* 32.1 (2017): 28 [36].

TABLE 3.19
Result of Intrasession Test-Retest with Single Body Fixed Sensor

Parameters	Pre-test Performance Mean ±SD	Retest Performance Mean ±SD
Gait Speed	0.60±0.18	0.60±0.20
Cadence	90.1±15.3	91.7±16.7
Step Length	39.4±9.4	38.9±9.7
Step time	0.69±0.13	0.68±0.13

Source: Werner et al. *Sensors* 20.17 (2020): 4866 [38].

3.4.2.4   Case Study of Dementia Patients

Dementia is a term used to describe the symptoms affecting memory and thinking capability resulting in inabilities which would disturb daily life. Considering the issues in coordination and motor functions, a few case studies describing the relation of variation in gait pattern and dementia are mentioned.

- Source: Lee et al. reviewed impaired cognitive function and its linking with daily activity monitoring, including loss of balance. Older adults diagnosed with dementia are considered for instrumented analysis, and a 10-meter walk was used, gait parameters their correlation were established and tested details are mentioned in Table 13.20 [39].

Through the test results, it can be stated that the association between gait parameters, balance and daily activity performance are closely related in the case of dementia [39].

- Source: Mc Ardle, Ríona, et al. Moving ahead of laboratory analysis, the effect of a real-world environment was tried with patients with a subtype of dementia and influence of them on gait parameters. For the gait parameter recording purposes, a triaxial accelerometer was used. The performance of the subject within a laboratory environment and real-world environment are tested for asymmetry, rhythm and postural control. Observation highlights the important perception about recording gait parameters in the laboratory environment and real word in that a different metric needs to be developed in gait variation assessment for a real-world scenario, as major gait impairment in controlled laboratory conditions is showing better distinguishing factors [40].

3.4.2.5   Case Study of Asymmetrical Walk

Variations in maintaining symmetry of walking are due to different reasons, including strength of muscle, weight, age, etc., but contribution in asymmetry due to continuous use of a handheld device is another matter to think about [41].

TABLE 3.20

Correlation Between Gait Parameter and BBS, MWT and MBI [39]

Parameters	Berg Balance Scale	10-Metre Walk Test	Modified Barthel Index
Velocity	0.341	0.488	0.516
Cadence	−0.032	0.108	0.046
Step Length	0.400	0.475	0.586
Stride length	0.372	0.455	0.580
Walk ratio	0.383	0.362	0.556

Source: Lee et al. *Geriatric Orthopaedic Surgery & Rehabilitation* 11 (2020) [39].

TABLE 3.21

Symmetric and Asymmetric Observations

	Method	Symmetric Gait Observation	Asymmetric Gait Observation
Subject 1	Stride Duration	−0.99±4.03	−0.56±1.44
	Swing Duration	−1.05±4.62	−33.38±6.71
Subject 2	Stride Duration	0.15±1.98	2.16±2.39
	Swing Duration	2.02±4.87	−9.44±4.26
Subject 3	Stride Duration	0.90±1.34	0.30±0.98
	Swing Duration	0.04±2.44	5.71±4.52

Source: Jeong et al. *Sensors* 21.11 (2021): 3750.

- Source: Jeong et al. Using spatiotemporal parameters of identifying asymmetry walking with dynamic time warping distance and time series analysis was proposed. Recording of parameters is done with pressure sensors and gyroscope. Table 3.21 indicated the mean, and standard deviation values observed [42].

The testing results are obtained with a simulated asymmetry walk, and using dynamic time warping, the algorithm distance is calculated. On the basis of statistical values, such a technique can be used for classification of hemiplegic gait [42].

3.5 WELLNESS WITH TECHNOLOGICAL SUPPORT

People take advice from a financial planner or tax consultant for their financial health. Over last decade there are improvements to have such consultants in personal health analysis through routine tests and follow-up in consultation with the family physician. Now, with such variations in lifestyle, we need to think about the feasibility of technology support in daily wellness maintenance. Definitely, the answer to this question is big yes! As per the latest statistics there are millions of users across India who uses a fitness band or application daily. The increased number of Fitbit or Apple fitness bands covering the market of wearable sensor technology is showing tremendous growth. Covering all types of age groups they are providing way a different vision of health awareness to users. After checking the success stories of using fitness bands through available testimonials, getting glimpses of what is happening in such a domain and its possible extent can be imagined [43–44].

3.5.1 NEED OF GAIT ANALYSIS FOR WELLNESS

As discussed in a prior section of the chapter, gait analysis has a tremendous contribution in clinical applications, contributing in surgical decisions in case of cerebral palsy, geriatric care to reduce fall risk with prediction, rehabilitation, human recognition and identification to understand variations from expected normal, etc. Inclusion of these technical concepts are helping even now in digital forensics and visual representation in augmented and virtual reality. Extending its applicability to monitoring wellness would be the great opening towards pre-habilitation. As always, recommended preventive care avoids losses to a great extent. To apply this thought to verify and maintain fitness, would be a great contribution for people.

The most common practice for fitness, weight reduction, etc., are various ways of walking. The greatest advantage of walking is anyone can do it anywhere irrespective of age. Considering a few exceptions with limitation of mobility due to certain reasons, all can start to adopt a walking exercise immediately as per comfort level. Duration, distance or speed of walking will be a personal decision, just make sure to maintain your natural gait; each one has a typical gait pattern, but make sure your back and head are held in the appropriate position.

Simple perfect steps will benefit us to gain all the benefits from walking exercise. To achieve this, it is essential to understand the expected posture, stride, velocity, hand swing, use of appropriate shoe and such – all small concerns contribute towards the defined target. Setting and achieving your own target with perfect walking analysis will contribute to fitness and wellness.

Clinical gait analysis done after a certain interval will definitely provide the guideline to achieve the maximum out of the exercise. The detailed instrumental analysis associated with clinical support is crucial to assure the way of walking adopted by a person is appropriate. Certain prolong walking habits such as bending on one side, inappropriate foot-ground clearance of one leg, age-velocity relation, shifting of body weight from one leg to other abruptly, etc., may invite some issues at a minor level or may lead to major consequences. That's why getting the gait analysis done will provide a guideline to maintain or achieve fitness for everyone. The thought of extension of fitness in everyone need to be imbibe for its applicability in sports training.

3.5.2 PROCESS OF PREVENTIVE CARE

When it comes to the preventive care, the foremost factor for consideration is increasing awareness of this concept among people. People most likely want to avoid medical intervention, so, awareness drive is an essential point in this process. While describing its reference to the gait analysis as a preventive care, aspects are going to be different. Going with a simple example in the case of diabetic patients' gait, care is very important point as the gait of a diabetic patient and normal person differs [45]. Diabetes is a concern because of the impact it can have on lifestyle. Irrespective type I or II category of diabetic prolong affect if monitored continuously will definitely help in clinical process.

Irrespective of any disease condition or its relevance to gait alteration, we can give a thought of the importance of maintaining an appropriate gait with reference to demographic characteristics. Increased body weight of an individual gets associated with several musculoskeletal diseases, and alterations are seen in the frontal and transvers planes [46]. Thus, according to your gender, age, height, weight, region, habits of exercising, etc., this is correlated with defining your gait pattern. Otherwise, gait deviations might be observed through different body parts:

- Deviation in hip rotation
  a. Backward leaning of the trunk during loading phase
  b. Forward bending of the trunk during loading response
  c. Lateral trunk leans towards the stance
- Deviation in knee
  a. Flexed position of the knee during stance despite normal range of motion at the knee joint
  b. Excessive knee flexion during swing phase
  c. Reduced knee flexion during swing phase
- Deviation in ankle
  a. Foot slap
  b. Foot drop

These are a few examples which we can observe in our surroundings that are untreated due to lack of awareness. Getting the analysis done through an appropriate gait laboratory and consultation with a practitioner will definitely help us to avoid impairments due to inappropriate gait adapted for certain reasons. Getting the technological assistance is always recommended with clinical support to remain on the appropriate track. The wellness adaption with gait analysis is depicted in Figure 3.7.

3.5.3 TECHNOLOGICAL SUPPORT FOR A CLOSED-LOOP SYSTEM

With the help of technological advancements, health information retrieval is becoming possible which in turn is helping to achieve the wellness of human beings. The purpose of a closed-loop system is assurance of following the right track through mentoring. The nature of mentoring may change according to the need or condition of the person. When one is keen towards preventive care and able to use the latest technology, then distance monitoring of health activity is possible. With enormous options made available for data transfer, it is possible to transfer information and its further processing or use some module to process and transfer instructions. The Internet of Things is providing a range of connectivity and communication options.

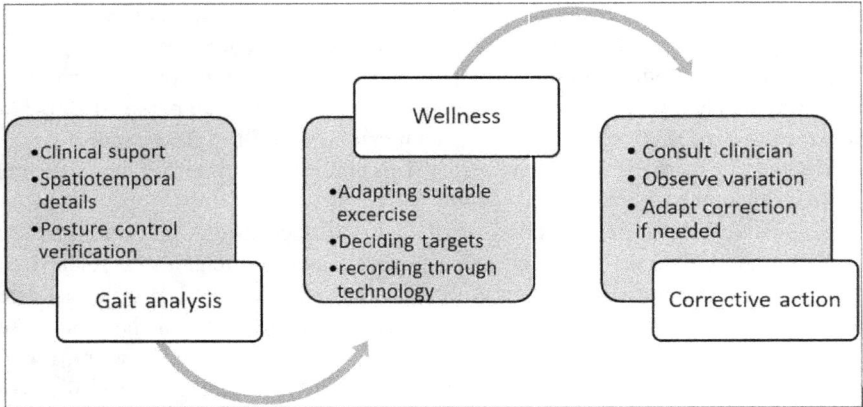

FIGURE 3.7   Process for wellness adaption through gait analysis.

All the fitness bands are tracking and keeping records of personal information. These fitness bands, when connected with mobile phones, provide basic analysis. Such a recorded database would be used for comparative analysis. Using alerts, notifications and messages like options for follow-up are suitable for quick review. Technological enhancements and their contribution in regaining health or in preventive care provides a great solution in achieving wellness.

3.6   CONCLUSION

Considering the personal healthcare aspect and technological blend for upgrading the lifestyle, use of appropriate tools needs to be as per recommendation of health experts. Awareness of gait monitoring and its long-term implications is normally observed in the process of rehabilitation. Using gait as a clinical tool in preventive care is highly recommended, and there are a lot of benefits that can be seen using it in sports for physical training of athletes. Opening the opportunity to use technology for the betterment of human health is most important and a possible option with advancements in health informatics. Considering the gait analysis as a tool in healthcare, the possible limitations need to be visualised. As reviewed in the technological options available for recording of the gait parameters, the typical demographic region a person belongs to, medical history, surrounding condition, etc., have a direct role in analysis. Thus, the system becomes person dependent. To overcome the limitations specified, the enormous emerging options in data science would be helpful to build the model for gait analysis in generalised phases. The challenges to work in the future on gait analysis starts with understanding numerous variations and dependencies. Creating a strong normative dataset for a different region would be the foremost point for technological deployment. Thus, this study provides the overview about the role, relevance and importance of gait analysis and related technological evolution in the domain and puts forward the concept of accepting it for preventive care in achieving wellness.

3.7 REFERENCES

[1] www.who.int/news-room/fact-sheets/detail/diabetes

[2] www.who.int/health-topics/digital-health#tab=tab_1

[3] Di Gregorio, Raffaele, and Lucas Vocenas. "Identification of gait-cycle phases for prosthesis control." *Biomimetics* 6.2 (2021): 22.

[4] Jacquelin Perry, M. D. *Gait analysis: Normal and pathological function.* New Jersey: SLACK, 2010.

[5] Whittle, Michael W. *Gait analysis: An introduction.* Butterworth-Heinemann, United Kingdom, 2014.

[6] Chen, Shanshan, et al. "Toward pervasive gait analysis with wearable sensors: A systematic review." *IEEE Journal of Biomedical and Health Informatics* 20.6 (2016): 1521–1537.

[7] Cook, Robert E., et al. "Gait analysis alters decision-making in cerebral palsy." *Journal of Pediatric Orthopaedics* 23.3 (2003): 292–295.

[8] Lee, Eng H., James C. H. Goh, and Kamal Bose. "Value of gait analysis in the assessment of surgery in cerebral palsy." *Archives of Physical Medicine and Rehabilitation* 73.7 (1992): 642–646.

[9] Gage, James R. "Gait analysis. An essential tool in the treatment of cerebral palsy." *Clinical Orthopaedics and Related Research* 288 (1993): 126–134. www.who.int/news-room/fact-sheets/detail/falls

[10] Montero-Odasso, Manuel, et al. "Quantitative gait analysis under dual-task in older people with mild cognitive impairment: A reliability study." *Journal of Neuroengineering and Rehabilitation* 6.1 (2009): 1–6.

[11] Schülein, Samuel, et al. "Instrumented gait analysis: A measure of gait improvement by a wheeled walker in hospitalized geriatric patients." *Journal of Neuroengineering and Rehabilitation* 14.1 (2017): 1–11.

[12] Rodrigues, Célio Fernando de Sousa, Fernando José Camello de Lima, and Fabiano Timbó Barbosa. "Importance of using basic statistics adequately in clinical research☆." *Revista brasileira de anestesiologia* 67 (2017): 619–625.

[13] David, Tomos W., David P. Marshall, and Laure Zanna. "The statistical nature of turbulent barotropic ocean jets." *Ocean Modelling* 113 (2017): 34–49.

[14] Armitage, Peter, Geoffrey Berry, and John Nigel Scott Matthews. *Statistical methods in medical research.* John Wiley & Sons, United States, 2008.

[15] Moe-Nilssen, Rolf, and Jorunn L. Helbostad. "Spatiotemporal gait parameters for older adults – An interactive model adjusting reference data for gender, age, and body height." *Gait & Posture* 82 (2020): 220–226.

[16] Kirtley, Chris, Michael W. Whittle, and R. J. Jefferson. "Influence of walking speed on gait parameters." *Journal of Biomedical Engineering* 7.4 (1985): 282–288.

[17] Menz, Hylton B., et al. "Reliability of the GAITRite® walkway system for the quantification of temporo-spatial parameters of gait in young and older people." *Gait & Posture* 20.1 (2004): 20–25.

[18] Duhamel, A., et al. "Statistical tools for clinical gait analysis." *Gait & Posture* 20.2 (2004): 204–212.

[19] Öberg, Tommy, Alek Karsznia, and Kurt Öberg. "Basic gait parameters: reference data for normal subjects, 10–79 years of age." *Journal of Rehabilitation Research and Development* 30 (1993): 210–210.

[20] Samson, Monique M., et al. "Differences in gait parameters at a preferred walking speed in healthy subjects due to age, height and body weight." *Aging Clinical and Experimental Research* 13.1 (2001): 16–21.

[21] Beauchet, Olivier, et al. "Guidelines for assessment of gait and reference values for spatiotemporal gait parameters in older adults: the biomathics and Canadian gait consortiums initiative." *Frontiers in Human Neuroscience* 11 (2017): 353.

[22] Alpaydin, Ethem. *Introduction to machine learning*. MIT Press, United States, 2014.

[23] Khera, Preeti, and Neelesh Kumar. "Role of machine learning in gait analysis: A review." *Journal of Medical Engineering & Technology* 44.8 (2020): 441–467.

[24] Zheng, Yuncheng, et al. "SVM-based gait analysis and classification for patients with Parkinson's disease." In *2021 15th International symposium on medical information and communication technology (ISMICT)*. IEEE, United States, 2021.

[25] Wang, Lei, et al. "Two shank-mounted IMUs-based gait analysis and classification for neurological disease patients." *IEEE Robotics and Automation Letters* 5.2 (2020): 1970–1976.

[26] *Logistic regression: NCSS statistical software*. https://www.ncss.com/wp-content/themes/ncss/pdf/Procedures/NCSS/Logistic_Regression-Old_Version.pdf

[27] Schniepp, Roman, et al. "Fall prediction in neurological gait disorders: differential contributions from clinical assessment, gait analysis, and daily-life mobility monitoring." *Journal of Neurology* (2021): 1–14.

[28] Gillani, Syeda Iqra, Muhammad Awais Azam, and M. Ehatisham-ul-Haq. "Age estimation and gender classification based on human gait analysis." In *2020 International conference on emerging trends in smart technologies (ICETST)*. IEEE, United States, 2020.

[29] Nam Nguyen, Quoc Duy, An-Bang Liu, and Che-Wei Lin. "Development of a neurodegenerative disease gait classification algorithm using multiscale sample entropy and machine learning classifiers." *Entropy* 22.12 (2020): 1340.

[30] Henderson, Benn, et al. "Effects of intra-subject variation in gait analysis on ASD classification performance in machine learning models." In *2020 31st Irish signals and systems conference (ISSC)*. IEEE, United States, 2020.

[31] Charbuty, Bahzad, and Adnan Abdulazeez. "Classification based on decision tree algorithm for machine learning." *Journal of Applied Science and Technology Trends* 2.01 (2021): 20–28.

[32] Damiano, Diane L., and Mark F. Abel. "Relation of gait analysis to gross motor function in cerebral palsy." *Developmental Medicine & Child Neurology* 38.5 (1996): 389–396.

[33] Chang, Franklin M., et al. "Effectiveness of instrumented gait analysis in children with cerebral palsy-Comparison of outcomes." *Journal of Pediatric Orthopaedics* 26.5 (2006): 612–616.

[34] Wren, Tishya AL, et al. "Efficacy of clinical gait analysis: A systematic review." *Gait & Posture* 34.2 (2011): 149–153.

[35] Roiz, Roberta de Melo, et al. "Gait analysis comparing Parkinson's disease with healthy elderly subjects." *Arquivos de neuro-psiquiatria* 68 (2010): 81–86.

[36] Pistacchi, Michele, et al. "Gait analysis and clinical correlations in early Parkinson's disease." *Functional Neurology* 32.1 (2017): 28.

[37] Pilotto, Alberto, Raffaella Boi, and Jean Petermans. "Technology in geriatrics." *Age and Ageing* 47.6 (2018): 771–774.

[38] Werner, Christian, et al. "Concurrent validity, test-retest reliability, and sensitivity to change of a single body-fixed sensor for gait analysis during rollator-assisted walking in acute geriatric patients." *Sensors* 20.17 (2020): 4866.

[39] Lee, Nam Gi, Tae Woo Kang, and Hyun Ju Park. "Relationship between balance, gait, and activities of daily living in older adults with dementia." *Geriatric Orthopaedic Surgery & Rehabilitation* 11 (2020): 2151459320929578.

[40] Mc Ardle, Ríona, et al. "The impact of environment on gait assessment: considerations from real-world gait analysis in dementia subtypes." *Sensors* 21.3 (2021): 813.

[41] Abid, Mahdi, et al. "Walking gait step length asymmetry induced by handheld device." *IEEE Transactions on Neural Systems and Rehabilitation Engineering* 25.11 (2017): 2075–2083.

[42] Jeong, Yeon-Keun, and Kwang-Ryul Baek. "Asymmetric gait analysis using a DTW algorithm with combined gyroscope and pressure sensor." *Sensors* 21.11 (2021): 3750.

[43] https://stories.fitbit.com/

[44] www.apple.com/apple-fitness-plus/

[45] Katoulis, Evangelos C., et al. "Gait abnormalities in diabetic neuropathy." *Diabetes Care* 20.12 (1997): 1904–1907.

[46] Sheehan, K., and J. Gormley. "Gait and increased body weight (potential implications for musculoskeletal disease)." *Physical Therapy Reviews* 17.2 (2012): 91–98.

4 Emerging Disruptive Technologies and Their Impact on Health Informatics

Venkatesh Krishna Murthy[1]

[1] Wharf Street Strategies Limited, London, United Kingdom

CONTENTS

DOI: 10.1201/9781003217107-4

4.1 INTRODUCTION

4.1.1 OVERVIEW AND IMPORTANCE OF THE TOPIC

Emerging technologies are widely used in various industries, including supply chain, manufacturing, IT, healthcare, etc., for enhancing their performance and providing intellectual benefits. This recent technological development has moved the business operations to the next level, where huge advancements have been identified in the healthcare industry [1]. Emerging technologies such as blockchain, IoT, artificial intelligence, wearable devices, augmented reality, etc., are widely used in healthcare organisations for enhancing medical informatics. Medical informatics is a new field in the healthcare sector that uses information technology for organising and analyzing multiple health records which will further help in improving the results of the healthcare industry. It deals with devices, resources and methods used for storing, retrieving and acquiring medical data [2].

Disruptive medical innovations is a concept which mainly focuses on customer needs and help in diagnosing diseases prior to their occurrence [1]. Wireless patient monitoring devices, mobile health, telemedicine and Internet of Things (IoT)–based solutions are the most commonly used disruptive medical innovations for maintaining patient monitoring practices and disease management. This research report plays a significant role in identifying the importance and benefits of using emerging technologies in healthcare industries. In this current COVID-19 pandemic, the death rate has been increasing, which is monitored using IoT devices, which will further help in obtaining relevant data for doctors about patients suffering from fatal diseases [3].

Apart from this, healthcare sectors faced various challenges in maintaining patient records, monitoring or tracking medical equipment, inappropriate method of curing diseases and many more. This research study has been conducted to eliminate the challenges faced by healthcare organisations with the use of disruptive technological innovations. The use of artificial intelligence (AI), IoT, blockchain, predictive analysis, wearable devices and visualisation have enhanced the healthcare organisation's operations and helped in curing fatal diseases in an easy and fast manner. All this information will be demonstrated efficiently in this research study and help in determining the benefits of disruptive technologies in the healthcare industry.

4.1.2 RESEARCH AIM AND OBJECTIVES

In order to accomplish this research study, the primary motive is to analyse the benefits of advanced technologies along with their impacts on health informatics. This will help in providing efficient healthcare services to patients with the development of appropriate information technology systems. Along with this, emerging technologies will also help in curing diseases by predicting them earlier and by providing relevant medical care to patients. To achieve this primary aim of the research study, multiple objectives are formulated which are defined as follows:

- To identify challenges faced by healthcare organisations.
- To analyse the importance of blockchain in enhancing clinical trials.
- To demonstrate use of wearables and predictive analytics in the healthcare sector.

- To determine the importance of IoT and augmented reality in medical equipment tracking and surgery, respectively.
- To identify and define probabilistic methods used in healthcare.

4.1.3 RESEARCH QUESTION

Research aims and objectives are formulated in this research study, where on the basis of these objectives, research questions are defined which will be answered throughout the whole research study.

RQ1: 'What are the challenges faced by healthcare industries?'
RQ2: 'What are the disruptive technological innovations used in healthcare organisations?'
RQ3: 'How can blockchain, IoT and augmented reality help in enhancing the performance in the healthcare industry?'
RQ4: 'What probabilistic methods and predictive analysis help in increasing healthcare operations?'

4.2 LITERATURE REVIEW

4.2.1 LITERATURE ON THE BASIS OF THEMES

4.2.1.1 Theme 1: Blockchain to Enhance Clinical Trials

[4] aimed to provide the deep insights about the use of disruptive technologies in the healthcare systems as well as in environment. The author also tried to investigate the use of latest technologies in the research and development of pan-Canadian monitoring and surveillance activities associated with the environmental impacts on health in the healthcare system. Further, the author highlighted that there can be various disruptive technologies that can be used in the implementation of these activities. Such technologies include data science, blockchain, AI, IoT, mobile health, machine learning, etc., that can be used in multiple domains such as in air quality monitoring and influenza surveillance. In order to accomplish the objectives of this research, the author has conducted a narrative literature review and descriptive analysis. In addition to it, the UbiLab team has conducted three rounds of external group discussions to identify the most relevant studies and technologies. Several use cases were developed to integrate the disruptive technologies such as AI, blockchain, machine learning, IoT, etc., in the brainstorming sessions. To know the significance of these disruptive technologies in the health and environment research, the author has searched the relevant articles from the scholarly databases IEEE Xplore, Research Gate, Scopus, etc. Only a few studies were included for this examination – those that met the inclusion criteria. Apart from this, the current study has examined the various benefits of implementing blockchain to stakeholders, doctors, researchers, insurance payers and pharmaceutical companies. The author has also described some major challenges related to patient security in this study. Similarly, this study provides an emphasis on the exploration of other disruptive technologies in healthcare and environment. Furthermore, the author recommended a software architecture in relation to the problem faced by pan-Canadian activities, which comprised various layers such as device, privacy and security, applications, data and communication. See Figure 4.1.

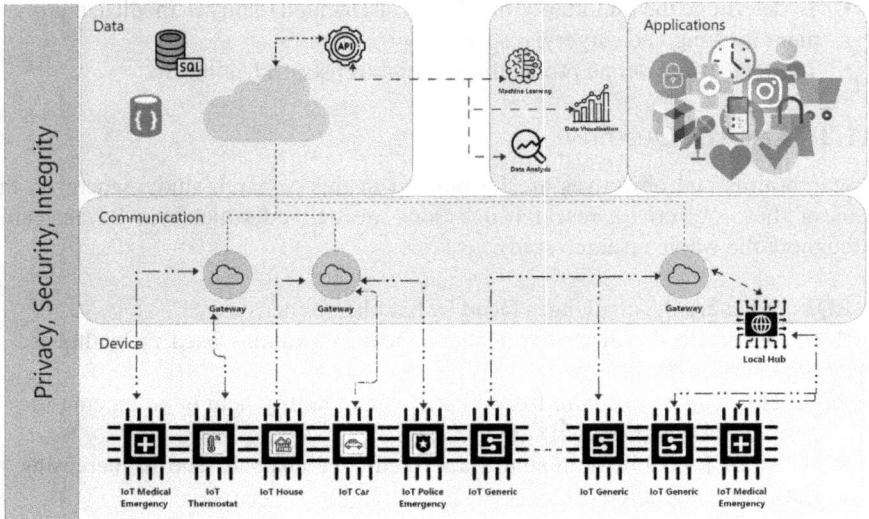

FIGURE 4.1   Recommended architecture for Pan-Canadian activities related to environment and healthcare systems [4].

According to the author, the recommended architecture can be used in monitoring the air pollution in schools and, automated environmental control and to analyse the death and disease patterns in healthcare systems with time. By concluding this study, the author mentioned that these disruptive technologies (AI, IoT and blockchain) have great potential and capabilities to integrate the healthcare and environmental data, as well as to be a part of the pan-Canadian systems. Moreover, the architecture proposes in this research can provide useful information related to monitoring and activities for future researches.

4.2.1.2   Theme 2: Visualisation, Knowledge Discovery and Predictive Analytics in Healthcare

[5] mainly emphasised the interpretability and explainability of the machine learning techniques to analyse their impact on the healthcare and medicine sectors. The author has addressed the interpretability and explainability by model and data visualisation (Figure 4.2). In addition, the author has elaborated the problems associated with the interpretability and explainability that can be solved by machine learning and computational intelligence technology. Further, the author has viewed the human cognitive problem associated with interpretability. Finally, the author has demonstrated a human analyst-computer machine learning interpretability cycle. Apart from this, the current research reviewed the visualisation as a tool for interpretable machine learning.

In this study, the author has explored the major challenges associated with the adoption of interpretable machine learning in healthcare and medicine. For instance, use of machine learning (ML)–based electronic health record (EHR) systems in

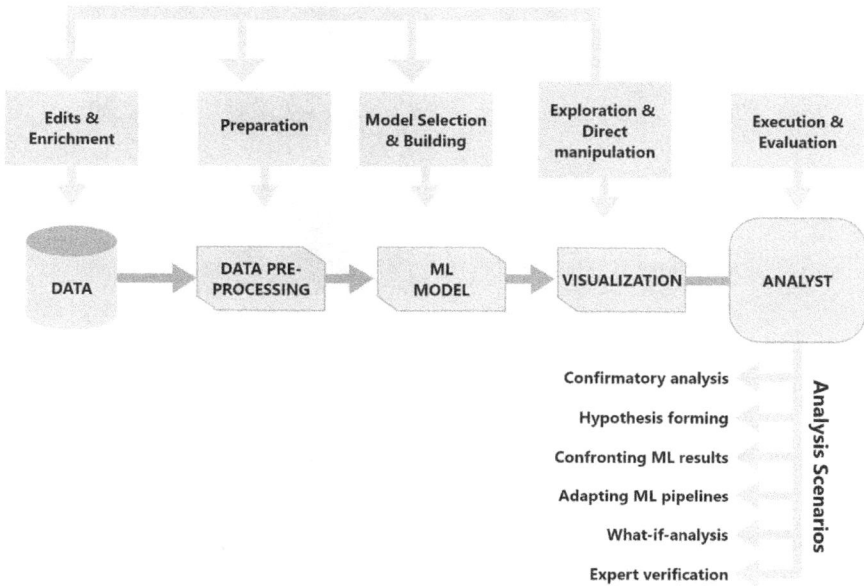

FIGURE 4.2 Human analyst-computer machine learning interpretability cycle by visualisation [5].

the healthcare industry have been analysed, which facilitate the medical staff and patients to access the clinical and patient data remotely in any format. The author has also identified visualisation as a problem in the healthcare and medicine industry. A case study related to interpretability from the neuro-oncology domain has been included in this study to illustrate the necessary things required by medical experts from data analysts. By analyzing this case study, the author has extended the previously developed human analyst-computer machine learning interpretability cycle. The results of this study depicted that medical experts need to widen the scope in the analytical process to ensure the interpretability. Furthermore, the author concluded that data analysts and medical experts should adhere to formal protocols while interacting with each other.

4.2.1.3   Theme 3: Wearable and Implantable Technologies

[6] illustrated the use of wearable and implantable medical devices and sensors in biomedical applications to monitor and prevent diseases (Figure 4.3). Additionally, the author has analysed the materials used in the fabrication of these kind of sensory devices as well as standards for wireless and mobile applications. Further, the author has explored such kind of medical devices that are commercially available, developments, regulatory and technical issues associated with these devices and future trends. This study demonstrated that such kind of wearable and implantable devices measures various other parameters of patients' daily activities and actions including sleep patterns, calories burned, steps taken, activity levels and eating habits.

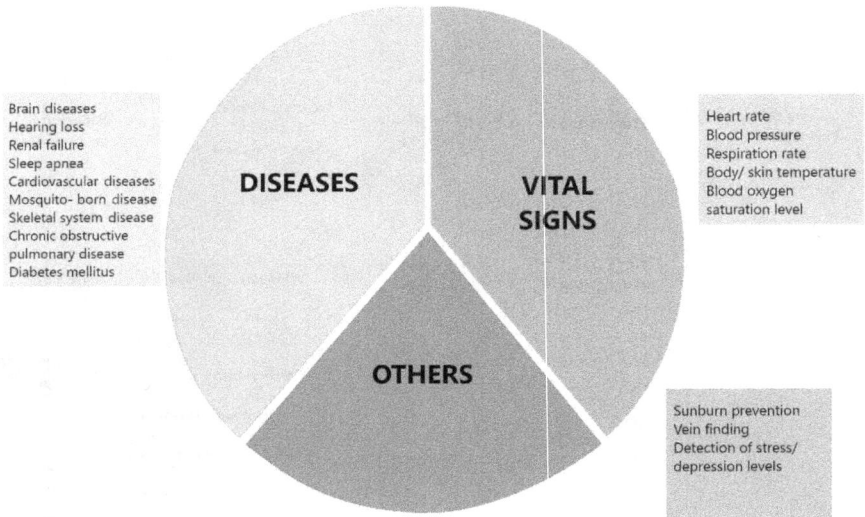

FIGURE 4.3   Biomedical applications of wearable devices [6].

Apart from this, the author has included some examples of the commercial wearable sensor devices along with the psychological parameters. Such mobile technologies lead to the easy diagnosis of diseases and disabilities so that patients are provided with the most suitable treatments. Thereafter, this study highlighted use cases of wearable devices. It may include sleep apnea, diabetes mellitus, brain diseases, chronic obstructive pulmonary diseases, mosquito-borne diseases, vein finding, etc. Furthermore, the author has identified the parts of body where these devices can be implanted and worn. Material technology used in the fabrication of wearables incudes smart textiles and stretchable electronics. Various standards provided by ISO, IEC, IEEE, AAMI, ANSI, etc., can be considered to design such wearable or sensory devices in the biomedical field. Physically, these devices are small in size and can store large amounts of data. Therefore, the chances of data loss and data hacking could be greater. Also, the issues of misalignment of wearable devices also yielded inaccurate results. In the future, the author would focus more to enhance the durability and robustness of the wearable devices.

4.2.1.4   Theme 4: IoT-Enabled Medical Equipment Tracking

[7] provides a systematic review of the examination of physical activity recognition measures (PARM)–related studies from the perspective of a novel 3D dynamic physical activity collection as well as a validation model based on IoT (Figure 4.4). The ultimate goal of PARM technology is to identify the intensity, duration and type of various activities as well as quantification of the parameters like energy expenditure associated with it. In order to accomplish this study, the author has adopted a survey analysis methodology to analyse a lifelogging data validation model lifelogging

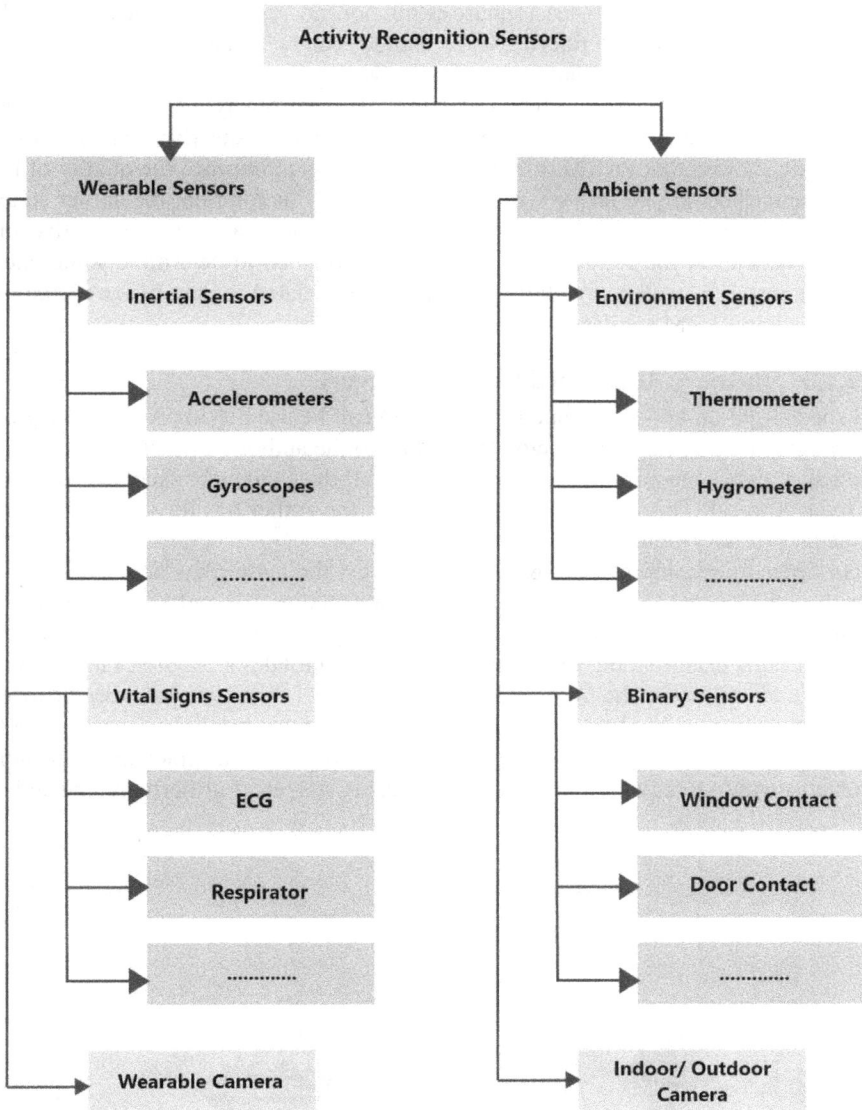

FIGURE 4.4 Categorisation of PARM sensors [7].

physical activity validation (LPAV)-IoT. Further, the author illustrated the concept of an IoT-based data fusion model of PARM in a diagrammatic format. According to this study, activity recognition sensors can be categorised into two major groups as wearable sensors and ambient sensors, which are then divided into sub-categories.

Likewise, data fusion categories of PARM include probabilistic, knowledge-based theory, statistics, evidence reasoning, etc., categories under which Bayesian analysis,

K-nearest neighbour (KNN), least square estimation, artificial neural network (ANN), genetic algorithm, Kalman filtering, etc., methods can be included. Despite that, the author has specified the advantages and disadvantages of the data fusion methods identified earlier. Data fusion methods have also been analysed from device and person perspective as well as from timeline and person perspectives. The results of this study showed that PARM offered various benefits to improve the quality of life of persons who were suffering with chronic diseases. In addition, the author stated that PARM technology–based methods also helped to maintain fitness for active and healthy people. In the future, this study can be extended to determine some latest research trends as well as to address the challenges related to data fusion technique in IoT enable PARM studies.

4.2.1.5　Theme 5: Augmented Reality in Surgery

[8] sheds light on how augmented reality (AR) can be used to improve the surgical procedures in the healthcare sector. According to the author, AR technology can be used as a replacement of surgeons by resolving all the challenges faced by surgeons in today's world. Through a schematic diagram, the author has illustrated the basic principles of AR (Figure 4.5).

In order to accomplish the research objectives, the author has adopted a literature-based analysis. In order to select the relevant studies, the author has used many online databases like Scopus and PubMed using augmented reality and surgery keywords. In this examination, the author has selected a total 808 studies, out of which 417 were identified for the final analysis. The results of this study have been carried out in response to AR basic principles, image alignment methods, operative field monitoring, AR for education and cooperation, use in clinical practices, precision, problems with AR, advanced image in fusion using AR, etc. Furthermore, the author

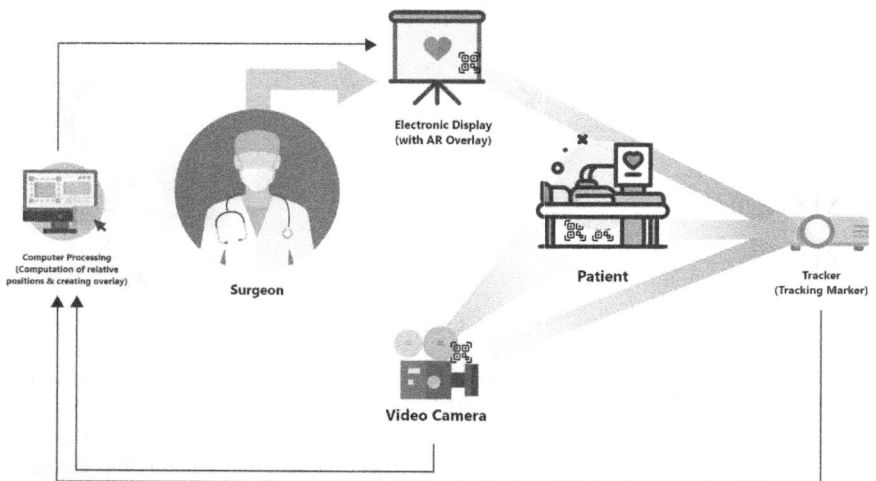

FIGURE 4.5　AR basic principles [8].

concluded that AR-based healthcare systems can be used as an alternative to the traditional navigation techniques along with precision, safety and clinical practices. Moreover, AR can also be used to solve the problems faced in the current researches regarding medical and technology. In the future, AR can be used as an advanced human-computer interface that works in symbiosis with surgeons yielding into better results. Moreover, cost-effectiveness and achieving maximum potential should be included in the further enhancements of AR.

4.2.1.6 Theme 6: Probabilistic Methods in Healthcare

[9] proposed an ontology-based monitoring system, namely Hapicare, that uses uncertain reasoning to evaluate the patients' current actions by analyzing their minimum sensing actions. The main motive behind conducting this research was to provide and improve the quality of life with less cost investments on medical care. While explaining the Hapicare system the author stated that this system was based on the expert knowledge working memory and Bayesian inference system. Additionally, the author has illustrated the architecture of this model diagrammatically.

The proposed system comprises various components including ontology, Bayesian belief network (BBN), rule engine and engine. Detailed descriptions about these components have been included in this study in an elaborative manner. In order to collect the information from the real world, a rule engine performed several tasks such as BBN activation, examination activation, reaction activation, feedback governance, customisation, etc. The rule engine is considered as the most important part of this system and selected by following the two criteria i.e. legibility and performance. The agent acts as a monitoring interface between two interactive parties. Apart from this, the author has demonstrated the workflow of the Hapicare system involving every constituting component.

Referring to a case study, the author has provided all details regarding the practical implementation of the proposed system to analyse the current situation and actions of patients. By concluding this study, the author mentioned that to solve the problems of data uncertainty and reasoning, the author sifted probabilistic reasoning. In the future, the author aimed to work on the security issues associated with the data availability in this system.

4.2.2 RESEARCH GAPS

This report includes a comprehensive literature review on the identified topic i.e. the significant role of disruptive technologies in the healthcare sector that uncovers the applications of such technologies in the biomedical or healthcare sector. By analyzing the previously reviewed studies, various issues or gaps in the current study have been identified (Figure 4.6). These research gaps may include privacy and security of the patient data on publicly available platforms or healthcare systems, problems in data visualisation, fear of data loss and hacking, lack of domain knowledge and expertise, issues of data uncertainty and reasoning, etc. In order to resolve these shortcomings, the author has presented some relevant solutions in the literature analysis. In order to develop new solutions, it is highly recommended to expand the current literature findings using latest technologies in the medical sector.

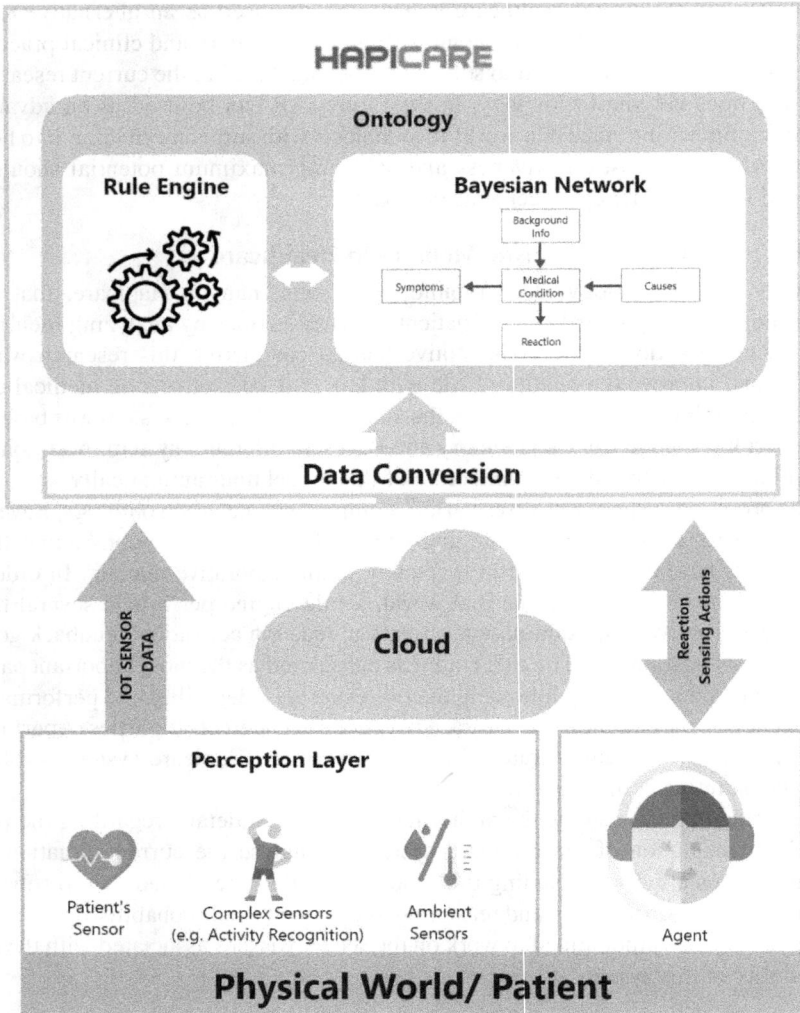

FIGURE 4.6   Architecture of the Hapicare system [9].

4.2.3 Summary

By summarising the findings of this literature analysis, it can be seen that disruptive technologies such as AI, blockchain, IoT, ML, AR, and probabilistic methods can be used in the medical sector for diagnosis and patient treatment in an effective manner. In this literature analysis, various state-of-art methods used in the medical field have been envisioned to analyse the challenges associated with them. According to the literature findings, blockchain technology can be used for monitoring and surveillance of patient actions to provide the appropriate treatment. Augmented reality helped to

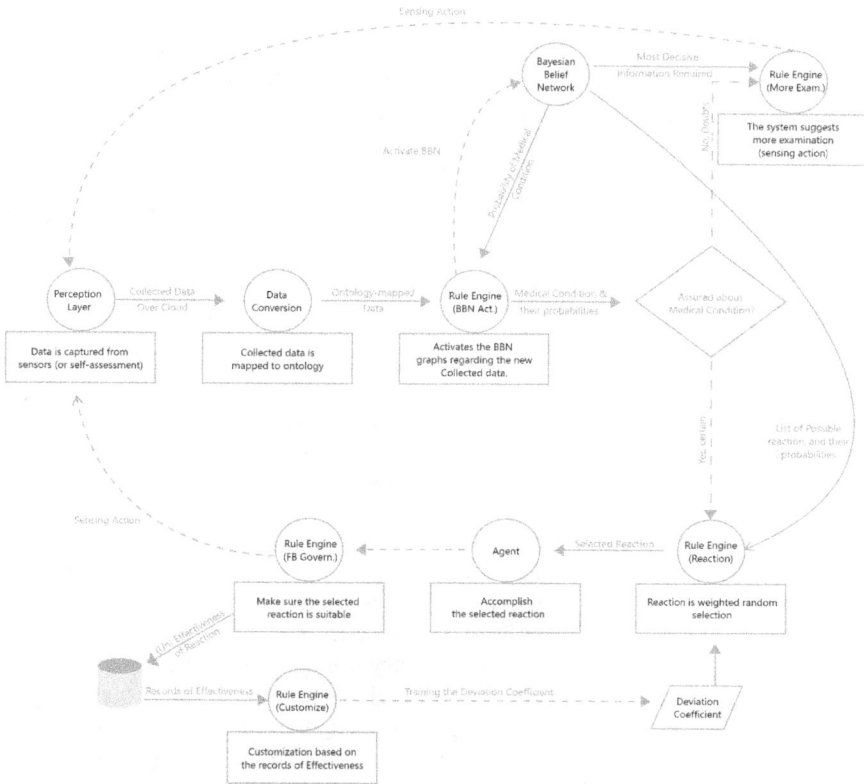

FIGURE 4.7 Workflow of Hapicare system [9].

analyse the human actions by sensing their emotions and conditions. In addition, from the findings of literature, it has been seen that physicians, medical experts and data analysts should adhere to the protocols while interacting with each other to avoid the issues associated with interpretability and explainability (Figure 4.7). Also, various limitations and research gaps are included in this study, which can be resolved by extending the current research using certain technological methods in the future.

4.3 METHODOLOGY

4.3.1 RESEARCH METHOD

A qualitative research methodology is used for accomplishing the research objectives and research questions in context with emerging disruptive technologies and their impact on health informatics. The reason for choosing this research methodology is that the results obtained from this methodology allow deeper understanding of phenomena, experiences and context regarding the research domain [10]. Along with this, experiences and viewpoints of other researchers are also identified with the use of this research methodology. In order to accomplish this research methodology, secondary data is collected. This data is already available in the form of research journals, articles, government publications, official reports and other official websites. The data will be collected from these resources and will be analysed on the basis of different techniques and methods used for obtaining relevant and valuable information. In addition to this, theme-based analysis will be performed for collecting valuable information regarding the research domain.

4.3.2 DATA COLLECTION AND ANALYSIS

The research methodology selected for conducting this research study is qualitative research methodology, and secondary data is collected for achieving research aims, objectives and research questions. Secondary data is collected because it will help in understanding the research gaps, techniques and methods used by previous researchers for overcoming the problems faced by healthcare organisations. The data is collected from online digital repositories which may include, IEEE, ScienceDirect, Emerald, SpringerLink, Mdpi, Taylor & Francis and many more. The data will be collected on the basis of formulated research objectives and research questions so as to obtain appropriate results regarding the research domain, emerging disruptive technologies and their impact on health informatics. In this research study, different challenges faced by the healthcare industry are identified and use of emerging innovative technologies in eliminating these challenges are listed. Most probably, the focus of this research study is on blockchain, augmented reality, predictive analysis, IoT, probabilistic methods and wearable devices. To collect only relevant and valuable information regarding the research domain, theme-based analysis will be performed which will collect data on the basis of identified emerging technologies, defined earlier.

4.4 FINDINGS

4.4.1 CHALLENGES FACED BY HEALTHCARE ORGANISATIONS

Healthcare organisations deal with very sensitive data which is required to be preserved or protected from different cyberattacks. The most common challenge faced by the healthcare sector is loss of data privacy through data breach or any other cyberattack. The use of EHR systems helped the healthcare professionals in decreasing manual errors and improving efficiency in business operations but the use of this system also initiated multiple challenges [11, 12]. The loss of data integrity affects the organisation's brand and customer's trust because of which various customers do not prefer to share their personal information. Apart from this, if data of any patient has been tampered with, they could get the wrong medications which would be difficult to eliminate. It has been identified that most of the healthcare sectors have vulnerable and weak security systems which cannot protect the data from cyberattacks. According to the Health Information Protection and Privacy Act (HIPPA), an

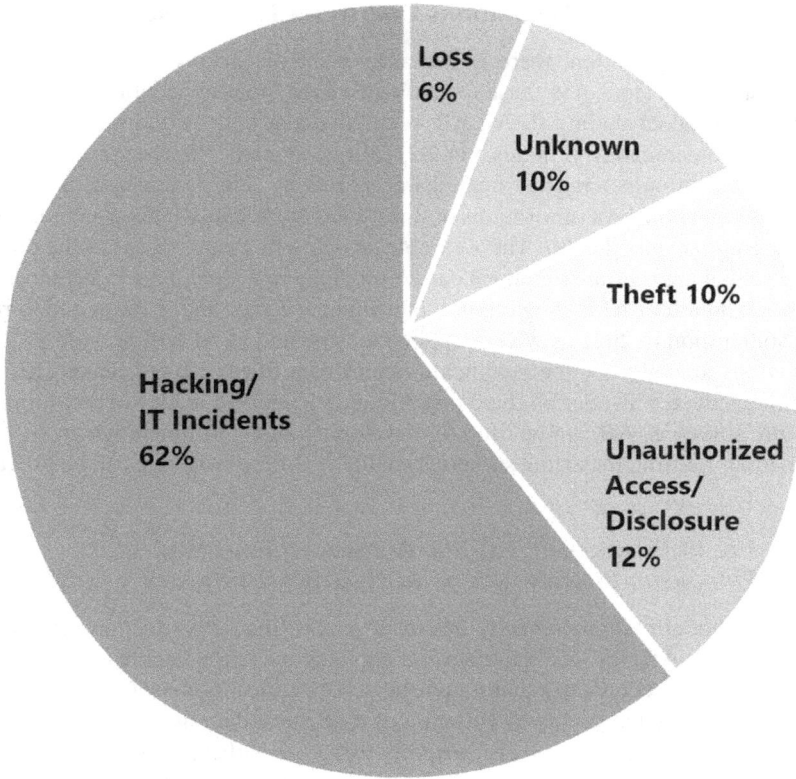

FIGURE 4.8 Type of data breaches in the healthcare sector [13].

online survey journal conducted with data from 2009 to 2018, it has been identified that most of the cyberattacks occurred in 2018 and the main cause of data breach is through information technology [13]. Figure 4.8 illustrates the other causes of data breaches in healthcare organisations.

COVID-19 led to various challenges for health systems across the United States in 2020. There was a huge increase in the number of COVID-19 patients because of which no appropriate treatments are provided and because of which a lot of people died. Hospital services including beds, hospital stay length, ventilators and other hospital equipment are decreased; therefore, hospital staff realised that there is a requirement for an efficient monitoring and tracking system which will ensure that equipment at stake can be renewed as soon as possible [14]. Besides this, the US healthcare systems also have other problems which include poor amenable mortality rate, difficulty in finding a doctor, lack of insurance coverage, inefficiencies, preventable medical errors, lack of transparency, high costs of care and nursing and physician shortage.

4.4.2 TECHNOLOGICAL INNOVATIONS USED IN THE HEALTHCARE INDUSTRY

In this era of digitisation, there is a development of various technologies which help in multiple sectors, and these technologies have great impact on the healthcare organisations. Blockchain, IoT, AI, AR, predictive analysis, virtualisation, wearable devices, nanotechnology, robotics, virtual reality and many other techniques or technologies help in enhancing the healthcare operations. The innovation of wearable devices is one of the best innovations of this digital era because it helps in monitoring and tracking patients' health. The wearable device will send a signal to the doctor's system so that appropriate treatment can be provided to the patient for curing various diseases. The use of AI is growing in the healthcare sector and is estimated to reach up to $6.6 billion in 2021 as well as applications related to AI will provide $150 billion savings annually for the healthcare department of the United States [15]. The research conducted also highlighted that AR and virtualisation help in providing better future surgeons. AR can be used for developing an environment which will help in providing training regarding surgeries so that real-time surgeries can be executed.

4.4.3 USE OF BLOCKCHAIN, IoT AND AUGMENTED REALITY IN ENHANCING PERFORMANCE IN THE HEALTHCARE INDUSTRY

In todays' modern technologically advanced world, disruptive technology such as blockchain, AI, AR, IoT, etc., have several applications in the healthcare sector. The adoption of such technology facilitated the secure transmission of patient medical information and management of voluminous amount of data in an efficient manner. Various medical organisations are currently using e-healthcare systems, which provide remote access to a patient's medical records, continuous monitoring and provide them with suitable treatment at the time of emergency. Blockchain in the healthcare system provides protection to patients' medical data using encryption mechanisms and to diagnose disease by analyzing patterns [16]. Various big organisations around the world have implemented blockchain-based techniques in healthcare systems. For instance, Guardtime organisation in California, USA, provides help to the government and healthcare companies to implement blockchain in the healthcare systems of Estonia. Guardtime also used blockchain technology in healthcare to cure several diseases by creating a central ecosystem for patients, where patients and doctors can access the patient's medical records remotely and take reference from doctors and pharmacists as well as facilitate personal care and easy diagnoses [17]. In addition to it, IoT in the medical and healthcare sector is regarded as the Internet of medical things due to its major contributions to healthcare. IoT-enabled devices offer various healthcare-related services such as remote monitoring of patients, automatic monitoring of glucose level in the human body, depression and mood swings monitoring, monitoring of heart rate and hand hygiene and many more other applications. IoT applications in healthcare are referred to as HIoT and provide various applications such as electrocardiogram (ECG) monitoring, blood pressure monitoring, hospital operation management, monitoring of oxygen saturation levels, nurse assistant robots, etc. [18]. Similarly, AR is serving the healthcare and medical sector by integrating the digital information into a patient's real-world environment. AR in healthcare can be used in several use cases such as reconstruction of tumours in 3D view, in surgical visualisation, disease simulation and surgical procedures, etc. [19].

4.4.4 USE OF PROBABILISTIC METHODS AND PREDICTIVE ANALYSIS IN INCREASING PERFORMANCE OF HEALTHCARE OPERATIONS

Probabilistic methods can be used in the healthcare sector to reduce the costs associated with reflex testing in healthcare. Probabilistic methods help the medical experts to analyse the activities and actions of patients at any time by sensing their emotions with the help of sensory devices. In addition to it, this technology helps the doctors and nurses to detect the sign of patient deterioration and provide them with the most suitable treatment at that time. These methods can also help to identify the patients at risk at their homes and assist them with home remedies and personal care ways. Predictive or probabilistic methods use data from EHRs, medical alert devices and fall detection pendants to identify the risk of an emergency in patients staying at home. Apart from the medical care, probabilistic methods can also be used to identify the requirements of medical equipment maintenance prior to leaving any negative impact [20]. Wearable or sensory devices also helped in continuous monitoring of patients to provide them medical care from experts before deterioration. ML-based probabilistic models helps predict the patient condition and analyse responses. Moreover, probabilistic methods help patients and medical experts to make better plans for patient healthcare in the future and make better decisions incorporating uncertainties. ML-driven probabilistic methods also contributed to the drug discovery process by simulating the use case scenarios. Other applications of probabilistic methods include diabetes-related policies learning and censoring, analyzing the impacts of HIV treatments, etc. [21].

4.5 DISCUSSION AND IMPLICATIONS

The healthcare industry plays a significant role in the development of a country as it will help in ensuring a strong economy. With increases in the development of emerging technologies, various areas in the healthcare industry are demonstrated which requires more attention. Along with this, there are some disruptive medical innovations which help in managing, monitoring or tracking patients and diseases. These technologies may include IoT, wireless patient monitoring system, telemedicine, etc. In this current era, technology is used everywhere because of its vast benefits or advantages. Similarly, emerging technologies such as wearable devices, IoT, AI, blockchain, etc., play a significant role in the development of treatments and information systems in healthcare sectors. Through the conducted research study it has been demonstrated that disruptive technologies have a capability in integrating environmental and healthcare data efficiently for maintaining sustainability [4]. Wearable devices help in monitoring patient movements and their medications, which help in preventing them from developing severe diseases. There are various parameters which are measured, including calories burned, activity levels, sleep patterns, steps taken and eating habits [6]. This will help in providing appropriate medication to patients so that diseases can be cured efficiently. Ava, GymWatch, KardiaMobile,

Motiv, Apple Watch, Fitbit, Garmin, Owlet, My Skin Track UV, TempTraq and Withings are some of the wearable devices which help in tracking and monitoring blood pressure, heart rate, ECG, fever, a baby's progress, fertility, ovulation, etc.

The use of IoT-enabled devices help in enabling healthcare professionals, which will help in connecting patients proactively. The primary motive of using this technology is to keep track of medical equipment such as defibrillators, oxygen pumps, wheelchairs and nebulisers. Along with this, there are various monitoring devices, including glucose monitoring, hand hygiene monitoring, connected inhalers, remote patient monitoring, heart rate monitoring, depression and mood monitoring and ingestible sensors [22]. Similarly, blockchain technology also helps in monitoring patients' actions which will further help in providing the right treatment to patients. The primary motive of using blockchain is to determine database management systems which further include robust data, unchangeable data, traceable data and provide access only to authorised users and protect the system from unauthorised users. It has been identified that smart contracts can be used for storing sensitive data and that data will be stored in encrypted form. This encrypted data is not visible to any normal user, and a decryption key will be used for accessing encrypted data.

AR is another technology which is used by healthcare professionals for providing training to new surgeons by creating a virtual environment which will further result in conducting the surgeries successfully [8]. Along with this, there are some other areas in the healthcare industry where AR is used which includes medical imaging, dentistry, medical education, training to nurses, remote surgical expertise, pediatric magnetic resonance imaging (MRI) evaluation and visualisation of peripheral vasculature. In addition to this, the research study highlighted that probabilistic methods also help in analyzing the activities of patients by sensing their emotions by using sensory devices. In order to predict the actions and treatment plans for a particular disease, EHRs are used which include every detailed information regarding the patient [20]. This research study will help the readers to gain knowledge regarding the importance of emerging technologies in the healthcare sector.

4.6   CONCLUSION

In a nutshell, this research study demonstrated the use of emerging technologies and their impact on health informatics. Data is the most important component which is to be protected from cyberattacks; therefore, the use of emerging technologies will help in preventing the loss of data. Medical informatics is a system of organising and managing information in an efficient manner so that data can be stored and retrieved in an efficient manner. The results obtained from this current research study highlighted that AI, IoT, predictive analysis, wearable devices, virtualisation, etc., are some of the advanced technologies which help in overcoming all the identified challenges in healthcare industries. Apart from this, the research study highlighted that the use of a literature review in analyzing the importance and benefits of advanced technologies is an excellent way of gathering information. The research questions and research objectives formulated for this research study are achieved efficiently by providing appropriate information regarding the research domain. In context with this, AI is a vast technology which helps in predicting the severity of a disease, whereas AR helps in providing training to new surgeons so that surgeries can be performed successfully.

4.7 REFERENCES

[1] A. Sapci and H. Sapci, "Digital continuous healthcare and disruptive medical technologies: m-Health and telemedicine skills training for data-driven healthcare", *Journal of Telemedicine and Telecare*, vol. 25, no. 10, pp. 623–635, 2018. Available: 10.1177/1357633x18793293 [Accessed 27 October 2021].

[2] Y. Kim and D. Delen, "Medical informatics research trend analysis: A text mining approach", *Health Informatics Journal*, vol. 24, no. 4, pp. 432–452, 2016. Available: 10.1177/1460458216678443 [Accessed 27 October 2021].

[3] M. Abdel-Basset, V. Chang and N. Nabeeh, "An intelligent framework using disruptive technologies for COVID-19 analysis", *Technological Forecasting and Social Change*, vol. 163, p. 120431, 2021. Available: 10.1016/j.techfore.2020.120431 [Accessed 27 October 2021].

[4] F. M. Bublitz et al., "Disruptive technologies for environment and health research: An overview of artificial intelligence, blockchain, and internet of things", *International Journal of Environmental Research and Public Health*, vol. 16, no. 20, p. 3847, 2019. Available: 10.3390/ijerph16203847 [Accessed 26 October 2021].

[5] A. Vellido, "The importance of interpretability and visualization in machine learning for applications in medicine and health care", *Neural Computing and Applications*, vol. 32, no. 24, pp. 18069–18083, 2019. Available: 10.1007/s00521-019-04051-w [Accessed 26 October 2021].

[6] H. Koydemir and A. Ozcan, "Wearable and implantable sensors for biomedical applications", *Annual Review of Analytical Chemistry*, vol. 11, no. 1, pp. 127–146, 2018. Available: 10.1146/annurev-anchem-061417–125956 [Accessed 26 October 2021].

[7] J. Qi, P. Yang, L. Newcombe, X. Peng, Y. Yang and Z. Zhao, "An overview of data fusion techniques for Internet of Things enabled physical activity recognition and measure", *Information Fusion*, vol. 55, pp. 269–280, 2020. Available: 10.1016/j.inffus.2019.09.002 [Accessed 26 October 2021].

[8] P. Vávra et al., "Recent development of augmented reality in surgery: A review", *Journal of Healthcare Engineering*, vol. 2017, pp. 1–9, 2017. Available: 10.1155/2017/4574172 [Accessed 26 October 2021].

[9] P. Vávra et al., "Recent development of augmented reality in surgery: A review", *Journal of Healthcare Engineering*, vol. 2017, pp. 1–9, 2017. Available: 10.1155/2017/4574172 [Accessed 26 October 2021].

[10] J. Cleland, "The qualitative orientation in medical education research", *Korean Journal of Medical Education*, vol. 29, no. 2, pp. 61–71, 2017. Available: 10.3946/kjme.2017.53 [Accessed 27 October 2021].

[11] J. Cuenca, "Cybersecurity challenges in healthcare industries", Doctoral dissertation, Utica College, 2017.

[12] H. Kordestani et al., "Hapicare: A healthcare monitoring system with self-adaptive coaching using probabilistic reasoning", *2019 IEEE/ACS 16th International Conference on Computer Systems and Applications (AICCSA)*, 2019, pp. 1–8. Available: https://doi.org/10.1109/AICCSA47632.2019.9035291.

[13] A. Pandey et al., "Key issues in healthcare data integrity: Analysis and recommendations", *IEEE Access*, vol. 8, pp. 40612–40628, 2020. Available: 10.1109/access.2020.2976687 [Accessed 27 October 2021].

[14] G. Berlin, S. Singhal, M. Lapointe and J. Schulz, "Challenges emerge for the US healthcare system as COVID-19 cases rise", *McKinsey & Company*, 2020. [Online]. Available: www. mckinsey.com/industries/healthcare-systems-and-services/our-insights/challenges-emerge-for-the-us-healthcare-system-as-covid-19-cases-rise [Accessed 27 October 2021].

[15] M. Roth, "6 Innovations that are propelling health systems into the future", *Health-leadersmedia.com*, 2021. [Online]. Available: www.healthleadersmedia.com/innova-tion/6-innovations-are-propelling-health-systems-future. [Accessed 27 October 2021].

[16] S. Daley, "How using blockchain in healthcare is reviving the industry's capabilities", *Built In*, 2021. [Online]. Available: https://builtin.com/blockchain/blockchain-health-care-applications-companies [Accessed 27 October 2021].

[17] R. Krawiec, D. Housman, M. Filipova, F. Quarre, D. Barr and A. Nesbit, "Blockchain – A new model for Health Information Exchanges", *Deloitte*, 2021. [Online]. Available: https://www2.deloitte.com/us/en/pages/public-sector/articles/blockchain-opportunities-for-health-care.html. [Accessed 27 October 2021].

[18] B. Pradhan, S. Bhattacharyya and K. Pal, "IoT-based applications in healthcare devices", *Journal of Healthcare Engineering,* vol. 2021, pp. 1–18, 2021. Available: 10.1155/2021/6632599 [Accessed 27 October 2021].

[19] A. Sosna, "The benefits of AR in healthcare – MedCity News", *MedCity News,* 2021. [Online]. Available: https://medcitynews.com/2019/09/the-benefits-of-ar-in-healthcare/ [Accessed 27 October 2021].

[20] J. Maltha, "Predictive analytics in healthcare: three real-world examples", *Philips*, 2021. [Online]. Available: www.philips.com/a-w/about/news/archive/features/20200604-predictive-analytics-in-healthcare-three-real-world-examples.html [Accessed 27 October 2021].

[21] I. Chen, S. Joshi, M. Ghassemi and R. Ranganath, "Probabilistic machine learning for healthcare", 2021. Available: https://doi.org/10.1146/ [Accessed 27 October 2021].

[22] M. Javaid and I. Khan, "Internet of Things (IoT) enabled healthcare helps to take the challenges of COVID-19 Pandemic", *Journal of Oral Biology and Craniofacial Research*, vol. 11, no. 2, pp. 209–214, 2021. Available: 10.1016/j.jobcr.2021.01.015 [Accessed 27 October 2021].

5 Scaling Up Telemedicine in India

Moving Towards Intelligent Healthcare via Disruptions

Sushant Bhargava[1]

[1] Indian Institute of Management, Lucknow, Lucknow, India

5.1 INTRODUCTION

The evolution of healthcare has taken on new and unprecedented directions with the introduction of 'intelligent' and 'learning' technological aids, prompting considerable research into novel applications and more benefits for patients [1]. The revolution in information communication technology (ICT) has gained rapidly during recent decades, and no aspect of human life has remained untouched from it. For healthcare, ICT has revolutionised the user interface/user interaction (UI) components and the requirement for human intervention continues to decline progressively for more and more complicated clinical interventions [2–3]. Since good health is a

DOI: 10.1201/9781003217107-5

primary need for every human being, an increase in the availability of affordable aids in technological tools encourages growth in their adoption among the masses. Users generate an information deluge of details (or *data*) which earlier required meticulous manual organisation and analysis (into *information*) and can now be cast into usable forms almost instantaneously using automation algorithms. A specialised branch of study called health informatics is dedicated to the use of this information and has grown parallelly with ITC in the generation of ideas and applications even for specific contexts [4–5]. New and cutting-edge developments in health informatics include those in the areas of investigative details such as prognostic or diagnostic/prognostic reporting and interpretations. Hybrid fields in the medical sciences which include biomedicine, genomics and general/public health praxis have reached new levels of sophistication with the use of computational tools and models such as block-chain, fuzzy logic and neural networks [6–8]. Situated at the intersection of healthcare and technology, these areas have received considerable scholarly development over the past few years. This is much needed because of the flurry of widespread new challenges that have arisen to directly or indirectly affect public and individual health, and robust new conceptualisations are needed to develop suitable applications and knowledge to contextualise the on-ground developments.

Instances of health emergencies and other destabilising events have become increasingly common in the past few decades. On the one hand are social/civil movements which have marked changes in political regimes, while on the other are pandemics and climate catastrophes which have caused restrictions on peoples' free movement and economic activities (see [9–10] for finer discussions). Every health emergency that finds the world unprepared is a lesson in the need to dramatically scale up the systems at the national, regional and world levels in order to serve all of humankind sustainably and effectively. The impact of these crises is uniform irrespective of the economic or developmental status of a country. Thus, it is expected that from among the countries those moving faster towards solutions should help those unable to do so, so that all can stay safe and maintain at least minimally sufficient health standards. The year 2020 proved to be a major shift in the world order and a watershed year which tested the limits of world cooperation. The COVID-19 pandemic, deemed the worst health crisis in about a century, spread far and wide. It morphed from a danger to health and life owing to its short- and long-term effects, to a danger for the socio-economic stability of the affected countries owing to its unique epidemiology and precipitous measures required to control the infection rate. A COVID-19 'wave' is typically marked by incidence of a large number of infections through relatively short periods of time (days or weeks), which overwhelms the continuously strained infrastructure and support systems. The 'new normal' ushered in by the pandemic has changed the world as we know it. Healthcare, which was usually marginalised in policy and funding [11–14], has now taken centre-stage in decision-making. Some unique features are observable during health emergencies in countries having large populations and/or population densities, such as India.

Located in the South Asian region, India is home to the world's second largest population. Healthcare facilities in Asia generally compare poorly with those in more advanced economies from Europe or North America [15–16]. A number of other Asian countries also have higher populations as compared to those from other continents. Healthcare in populous countries is characterised by availability of lesser nuanced facilities which discourage distinctive diagnoses and limited or infrequent access to well-maintained infrastructure or skilled personnel. For instance, India had 0.7 doctors, 1.3 nurses and 1.1 hospital beds per 1000 people according to some estimates made in the year 2017 [17]. Additionally, there are global and regional policy pressures which affect the pace of developments in healthcare protocols and infrastructure. On the contrary, healthcare decisions are largely governed by popular or political positioning, and fragmentation of efforts impedes an integrative approach. Therefore, India and many other Asian countries demonstrate a prevalence of traditional systems of medicine and treatment which are ill-suited to the treatment of new and disruptive challenges to human health [18–19]. This reliance on age-old systems is compounded by the absence of preventive or consultative care in the non-urban areas especially in India, thereby entering a self-feeding cycle of neglect. Yet medical tourism thrives in the Indian subcontinent which testifies to the capability of the healthcare system and the potential which can be realised by taking it to unconnected areas. Intelligent healthcare solutions, where the role of the doctor is minimal during interventions and through which hospital admissions can be minimised, are extremely valuable from the perspective of India and other Asian countries.

How has a disruptive health emergency like COVID-19 affected the usage, adoption and development of healthcare-focussed computational intelligence? This chapter answers by tracing paths of growth for intelligent healthcare in India through the patterns of increase in usage of telemedicine1 observed during the COVID-19 pandemic. The context of India is important because a) it has immense potential for developing tools for contributing to Intelligent Systems in healthcare, and b) scaling up existing systems should offer interim relief to other healthcare systems across the world which are struggling to recover from disruptions such as the health emergency which has resulted from the COVID-19 pandemic. Scalable systems are the gold standard for investment intensive and critically important infrastructural facilities such as healthcare. Healthcare must additionally preserve cost-efficiency in a country like India where income levels are relatively low and accessibility to even well-established infrastructure remains a challenge. Further, integrating traditional healthcare systems with modern and technologically advanced facilities while preserving its inherent approachability and connect is the need of the hour. Presentation of exemplars of successful efforts which achieve these stated objectives, as done in this study, is helpful for emulation and groundwork in countries where healthcare systems continue to bear the full brunt of crises such as the pandemic, while being in the foundational or nascent stages of development. Additionally, the study lays out parameters for quantifying and prudently dividing the tasks involved in scaling up healthcare systems, especially using the aids of telemedicine and technology.

5.2 LITERATURE REVIEW (STATE OF HEALTHCARE IN INDIA – PRIMING FOR DIGITAL SOLUTIONS)

Indian healthcare has undergone major changes since the country gained independence from the British rule in the year 1947. The Indian healthcare system now consists mainly of the public and private sectors, with the private sector offering better services. This is because of the larger availability of funds in the private sector and its ability to charge patients more for the same services, in comparison with the public sector's lower allocation of funds and orientation towards public welfare which causes it to subsidise services. As healthcare delivery creates and meets new benchmarks, demand from patients for scarce and quality facilities rises concurrently, placing those facilities under strain and pushing up prices. Growing awareness about the selective availability of facilities in a limited number of (urban) centres causes (non-urban) patients to migrate for treatments, causing unsustainable demographic pressures on those centres. Viability of achieving parity in quality of healthcare through digital means, especially in the case of Asian countries, has already been highlighted in a number of different contexts by a number of researchers [20–24]. For disruptive emergencies in the league of COVID-19 pandemic, the strain on an already rudimentarily equipped healthcare delivery system can be relieved using digital means. Digital means have played a critical role during the COVID-19 pandemic, since visits to hospitals were not allowed during movement restrictions and the need for doctoral consultations was higher as the symptoms evolved [25].

Healthcare delivery is also a business which follows the rules of demand, supply, price fixation, quality, reach and competition. The digital means which can enable and enrich healthcare systems for better delivery should have certain dimensions [26]. They include a) protocols (for secure exchange of patient information and inputs in real time over different media), b) interfaces (to provide information at a glance in meaningful formats for all stakeholders, including doctors and third-party providers), c) networks (of both people and sensors or touchpoints for connections among components) and d) analysis methods (to ensure timely predictions based on numerical analyses of past data and smooth running of systems/delivery through timely human intervention). These dimensions form synergetic factors which come together as an ecosystem to create sufficient conditions for survival of solutions and applications to leverage the market conditions. There are also some salient requirements which contribute to the proliferation of digital solutions in the Indian healthcare space by creating appropriate environment for the dimensions to come together. Though a consideration of specific technologies is possible, the discussion here is limited to five specific overarching themes from the perspective of healthcare in India.

5.2.1   CHANGE IN MINDSET

Any form of change or technological change requires the consumers to alter their mindsets to some extent. Positive messaging from trusted sources goes a long way in assuaging initial doubts. At times, early adopters also serve this function of removing barriers. In the case of healthcare, the doctor-patient relationship is fundamentally altered with the use of digital technologies. Therefore, communication between these two parties (at the very least) and concerns about the safety of the patient are required for building a robust ecosystem [27–28]. In the Indian social conditions, these concerns are also primary since health interactions and decisions are highly personalised (i.e. dyad-based and devoid of external parties such as insurers), which may result in significant barriers to adoption of telemedicine and digital health.

5.2.2   CHANGE IN INFRASTRUCTURE

India's healthcare services and healthcare service providers (especially from the public sector which serves larger masses residing in non-urban areas) do not have much to offer or enjoy in infrastructural facilities. Digital solutions can overcome these issues only if the availability of minimal standards in another kind of infrastructure are ensured – digital infrastructure. The potential of India's professionals in delivering economic, innovative and technologically superior solutions has not gone unnoticed by the world. In fact, India's economic growth has largely been fuelled by these professionals. Though India is progressing towards becoming a hub of technological development and manufacturing, its expertise and prowess are yet to benefit the cause of increasing penetration of digital services, which are critical to the delivery of digital solutions in healthcare.

5.2.3   CHANGE IN THE REACH OF TOOLS

Even with the absence of mental barriers and presence of infrastructure, pockets of the Indian landmass are marred by the crippling deficiency of a *digital divide*. This divide is caused by factors outside the ambit of healthcare (such as poverty levels or misinformation), but affect the state of India's health and healthcare delivery. The COVID-19 pandemic caused a rapid transition to digital technologies in all spheres of human work. But how far has this transition had an impact on access and equity, given the crippling constraint of the digital divide, still remains to be seen [29]. What is needed in the short term are efforts to bridge gaps between access and availability, since both are required for efficient delivery of healthcare services.

5.2.4   DESIGNING DIGITAL HEALTH

Digital solutions for healthcare have a number of design issues (that derive directly from the dimensions of the digital ecosystem discussed earlier) which need to be resolved in the respective country's context before implementation. India being a democracy, political concerns always tend to overshadow other logical and practical issues arising around digitisation and other upstream developmental initiatives. Even when there is sufficient will to change constructively, restructuring of health systems is required to implement digital solutions for healthcare. Digital solutions differ on key aspects from their real-world counterparts. This includes imprinting different branches of medical interventions, which require visual or physical inspection, over digital media. For India, the options of having these interventions or examinations digitally were nascent and could only find an impetus to develop once the pandemic took over. Therefore, efforts to find designs which work with other constraints and also integrate standards are still required. The designing efforts may also need to redefine the services being offered in order to be feasible or fruitful.

5.2.5   PLACE IN THE INFORMATION ECONOMY

India becoming digital would entail the generation of huge volumes of data and information. When harnessed properly, information from this large a number of people shapes up an information economy – where information drives other economic activities rather than the traditional means of production. Digital solutions in healthcare are a small part of the information economy, if one exists [30]. Consequently, a careful disambiguation of all the terms related to digital health is relevant for designing and focussing product development. Also, there is a need to specify what kind of care is being offered by a particular implementation – primary, secondary or tertiary. COVID-19 patients require primarily secondary or tertiary care, and this is where product development has taken place during the pandemic.

Given the generalised nature of the themes, the Indian trajectory to adoption of digital solutions in healthcare is relevant to all parts of the world looking to go a similar way. In fact, transition to digital solutions has become a necessity in the post-pandemic world. One of the sub-areas in which digital solutions form India have grown is *mobile health* (m-health). Mobile health is a delivery mechanism of telemedicine which uses handheld mobile devices and mobile or broadband internet connectivity. Usage of these devices has grown considerably post their introduction in the beginning of the 21st century. The products or applications in the mobile health space which have come out of India recently are summarised in Table 5.1.

5.3   FINDINGS (SCALING UP DIGITAL HEALTH – INCREASING HEALTH COVERAGE)

Scaling up drives volumes, which is the need of the hour for Indian healthcare and global healthcare systems. The world population is on an upward trajectory and it is becoming increasingly difficult to provide quality healthcare to all. While developing economies struggle to balance welfare considerations with economic growth, digital technologies have become viable alternatives in driving grassroot change.

TABLE 5.1
Summary of Leading m-Health Apps in India

Name of Mobile Application	Year of Launch	Description
Practo	2014	Medicine delivery/Lab appointments/Review of practitioners
1mg	2015	Medicine delivery/Record keeping/Lab appointments/ Consultations
Lybrate	2013	Review of practitioners/Consultations/Record keeping
MediBuddy	2000	Medicine delivery/Lab appointments/Consultations/Insurance
Curefit	2020	Consultations/fitness classes/therapy
Apollo 247	2020	Consultations/Medicine delivery
Netmeds	2015	Medicine delivery

Ensuring a basic digital infrastructure can act as a platform for many other types of developmental activities. Digital infrastructure scales up applications using it as a base by multiplying its communication and reach – placing it in the hands of billions of connected individuals. *Telemedicine, e-health* and *m-health*2 are the integration of technology and healthcare services [31–32]. They scale health services up by allowing access to healthcare remotely, especially when physical access is difficult or impossible because of geographical constraints (hence the moniker *remote healthcare*). They also remove economic barriers since technology which is widely available is usually cheap, and access to healthcare through this technology makes the pricey accessed services cheap. Instances and advancement of digital healthcare are the result of integrated progress of two branches of science. Hence, defining the field and integrating the available tools may prove difficult at times, involving a range of activities. A natural advancement of digital healthcare is *intelligent healthcare* which is based on predictive and learning algorithms that dynamically interact with and remedy patient concerns or needs without any practitioner intervention. It provides easily accessible options to ensure that a uniform health experience can be provided to the aging and fluctuating population having mobility across a large landmass.

According to some estimates, almost 70% of the Indian people live in non-urban areas which have lack of access and limited health infrastructure as defining features [33]. The difficulties faced by the people were compounded by the incidence of the COVID-19 pandemic when mobility of the population to outside areas, necessary to secure supplies and access to healthcare facilities, was restricted. As more people started falling into the clutches of the pandemic, help could only be made available through telemedicine. As mentioned earlier, the impact of digital healthcare in India was being gauged earlier too, but it became much clearer after the pandemic. India faced two major waves of infections when daily caseloads rose to hundreds of thousands [34–35]. The cases were mostly concentrated in urban areas during the first wave, but non-urban areas saw a rise in cases during the second one. Telemedicine served the purpose of a) extending healthcare to COVID-19 patients who did not require hospitalisation and b) extending healthcare services to other patients when it was not possible for them to reach a care facility because of the restrictions in non-urban areas during both the waves. Thus, telemedicine could be used to effectively scale up the facilities available in urban areas to others.

There was a marked government impetus to the building of required inputs for digital technologies form before the pandemic in India. India has a federal structure to its union, with powers divided between the state and the central governments. Both levels of government had been systematically encouraging and investing in digital infrastructure which came in handy during the pandemic disruptions. However, concerns with collection of Big Data and privacy/security of that data remained. This raises questions about the scope of any scale up which includes health informatics and/or Big Data directly or indirectly. The formation of a robust and foolproof ecosystem of digital health should then have some minimal set of measures against which developments can be gauged. These scope-determining measures should move in line with other disruptions and disruptive technological changes. The disruptive changes in technology have remained fairly stabilised since the occurrence of the pandemic and are likely to remain so until things are completely back to normal, when the 'need' for development in other stagnant spheres would promote more 'inventions.' Moreover, scaling up is only possible through technologies which have potential for wide rollout, and this should be reflected in the measures. Here, a mapping of five measures with specific needs of the ecosystem discussed earlier.

5.3.1 IoT (INTERNET OF THINGS) AND AI (ARTIFICIAL INTELLIGENCE) SOLUTIONS

This measure roughly corresponds to 'Change in Reach of Tools.' IoT and AI are tangential developments that contribute to scalability of intelligent healthcare systems and are therefore included as scope-defining measures the developments in which can be compared to those in digital healthcare.

5.3.2 BIOMEDICAL AND HEALTH INFORMATION SCIENCES

This measure roughly corresponds to 'Place (of digital healthcare) in the Information Economy.' Hybrid and data intensive sub-fields of the medical sciences have a direct bearing on the extent of the scaling up which can be achieved.

5.3.3 MONITORING BEHAVIOUR AND ACTIVITY

This measure roughly corresponds to 'Change in Mindset (of stakeholders.)' Monitoring offers benefits for measuring any possible resistance to the changes introduced and remaining proactive to mitigate them.

5.3.4 INVESTMENT IN WELLBEING-SUPPORTIVE TECHNOLOGY

This measure roughly corresponds to 'Designing Digital Health.' Any design of scalable solutions must have wellbeing considerations firmly embedded within them, so that preventive healthcare can be managed equally well and simultaneously.

5.3.5 INNOVATION IN SUSTAINABLE SOLUTIONS

This measure roughly corresponds to 'Change in Infrastructure.' Any scaling up should be measured against suitable standards of sustainability too. Big Data and informatics can easily become sources of misinformation and misuse, which are both lethal in any healthcare system/initiative.

While moving from wave one to wave two presents some interesting instances of the uses of telemedicine, there are clear advantages to scaling up in this manner for facing wave-'n' and beyond. The reach of telemedicine not only allows practitioners to service the ailing patients, but it also helps in spreading awareness among other residents so that future infections can be controlled and waves averted. Such an approach can be adopted for any health emergency in the future, when latest information and insights can be exchanged in real time and plans or decisions drawn. Thus, scaling up in healthcare becomes equivalent to increasing its range to include healthy habits, leading to preventive healthcare. Given the advantages offered by m-health, its extensions towards the treatment of other ailments have also been suggested [36–37].

Hence, disruptions have proved to be potent tools in accelerating the development of sophisticated information technologies to manage all aspects of healthcare. From the point of view of health informatics, scaling up through digital health includes the construction of accurate information supply chains, which are important in handling future disruptions too (healthcare or otherwise). Also important in scaling up, is promotion of regional (neighbourhood) partnerships through sharing of vaccine doses and medical expertise, which can again be made possible through telemedicine-based planning and execution as and when the need arises.

5.4 DISCUSSION AND THEORETICAL IMPLICATIONS

The explained mappings of essential observed technology-related features which make rapid scale-up possible with the healthcare ecosystem features are summarised in Table 5.2 for ready reference and clarity.

It is useful to look at these mappings in order to develop informed procedures, especially where government- or country-level interventions are concerned. The COVID-19 response has also shown how largely human responses to any crises can diverge from templates or predictions. This is because every crisis spills over or cascades to other seemingly unrelated domains in the modern world connected by technology. Just as it is impossible to promulgate technological solutions without the presence of a certain assumed minimal commonly available infrastructural facilities, it is also impossible to prevent reverse economic impact of healthcare crises on economies and long-term projections of growth for countries. Looking deeply into these cascading of effects can be taxing or prevented because of time constraints. However, a sensitivity towards these effects is necessary in the manner illustrated by the mappings. Hence, a scaling up without a design may be necessitated by external constraints, but must not happen at the expense of wellbeing of the consumers. Hence, theoretical developments on the topic become critical, since all implementations cannot be carried out in the field or on human subjects, even on a smaller scale. We consider some such implications here.

TABLE 5.2

Correspondence of Recommended Measures with the Salient Requirements of Scalable Healthcare Ecosystems

IoT (Internet of Things) and AI (Artificial Intelligence) Solutions	Change in Reach of Tools
Biomedical and Health Information Sciences	Place (of digital healthcare) in the Information Economy
Monitoring Behaviour and Activity	Change in Mindset (of stakeholders)
Investment in Wellbeing-Supportive Technology	Designing Digital Health
Innovation in Sustainable Solutions	Change in Infrastructure

In this chapter, we focus on the COVID-19 pandemic and issues faced during a scale-up of healthcare in its response. There are other issues in digital healthcare which persist and hinder its widespread adoption, especially in developing countries where purchasing power of the consumers and spending powers of the establishment are both limited. Healthcare systems fall under the purview of public health, and ethical issues in public health persist [38]. Just as ensuring synergies among goals of development is a moving target, so is keeping up with the fast pace of development in technology. Therefore, the challenges also morph as time progresses, and theory development makes sense of these changes [39]. However, the global nature of these challenges is unique as technology has also been seen by researchers as a great leveller across divides [40]. The platform economies phenomenon also touches upon healthcare and digital scale-up [41]. The challenge we have focussed on is one of digitalising as well as scaling up. The dual nature of this challenge makes it worthy of further exploration.

5.5   LIMITATIONS OF THE STUDY AND SCOPE FOR FUTURE WORK

This study looks at the example of a single country. Though informative from the theory and policy points of view, each country faces different limitations in the implementation of such solutions. This limitation can be overcome through the use of local surveys and ground-level data. Additionally, the country level of analysis is limited in allowing for a nuanced exploration of population specific responses. There are complications introduced by the diversity of the population and reception of the implementations in the case of healthcare. The recommendations made here may be limited in their applicability when time sensitive situations are in question. Also, analysis based on the response to a single pandemic does not take into account the specific requirements of others. Other limitations are embedded in the topic-enforced boundaries of the challenges that have been highlighted throughout the chapter – such as interoperability of solutions across geographies, market barriers and political willingness, brinksmanship or grandstanding.

Hence, future studies can focus on other developing countries or countries which have set examples in their COVID-19 healthcare emergency response. They can focus on means other than technology that can bolster and supplement the gains made by a widespread response based on technology. As explained earlier, the continuously changing nature of challenges and balancing the spillover effects of any technological change is fertile ground for future theoretical and empirical research both within and outside the domain of healthcare.

5.6   CONCLUSION

Health is not an absence of illness, and it is necessary to learn from the examples and experiences of others when it comes to caring for the health of one's own people. The Indian healthcare system and its scaling up as a result of the COVID-19 pandemic offers numerous and pertinent insights into the design and maintenance of effective solutions/systems with limited resources. Hence, its example can be used to construct strategies for meeting future (healthcare) disruptions. Developments in digital and virtual healthcare picked up steam during the COVID-19 pandemic. We find that digital healthcare has great welfare potential but continues to be driven by financial or policy considerations. Further, scaling up is the need of the hour to serve the health-related needs of the ever-growing population. Digital healthcare has emerged as a viable alternative in this regard too. However, further work is needed to resolve other considerations which may simultaneously arise at different levels of application such as regional or country levels [19, 42].

The future is owned by disruptions, and cutting-edge research in healthcare would only make the world a more habitable place. There is still much unbounded scope for work in ancillary technologies and discovery of uses based on growing awareness patterns in different societies. Of course, specific m-health and intelligent aids can be used for traditional functions and work continues in those directions. Integration of digital healthcare metrics with smart wearables and IoT is also an ideal and interesting direction to pursue, that could potentially ensure every connected person's automated monitoring and priority in attention as and when required. Work also continues on visualisation and knowledge discovery form the collected and voluminous data, and on using those attributes to generate predictive analytical outputs [43]. Smart integration with other areas of development and work on territorial limitations are topics within digital healthcare which deserve scholarly attention. In an age of disruptions, when progress has been hampered in most areas, health informatics has emerged as a fertile avenue for development, advancement into which will benefit humankind through intelligent and learning systems, products and services that can scale up delivery of healthcare for the wellbeing and sustenance of mankind. What is needed is a careful approach and a keen eye for opportunities which may be few and far between.

5.7 NOTES

1 Sometimes also known as e-health or m-health.
2 These terms are used interchangeably but actually differ in the use of the specific digital medium.

5.8 REFERENCES

[1] F. Ali *et al.*, "An intelligent healthcare monitoring framework using wearable sensors and social networking data," *Futur. Gener. Comput. Syst.*, vol. 114, pp. 23–43, Jan. 2021, doi: 10.1016/j.future.2020.07.047.
[2] R. Gururajan and A. Hafeez-Baig, "An empirical study to determine factors that motivate and limit the implementation Of ICT in healthcare environments," *BMC Med. Inform. Decis. Mak.*, vol. 14, no. 1, p. 98, Dec. 2014, doi: 10.1186/1472-6947-14-98.
[3] N. Zakaria, S. Affendi, and N. Zakaria, "Managing ICT in healthcare organization: Culture, challenges, and issues of technology adoption and implementation," in *Handbook of Research on Advances in Health Informatics and Electronic Healthcare Applications*, IGI Global, 2010, pp. 153–168.
[4] A. Friede, H. L. Blum, and M. McDonald, "Public health informatics: How information-age technology can strengthen public health," *Annu. Rev. Public Health*, vol. 16, no. 1, pp. 239–252, May 1995, doi: 10.1146/annurev.pu.16.050195.001323.

[5] P. A. Bath, "Health informatics: Current issues and challenges," *Information Science in Transition*, vol. 34, Facet, 2018, pp. 169–198.

[6] J. H. Holmes, "Methods and applications of evolutionary computation in biomedicine," *J. Biomed. Inform.*, vol. 49, pp. 11–15, Jun. 2014, doi: 10.1016/j.jbi.2014.05.008.

[7] Q. Zou, L. Chen, T. Huang, Z. Zhang, and Y. Xu, "Machine learning and graph analytics in computational biomedicine," *Artif. Intell. Med.*, vol. 83, p. 1, Nov. 2017, doi: 10.1016/j.artmed.2017.09.003.

[8] C. Cao *et al.*, "Deep learning and its applications in biomedicine," *Genomics. Proteomics Bioinformatics*, vol. 16, no. 1, pp. 17–32, Feb. 2018, doi: 10.1016/j.gpb.2017.07.003.

[9] A. Morgans and S. J. Burgess, "What is a health emergency? The difference in definition and understanding between patients and health professionals," *Aust. Heal. Rev.*, vol. 35, no. 3, p. 284, 2011, doi: 10.1071/AH10922.

[10] W. J. Ripple, C. Wolf, T. M. Newsome, P. Barnard, and W. R. Moomaw, "World scientists' warning of a climate emergency," *Bioscience*, vol. 70, no. 1, pp. 8–12, Nov. 2019, doi: 10.1093/biosci/biz088.

[11] A. Chandra, J. Holmes, and J. Skinner, "Is this time different? The slowdown in healthcare spending," Cambridge, MA, Dec. 2013, doi: 10.3386/w19700.

[12] M. Jakovljevic *et al.*, "Real GDP growth rates and healthcare spending – comparison between the G7 and the EM7 countries," *Global. Health*, vol. 16, no. 1, p. 64, Dec. 2020, doi: 10.1186/s12992-020-00590-3.

[13] E. F. Madden, S. Kalishman, A. Zurawski, P. O'Sullivan, S. Arora, and M. Komaromy, "Strategies used by interprofessional teams to counter healthcare marginalization and engage complex patients," *Qual. Health Res.*, vol. 30, no. 7, pp. 1058–1071, Jun. 2020, doi: 10.1177/1049732320909100.

[14] J. A. Razzak and A. L. Kellermann, "Emergency medical care in developing countries: Is it worthwhile?" *Bull. World Health Organ.*, vol. 80, no. 11, pp. 900–905, 2002, doi: 10.1590/S0042-96862002001100011.

[15] S. Zaidi, P. Saligram, S. Ahmed, E. Sonderp, and K. Sheikh, "Expanding access to healthcare in South Asia," *BMJ*, vol. 357, no. April, pp. 1–4, Apr. 2017, doi: 10.1136/bmj.j1645.

[16] N. Yeates and J. Pillinger, "International healthcare worker migration in Asia Pacific: International policy responses," *Asia Pac. Viewp.*, vol. 59, no. 1, pp. 92–106, Apr. 2018, doi: 10.1111/apv.12180.

[17] PwC India and CII, "How m-Health can revolutionise the Indian healthcare industry," 2017. [Online]. Available: www.pwc.in/publications/2017/how-mhealth-can-revolutionise-the-indian-healthcare-industry.html.

[18] C. Y. Luk, "The impact of digital health on traditional healthcare systems and doctor-patient relationships," *Innovative Perspectives on Public Administration in the Digital Age*, vol. i, 2018, pp. 143–167.

[19] Y. L. Park and R. Canaway, "Integrating traditional and complementary medicine with national healthcare systems for universal health coverage in Asia and the Western Pacific," *Heal. Syst. Reform*, vol. 5, no. 1, pp. 24–31, Jan. 2019, doi: 10.1080/23288604.2018.1539058.

[20] Y. Wang, Y. Liu, Y. Shi, Y. Yu, and J. Yang, "User perceptions of virtual hospital apps in China: Systematic search," *JMIR m-Health u-Health*, vol. 8, no. 8, p. e19487, Aug. 2020, doi: 10.2196/19487.

[21] R. K. Alsalamah, N. A. Almasoud, J. A. Alghtani, and M. A. Alrowaily, "The use of mobile application in primary health care in Saudi Arabia: A cross-sectional study.," *J. Fam. Med. Prim. Care*, vol. 9, no. 12, pp. 6068–6072, Dec. 2020, doi: 10.4103/jfmpc.jfmpc_1568_20.

[22] M. Dolezel and Z. Smutny, "Usage of e-Health/m-Health services among young Czech adults and the impact of COVID-19: An explorative survey," *Int. J. Environ. Res. Public Health*, vol. 18, no. 13, p. 7147, Jul. 2021, doi: 10.3390/ijerph18137147.

[23] M. Pikkemaat, H. Thulesius, and V. Milos Nymberg, "Swedish primary care physicians' intentions to use telemedicine: A survey using a new questionnaire – physician attitudes and intentions to use telemedicine (PAIT)," *Int. J. Gen. Med.*, vol. 14, no. July, pp. 3445–3455, Jul. 2021, doi: 10.2147/IJGM.S319497.

[24] O. Byambasuren, E. Beller, T. Hoffmann, and P. Glasziou, "Barriers to and facilitators of the prescription of m-Health apps in Australian general practice: Qualitative study," *JMIR m-Health u-Health*, vol. 8, no. 7, p. e17447, Jul. 2020, doi: 10.2196/17447.

[25] Y. Z. Almallah and D. J. Doyle, "Telehealth in the time of Corona: 'Doctor in the house'," *Intern. Med. J.*, vol. 50, no. 12, pp. 1578–1583, Dec. 2020, doi: 10.1111/imj.15108.

[26] G. Sainger, "Digital dimension of indian healthcare sector: A review," *Ann. Rom. Soc. Cell Biol.*, vol. 25, no. 3, pp. 1523–1528, 2021, [Online]. Available: www.scopus.com/inward/record.uri?eid=2-s2.0-85102990870&partnerID=40&md5=768cef3fa8e169af-4307241d68e5cbd0.

[27] M. Raj *et al.*, "Addressing evolving patient concerns around telehealth in the COVID-19 era," *Am. J. Manag. Care*, vol. 27, no. 1, pp. e1–e3, Jan. 2021, doi: 10.37765/ajmc.2021.88576.

[28] A. Kashgary, R. Alsolaimani, M. Mosli, and S. Faraj, "The role of mobile devices in doctor-patient communication: A systematic review and meta-analysis," *J. Telemed. Telecare*, vol. 23, no. 8, pp. 693–700, Sep. 2017, doi: 10.1177/1357633X16661604.

[29] J. E. Chang, A. Y. Lai, A. Gupta, A. M. Nguyen, C. A. Berry, and D. R. Shelley, "Rapid transition to telehealth and the digital divide: Implications for primary care access and equity in a post-COVID era," *Milbank Q.*, vol. 99, no. 2, pp. 340–368, Jun. 2021, doi: 10.1111/1468-0009.12509.

[30] K. D. Mandl, J. C. Mandel, and I. S. Kohane, "Driving innovation in health systems through an apps-based information economy," *Cell Syst.*, vol. 1, no. 1, pp. 8–13, Jul. 2015, doi: 10.1016/j.cels.2015.05.001.

[31] J. A. Rodriguez, J. R. Betancourt, T. D. Sequist, and I. Ganguli, "Differences in the use of telephone and video telemedicine visits during the COVID-19 pandemic," *Am. J. Manag. Care*, vol. 27, no. 1, pp. 21–26, Jan. 2021, doi: 10.37765/ajmc.2021.88573.

[32] I. de la Torre-Díez, M. López-Coronado, C. Vaca, J. S. Aguado, and C. de Castro, "Cost-utility and cost-effectiveness studies of telemedicine, electronic, and mobile health systems in the literature: A systematic review," *Telemed. e-Health*, vol. 21, no. 2, pp. 81–85, Feb. 2015, doi: 10.1089/tmj.2014.0053.

[33] C. Elbers and P. Lanjouw, "Inequality in rural India," vol. 2019, no. 4. UNU-WIDER.

[34] K. S. Reddy, "Pandemic lessons from India," *BMJ*, vol. 373, p. n1196, May 2021, doi: 10.1136/bmj.n1196.

[35] O. P. Choudhary, Priyanka, I. Singh, and A. J. Rodriguez-Morales, "Second wave of COVID-19 in India: Dissection of the causes and lessons learnt," *Travel Med. Infect. Dis.*, vol. 43, no. January, p. 102126, Sep. 2021, doi: 10.1016/j.tmaid.2021.102126.

[36] J. Nicholas, M. E. Larsen, J. Proudfoot, and H. Christensen, "Mobile apps for bipolar disorder: A systematic review of features and content quality," *J. Med. Internet Res.*, vol. 17, no. 8, p. e198, Aug. 2015, doi: 10.2196/jmir.4581.

[37] E. Widnall *et al.*, "User perspectives of mood-monitoring apps available to young people: Qualitative content analysis," *JMIR m-Health u-Health*, vol. 8, no. 10, p. e18140, Oct. 2020, doi: 10.2196/18140.

[38] C. Brall, P. Schröder-Bäck, and E. Maeckelberghe, "Ethical aspects of digital health from a justice point of view," *Eur. J. Public Health*, vol. 29, no. Supplement_3, pp. 18–22, Oct. 2019, doi: 10.1093/eurpub/ckz167.

[39] N. Cummins and B. W. Schuller, "Five crucial challenges in digital health," *Front. Digit. Heal.*, vol. 2, no. Dec., pp. 1–5, Dec. 2020, doi: 10.3389/fdgth.2020.536203.

[40] S. Kraus, F. Schiavone, A. Pluznikova, and A. C. Invernizzi, "Digital transformation in healthcare: Analyzing the current state-of-research," *J. Bus. Res.*, vol. 123, pp. 557–567, Feb. 2021, doi: 10.1016/j.jbusres.2020.10.030.

[41] S. Hermes, T. Riasanow, E. K. Clemons, M. Böhm, and H. Krcmar, "The digital transformation of the healthcare industry: Exploring the rise of emerging platform ecosystems and their influence on the role of patients," *Bus. Res.*, vol. 13, no. 3, pp. 1033–1069, Nov. 2020, doi: 10.1007/s40685-020-00125-x.

[42] C. A. Bowman, M. Nuh, and A. Rahim, "COVID-19 telehealth expansion can help solve the health care underutilization challenge," *Am. J. Manag. Care*, vol. 27, no. 1, pp. 9–11, Jan. 2021, doi: 10.37765/ajmc.2021.88571.

[43] M. Alcocer Alkureishi *et al.*, "Teaching telemedicine: The next frontier for medical educators," *JMIR Med. Educ.*, vol. 7, no. 2, p. e29099, Apr. 2021, doi: 10.2196/29099.

6 A Wearable ECG Sensor for Intelligent Cardiovascular Health Informatics

Dhanashri H. Gawali[1]*, Vijay M. Wadhai*[2]*,*
Minakshee Patil[3] *and Akshita S. Chanchlani*[1]
[1] Sant Gadge Baba Amravati University, Amravati, India
[2] D.Y. Patil College of Engineering, Pune, India
[3] Sinhgad Academy of Engineering, Pune, India

6.1 INTRODUCTION

As per the World Health Organization (WHO) estimate, 31% of deaths occurring worldwide are due to cardiovascular diseases (CVDs), out of which more than 75% of CVD deaths occur in low- and middle-income countries. Almost 80% of CVD deaths occur due to heart attack and stroke. CVDs remained the leading cause of death worldwide owing to various risk factors. Also, there is a potential threat of long-term impact on the cardiovascular system due to the recently emerged COVID-19 disease. Cardiovascular health informatics refers to the processing,

DOI: 10.1201/9781003217107-6

storage, transmission, acquisition and retrieval of cardiac information for the early detection, early prediction, early prevention, early diagnosis and early treatment of CVDs [1]. The major goal is to detect symptoms or risk factors at an early stage using wearable sensors with higher sensitivity. The electrocardiogram (ECG) plays a vital role in the diagnosis and management of CVDs. ECG data enable the diagnosis of many cardiovascular abnormalities, including numerous arrhythmias, atrial fibrillation (AF), premature contractions of the atria (PAC) or ventricles (PVC), myocardial infarction (MI) and congestive heart failure (CHF) [2]. A few arrhythmias such as MI are life-threatening, while rare and serious arrhythmias such as Brugada syndrome, arrhythmogenic right ventricular cardiomyopathy, long QT syndrome, hypertrophic cardiomyopathy, etc., are infrequent and only get detected on prolonged monitoring. This requires innovative solutions to monitor ECG signal over longer durations of time. Artificial intelligence (AI) techniques such as machine learning, deep learning and cognitive computing have the potential for rapid and accurate interpretation of large digital ECG data for early detection and diagnosis of CVDs [3].

With the rising penetration of smartphones, m-Health has been an emerging area of innovation to deliver personalised healthcare services at home or in non-clinical environments. The long-term ECG monitoring applications demand wearable sensors for patient data collection and processing in real time. Often such sensor nodes consist of a set of non-invasive physiological sensors connected wirelessly to a cell phone, which stores, transmits and analyses the physiological data and presents it to the user in an intelligible way [4]. m-Health-based wearable ECG sensors integrated with cloud-based artificial intelligence hold the promise of early detection, prediction, prevention, diagnosis and treatment of CVDs. Such systems enable monitoring of an individual unobtrusively and assist physicians to evaluate patient's health condition remotely. Earlier detection of a disease state leads to earlier intervention and treatment. Furthermore, AI techniques can eventually help establish prediction and prevention of CVDs based on the disease progression dataset. Figure 6.1 shows the general model of m-Health-based intelligent cardiovascular health informatics. Wearable sensors acquire ECG data over long durations; m-Health technologies support the collection, local storage, processing and transfer of the data over the cloud; and AI techniques assist in the automated, efficient and accurate interpretation of the large ECG data for early detection and diagnosis of CVDs. Physicians can use such systems to monitor individuals recovering from an existing health condition, those at risk and those experiencing some discomfort.

The main objective of this chapter is to introduce mobile health (m-Health)–based long-term ECG monitoring for intelligent cardiovascular health informatics and present an approach to develop a wearable ECG sensor suitable for the same. Section 2 describes the literature review of the m-Health platform for intelligent cardiovascular health informatics. It further presents the current state of the art of wearable sensors for intelligent cardiovascular health informatics. It briefly discusses key technology areas, challenges and opportunities in wearable sensor development. Section 3 elaborates an approach to design and develop a wearable ECG

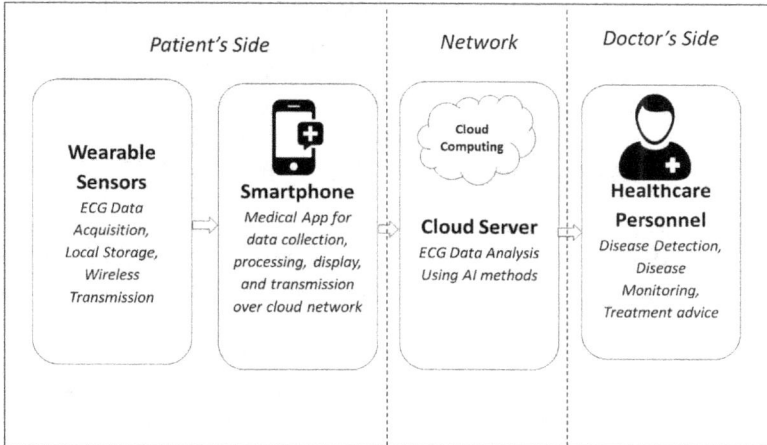

FIGURE 6.1   General model of m-Health-based intelligent cardiovascular health informatics.

sensor consisting of sensing element and sensor electronics suitable for m-Health-based intelligent cardiovascular health informatics. The experimental results and discussion are presented in Section 4. The key contributions of the chapter and concluding remarks are mentioned in Section 5. Finally, limitations of the study and scope for further research are presented at the end of the chapter.

6.2   LITERATURE REVIEW

Most of the world's population, including the most remote areas of Africa, Latin America and Asia, have access to mobile communication. This infrastructure offered societies an opportunity to transform their healthcare services [5]. A recent Indian scenario depicted extensive use of smartphones with 3G and 4G services, and their affordable prices encouraged both the data usage and adoption of m-Health services [6]. The following presents the current state of the art in the field of m-Health and wearable technologies for intelligent cardiovascular health informatics.

6.2.1   m-HEALTH-BASED INTELLIGENT CARDIOVASCULAR HEALTH INFORMATICS

Several m-Health-based clinical studies reviewed by Enone Honeyman et al. offered strong evidence of the general capabilities and features of m-Health that enable cardiac care involving monitoring and management of cardiac arrest, arrhythmias, MI and heart failure (HF) [7]. Furthermore, combining standard preventive measures with wearable sensors, m-Health technologies and cloud-based AI methods enabled intelligent cardiovascular health informatics to enhance CVD detection and prevention in high-risk patients [2–3,7–8]. Numerous research groups have been working on AI-based ECG analytics for intelligent cardiovascular health informatics [2, 9]. Deep learning (DL) methods have become popular among AI owing to their ability to identify novel relationships in the data independent of features selection. Numerous deep learning architectures used in ECG analytic studies for disease detection/classification, annotation/localisation, sleep staging, biometric human identification and denoising included convolutional neural networks (CNNs), recurrent neural networks (RNNs), combinations of CNNs and RNNs (CRNNs), deep belief networks (DBN), autoencoders (AEs), generative adversarial networks (GANs), fully connected neural networks (FCs) etc. [2, 10]. Several studies used ECG datasets available with the organisations in Brazil, the United States and China [9]. Most of the studies used open-source datasets such as MIT-BIH and PhysioNet; however, a few datasets were collected from healthcare devices. Many algorithms were derived using 12-lead ECG data, while a few studies demonstrated satisfactory performance with single-lead ECGs [9]. Various cardiac diseases can be detected based on short-term ECG data (few seconds or minutes) for the primary diagnostics, while long-term ECG (24 hours) can help to detect diseases with intermittent symptoms such as paroxysmal ventricular fibrillation (VF) and AF.

Although, DL methods offer many advantages, it suffers from implementation challenges. Wearable device technology, m-Health technology and AI methods have been investigated extensively, often individually, in the context of intelligent cardiovascular health informatics. However, evidences based on the combination of all of them are still lacking. DL methods perform efficiently with large training data and do not generalise well for the test data. They are computationally intensive; thus, their implementation on low-power embedded devices is a major obstacle in real-world applications. Cloud-based ECG analytics provide a solution to this at the expense of additional cost and latency. Recently emerged Edge AI technology relies on the user device hardware instead of cloud for processing of AI algorithms. It can bring the benefits of reduced latency, integration between wearable devices, reduced bandwidth, reduced costs, greater security and privacy of data. A hybrid architecture based on the balanced use of edge and cloud computing for AI algorithms can bring the trade-off between the accuracy of the diagnosis and the complexity of the model [11]. Furthermore, the success of the DL method depends largely on the adequate high-quality dataset suitable for the given task, which is another major obstacle. Most of the current investigations are based on old datasets collected over 40 years ago or recent high-quality database with short-term ECG recordings [2]. Thus, there is a need for a new high-quality long-term ECG dataset with annotations. In addition to long-term ECG monitoring, wearable devices can help in creating large datasets to support intelligent cardiovascular health informatics. The following section presents the innovations and current trends in wearable technology.

6.2.2   WEARABLE TECHNOLOGY FOR CARDIOVASCULAR HEALTH INFORMATICS

Wearable devices incorporating noninvasive physiological sensors, data processing modules and wireless data transmission capabilities are small, light, unobtrusive and designed to operate by unskilled users. The global wearable healthcare devices market is projected to reach USD 46.6 billion by 2025 from USD 18.4 billion in 2020, at a compound annual growth rate (CAGR) of 20.5% from 2020 to 2025 [12]. The growing adoption of mobile platforms with AI and 5G in emerging economies such as India, China and Brazil provide a wide range of opportunities. The wearable cardiac devices market is expected to grow by a CAGR of 24.2% up to 2026 from USD 1.2 billion in 2019 [13]. Wearable cardiac devices including patches, Holter monitors, ECG devices, mobile cardiac telemetry and wearable defibrillators provide real-time data to cardiac patients and doctors with continuous out-of-hospital monitoring of cardiac health, thereby minimising the cost and hospital visits. Wearables could be seamlessly integrated with clothing such as chest belt or T-shirt. Besides, it may be embedded in the objects such as chair, bed, vehicle, etc. [14]. The rising research efforts in the field leading to technological advancements will boost growth of wearable cardiac devices industry.

Technology innovations have been playing an important role in the development of wearable biosensors. For long-term physiological signal monitoring, textiles have been the preferred platform for sensors being the most natural materials close to the skin [15]. Textile-based ECG sensors were developed that can be worn as badges or patches [15–16]. Also, a textile-based integrated conformal patch antenna with system-level radio design along with textile-based ECG electrode design were suggested in the literature [15, 17]. However, it is essential to address mechanical resistance and the durability of the materials in a harsh environment for wide acceptance. Adhesives were often used to hold the electrodes in the place against the skin for long-term monitoring. Dry electrodes were preferred over wet electrodes as they seamlessly integrate into clothing. Use of innovative organic-inorganic hybrid materials, nanomaterials and nanostructures were suggested to achieve the desirable electrical and mechanical properties for dry electrodes [18–19]. Advancements in material science led the manufacturing of small, lightweight and high-efficiency batteries. Developments in miniaturised devices, embedded architectures and modern circuit design methodologies enabled an efficient signal acquisition, on-board processing and wireless transmission of bio-signals over longer durations of time [20–24]. Flexible sensors are best suited for wearable applications. Thus, flexible sensor circuits fabrication onto flexible substrates such as paper, plastic and cloth fabrics were suggested in the literature [25–27].

Various high integration technologies such as system-on-chip (SOC) and application-specific integrated circuit (ASIC) have been explored to achieve miniaturisation and low-power performance of the wearable device [20–24]. Recent trends in direct die/wafer, wafer/wafer bonding, optical interconnect, system in package (SiP), package on package (PoP), etc., offer the benefits of increased performance, low cost, smaller footprint, power management and time-to-market for the wearable devices [28]. With emerging thin-film technology, batteries are becoming ultra-thin, flexible, rollable, stretchable and more. For wearable sensors, high-energy thin-film batteries have the highest potential followed by printed rechargeable zinc battery [29]. Energy harvesting and wireless power transmission (WPT) methods can support even battery-less and energy-efficient solutions [30–32]. Acquiring power from the human body needs low-power integrated circuits and microchips that can harvest maximum energy from body movement, heat, vibration, electromagnetism, the piezoelectric effect, etc. WPT has recently emerged as a favourable alternative of supplying power to battery-free wearable devices. It can eliminate frequent battery replacements, minimise total weight and size of the wearable device and support long-term studies.

However, implementation of these approaches for wearable devices is still at the primary stage of research.

Despite technology innovations and emerging trends, the development of a wearable ECG sensor suffers from various challenges such as small form factor, robust and comfortable designs, longer battery life, privacy issues and affordable price. These devices need to be extremely accurate and reliable for long duration measurements. Embedding sensors and electronics into textiles imposes the challenge of creating comfortable, flexible and washable solutions. Interconnections and electronics must be robust and unobtrusive. The sensors must be light in weight, small in size, and should support the patient's movements. Energy management is a big challenge in order to ensure that the data are not lost during charging or battery replacement periods. The low-energy operation may lead to a challenge for the quality of the data captured.[32] Privacy of sensor data is important, as the contain sensitive information that should not be accessed or modified by an unauthorised person. It becomes critical when the device gets integrated into an m-Health platform. As platforms multiply and integrate with each other, security concerns become more complex [33]. The high initial cost of smart wearable devices is one of the major challenges. Hence, the growth of the wearable market highly depends on the cost that consumers can afford. Thus, a multidisciplinary approach with knowledge of various domains is highly needed for affordable, reliable, secure, user-friendly and robust wearable devices. The following section describes the methodology for the prototype-level design and development of the proposed wearable ECG sensor.

6.3 METHODOLOGY FOR WEARABLE ECG SENSOR PROTOTYPE DEVELOPMENT

Electrocardiography is a fundamental part of cardiovascular assessment and an essential tool for investigating CVDs. The electrical changes due to depolarisation and repolarisation of myocardial cells resulting in contraction and relaxation of cardiac muscle are recorded with electrodes placed on the limbs and chest wall [34]. Monitoring applications typically use one or two leads to reliably recognise each heartbeat and perform rhythm analysis. Here, we propose a wearable single-lead ECG sensor consisting of sensing element and sensor electronics suitable for m-Health-based intelligent cardiovascular health informatics as shown in Figure 6.2. The major goal was to achieve a wearable, miniaturised and energy-efficient solution. In the proposed system, innovative nanocomposite material based capacitively coupled biopotential electrodes were used as a sensing element, while a reconfigurable platform-based circuit formed the sensor electronics. The electrodes were attached to the skin surface to convert biopotentials into electric signal. Sensor electronics included the analog front end (AFE), processing module, data storage memory, wireless interface, battery and energy management module. The analog frontend converted the electrical signal into sensor data; the embedded processor supporting low-power modes efficiently processed it; and the processed data were transmitted to the smartphone device wirelessly using the Bluetooth technology supporting low-power operation. With the proposed solution it was possible to continuously monitor the ECG signal from a remote location for a prolonged period of time.

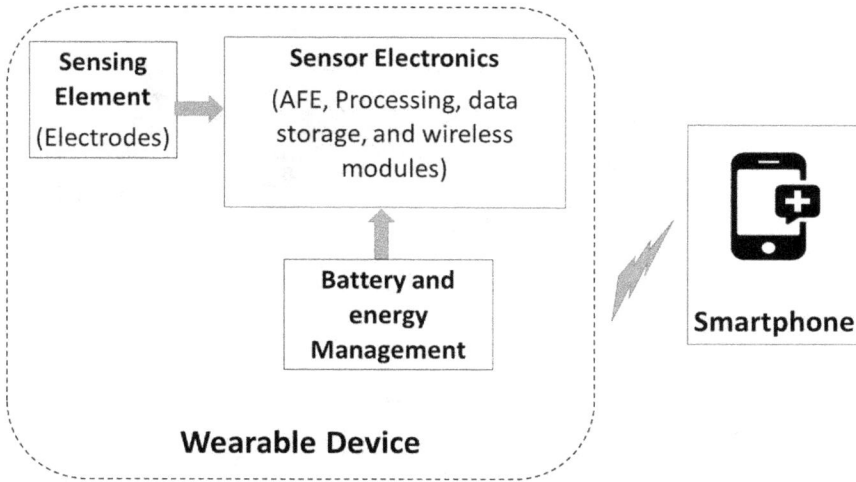

FIGURE 6.2 Block diagram of the proposed system.

6.3.1 BIOPOTENTIAL ELECTRODE DESIGN AND DEVELOPMENT

The major requirements of biopotential electrodes for long-term physiological monitoring include appropriate placement on the body, good electrical contact with the skin, good immunity to noise and motion artifacts, comfortable to wear without causing skin irritation, and it should not require skin preparation. The noncontact electrodes have recently been popular, which can sense signals with the sensor placed over clothing, where the cloth essentially acts as a dielectric material between metal sensor and skin. Dry capacitive electrodes are safe as no DC current flow through them; also, they do not suffer from half-cell potential. Thus, they are found suitable for mobile and long-term monitoring applications. However, they couple signals through a small capacitance (10s pF) [35–36]. Capacitive coupling has a disadvantage of degrading the low-frequency performance of the system. Hence, for adequate low-frequency response, the capacitance value must be high enough. Thus, electrodes with large specific surface area but less actual area are required to enhance the coupling capacitance. A higher value of capacitance can be achieved by reducing the thickness of dielectric material, increasing the dielectric constant of dielectric material, and increasing the area of electrode. A flexible polymer matrix nanocomposite material-based electrode with suitable electrical and mechanical properties are potential candidates to meet these requirements. Using them in capacitive arrangements would be beneficial to enhance skin electrode impedance as they tend to increase the value of capacitance. Figure 6.3 shows the proposed electrode structure with approximate dimensions. To meet the requirements, flexible material such as poly-dimethyl-siloxane (PDMS) with barium titanate (BaTiO3) nanoparticles (nanoBaTiO3) and silver nanowires (AgNW) as fillers were used as a dielectric and metal layer, respectively.

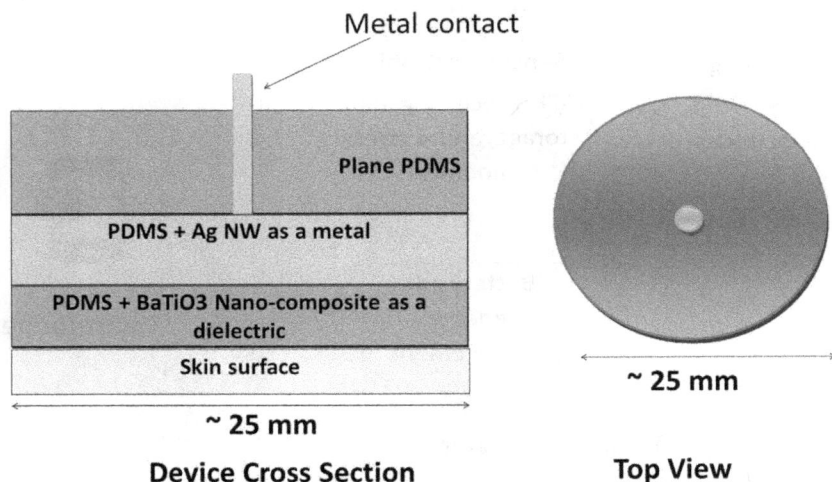

FIGURE 6.3   The proposed electrode structure.

AgNW were synthesised using polyol process [37–38]. Ultraviolet-visible spectroscopy was performed to confirm the optical signature of silver nanowires followed by the scanning electron microscopy (SEM) for structural characterisation. PDMS +n anoBaTiO3 was prepared by mixing BaTiO3 nanoparticles with a polymer matrix (PDMS) [39]. The process used for forming the electrode structure is shown in Figure 6.4(a). Initially, PDMS + nanoBaTiO3 was cast onto a precleaned glass substrate using a spin coater, followed by curing at 65°C for 12 h. Next, AgNW were deposited on top of the PDMS + nanoBaTiO3 film, and the liquid PDMS was cast on the AgNW film such that the nanowires get buried in the PDMS. While the PDMS was in liquid form, a metal snap connecter was inserted in the PDMS so that it touches the AgNW film. It was allowed to cure for 12 h at 65°C. When peeled off the substrate, the AgNW film was bonded to the PDMS + nanoBaTiO3 film. This process is scalable for preparing multiple electrodes as shown in Figure 6.4(b). Multiple electrodes were obtained by using a sharp cutter. The electrical and microscopic characterisations were performed using Lifetime Clinical Record (LCRQ) metre and SEM, respectively. The final device structure is as shown in Figure 6.4(c).

6.3.2   Sensor Electronics Design and Implementation

To make the sensor energy-efficient and of a small size, it is inevitable to use a highly integrated and low-power platform for the system implementation. Complementary metal oxide semiconductor (CMOS) technology based programmable system on chip (PSoC) is a highly integrated system with a CPU, analog and digital blocks to configure mixed-signal circuits, and an internal oscillator in a single Integrated Circuit (IC) package [40]. It is equivalent to an ASIC with no fabrication process involved for creation of custom configuration. Also, it resembles field

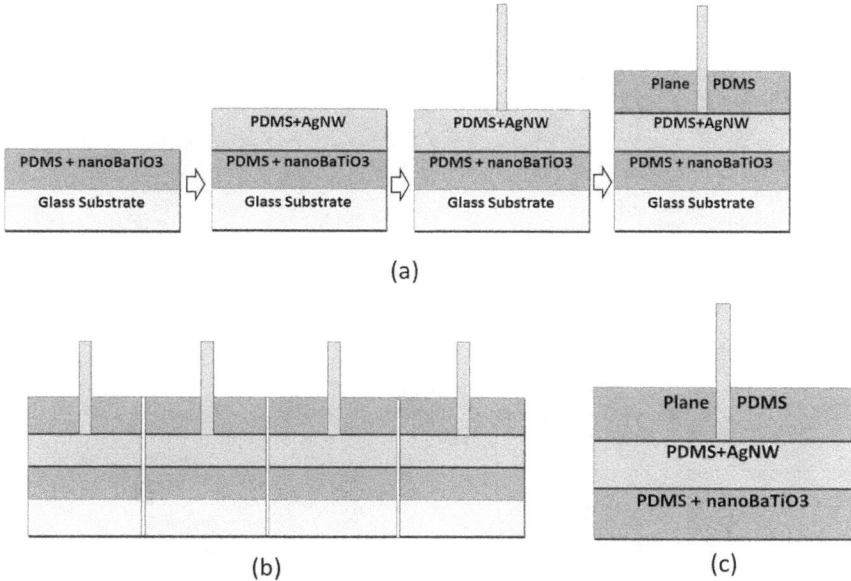

FIGURE 6.4 The electrode fabrication process flow (a) Electrode Structure, (b) Preparing multiple electrodes and (c) Final device Structure.

programmable gate array (FPGA) technology, as it gets configured on power-up. Among PSOC device families, a 32-bit three-stage pipelined ARM Cortex-M3 processor–based PSOC-5LP provides wide functionality with low-power performance. Thus, it allows designers to reduce the number of external discrete components and the system size.

6.3.2.1 System Design

The proposed single-lead PSoC-based ECG sensor was capable of acquiring and transmitting ECG data to a smartphone using radiofrequency (RF) communication. Figure 6.5 shows the system block diagram. It uses three electrodes: right arm left arm and left leg (RA, LA and LL). To get the best results, electrodes were placed on the chest wall equidistant from the heart (rather than the specific limbs). The AFE, along with embedded signal processing, was integrated at the chip level using a reconfigurable platform, and Bluetooth-based wireless transmission of ECG data was demonstrated. The received data were available for storage and viewing for health monitoring purpose in the smartphone application. Here, the smartphone acts as a central node for receiving, storing and display of health data, which may further be sent over the cloud using internet services for further analysis.

Table 6.1 shows specifications of the proposed sensor electronics based on various design considerations. It includes specifications for various system blocks such as electrodes, biopotential amplifier, ADC, filter, etc.

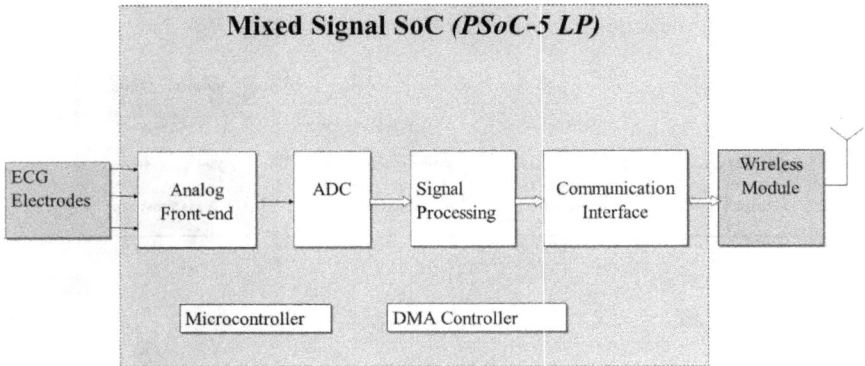

FIGURE 6.5   The proposed system block diagram.

TABLE 6.1
The Proposed System Specifications

S. N.	Particulars	Design Specification
1	Number of leads	Single lead – II
2	Electrode type	Nanocomposite based capacitive electrodes (three)
3	Power supply/battery	Single DC power supply +3.3 V
4	Biopotential amplifier gain	~250
5	Biopotential amplifier CMRR	80–100 dB
6	ADC type	Delta-sigma ADC
7	ADC resolution	16-bit
8	ADC sampling rate	500
9	Filter cutoff frequency for low pass, high pass and notch	150 Hz, 0.5 Hz and 50 Hz
10	Processing unit	ARM Cortex M3
11	Communication interface	RF-BLE
12	Display device	Smartphone screen

The ECG signal amplitude is in the range of a few millivilts, typically 1.5–2.5 mV, while the useful signal bandwidth ranges between 0.05 and 150 Hz. Thus, low-amplitude and low-bandwidth signal acquisition needs careful design considerations for biopotential measurement [41]. Furthermore, these signals are often corrupted by environmental and biological sources of interference, such as 50/60-Hz noise from powerline interference, electromyography (EMG) from muscles, motion artifact from the electrode and skin interface and possibly other interference from the operating room [42]. To achieve a clean ECG, essential design requirements include appropriate amplification and filtering.

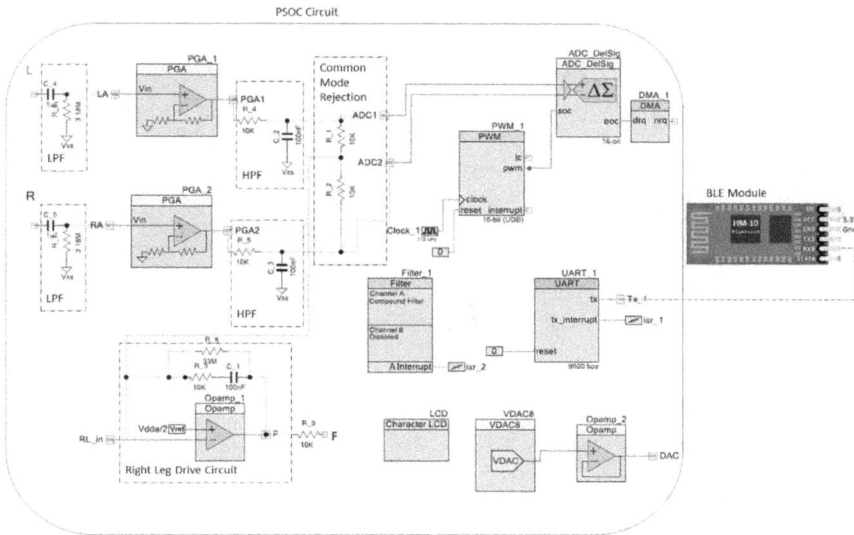

FIGURE 6.6 The overall system design.

The proposed system design was created in PSoC Creator 4.1 IDE and implemented in the PSoC 5 LP family device. The overall design of sensor electronics using mixed signal SoC platform is shown in Figure 6.6. Biopotential amplifier with high input impedance, high common-mode rejection ratio (CMRR), low noise, suitable frequency response and stability against temperature and voltage fluctuations are crucial elements of the sensor electronics. In the proposed prototype, it is designed using two programmable gain amplifiers (PGAs) and an ADC front-end buffer as shown in Figure 6.6. The delta-sigma ADC had a differential amplifier front end with very high input impedance and CMRR. Gain of both PGAs and ADC were set to 16 and 8, respectively, which amplified the differential signal by a factor of 128. The delta sigma ADC provided a low-power and low-noise front end for precision measurements, suitable for low-speed high-resolution (16 to 20 bits) applications.

For signal filtering, a band pass filter was designed using passive low pass and high pass filters to pass frequencies raging between 0.5 and 150 Hz whilst blocking off other frequencies. Power line noise was removed by a notch filter implemented in the digital domain using a two-stage finite impulse response model (FIR) filter by customising the filter block in PSoC. It included a 50-Hz notch filter followed by a band pass filter with 76-Hz centre frequency and 150-Hz bandwidth. A hamming window was used for both the filters. Figure 6.7 shows the filter response of two-stage FIR filter. The 16-bit ADC and digital filter processed the data with better dynamic input range. In order to fulfill data rate requirements of the filter, ADC data conversion was controlled using a pulse width modulation (PWM) block. The soc (start of conversion) signal of ADC was driven at the required rate. An end of conversion (eoc) signal of ADC enabled DMA transfer for filtering operation at the right time.

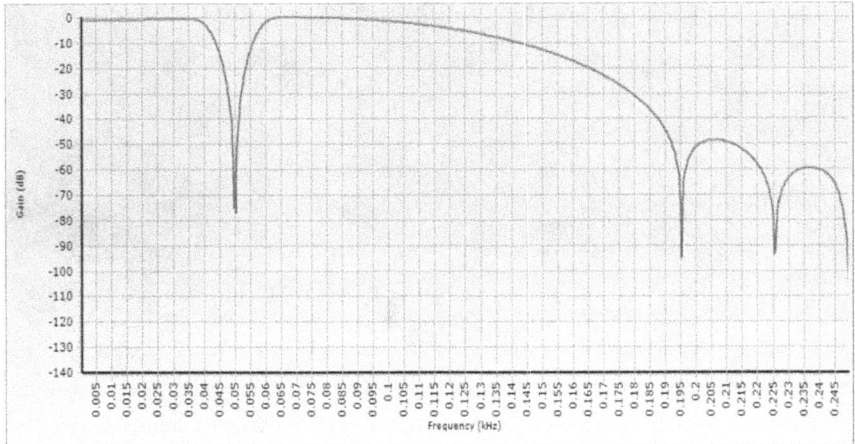

FIGURE 6.7   The filter response of the two-stage FIR filter.

The data moved from ADC to the filter via direct memory access (DMA)⁰ without involving processor resources.

Filtered signal data were applied to a digital to analog converter (DAC) for the signal measurements in the analog domain. Furthermore, a universal asynchronous receiver-transmitter (UART) was used for sending filter data to a Bluetooth module for serial communication. It was set in transmit mode with a 9600 baud rate. HM-10, a Bluetooth low energy (BLE) serial module based on Bluetooth version 4.0, was used for establishing a relatively short-range, continuous wireless connection with low-power operation.

6.3.2.2   System Implementation

Figure 6.8 shows the prototype implementation comprising a PSoC-based pro-type board, BLE module, a few passive components, battery, solar panel and energy harvesting module. A CY8CKIT-059 PSoC 5LP prototyping kit was used for the implementation of sensor electronics for the proof of concept of a wearable ECG sensor. It provides a low-cost, small-size and low-power platform to easily develop and integrate the PSoC 5LP device into the end system. The system was made ener-gy-efficient by using low-power system components, low-power system implemen-tation approach and energy harvesting technology. The key was to use minimum hardware resources to save power. The proposed system implemented optimised hardware design for ECG signal acquisition without limiting the functionality. The overall current draw was reduced to a great extent by using low-power modes imple-mented with other power-saving features and techniques at the circuit, system and algorithm level.

Being a wearable device, it needs a battery as the primary source of power. Lithium-ion (Li-ion) and lithium-ion polymer (LiPo, Li-Po, LIP, Li-poly) batteries have become the most popular for wearables due to higher capacity and smaller

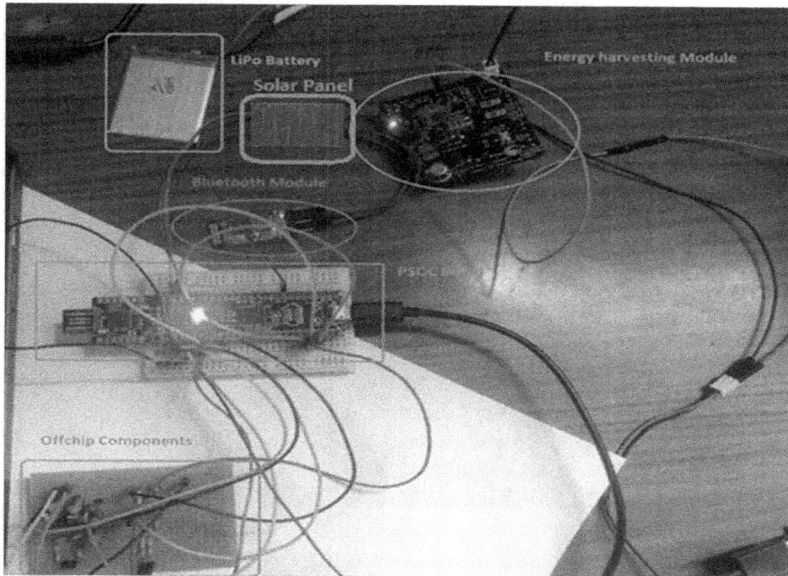

FIGURE 6.8   The proposed sensor electronics prototype implementation.

form factors. The proposed system explored an energy harvesting method for supporting the life extension of a primary battery. The idea was to harvest ambient light energy using a solar-based energy harvesting method. It was possible to obtain slight amounts of power generation from compact solar cells under low-brightness environments of approximately 100 lx. Panasonic AM-1801, a series solar module sensitive to indoor light energy, and a power management IC (S6AE102A/103A)–based module consuming ultra-low current were used for the energy harvesting. It stored the power generated by solar cells to an output super-capacitor using built-in switch control, and it turned on the power switching circuit while the capacitor voltage was within a preset range for supplying energy to a load [43]. When the power generated from solar cells was not enough, the energy was supplied from the primary battery.

6.4   RESULTS AND DISCUSSION

Here, we describe the testing, results, and discussion on performance evaluation of the proposed ECG sensor. It involves results based on biopotential electrode characterisation and ECG sensor electronics output and performance. It further presents theoretical implications of the proposed system.

6.4.1   Biopotential Electrode Characterisation

Microscopic characterisations were performed using SEM for the electrode, whereas electrical characterisation was performed with the LCR-Q metre. A PDMS-based

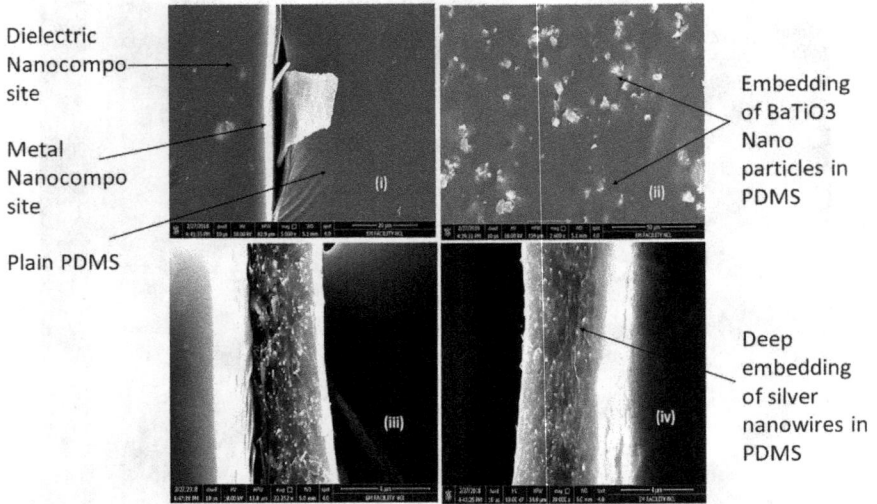

FIGURE 6.9   SEM images of the electrode showing (i), embedding of BaTiO3 nanoparticles (ii), and deep embedding of silver nanowires (iii and iv) in the PDMS material.

electrode structure was confirmed with SEM analysis. A vertical cross section of the ECG electrode was prepared with the help of a sharp metal razor for an image analysis. Figure 6.9 shows the layering of various materials in the electrode structure with (i), embedding of BaTiO3 nanoparticles (ii), and deep embedding of silver nanowires (iii and iv) in the PDMS material. SEM image in Figure 6.9 shows thin silver nanowires film is sandwiched between PDMS + nanoBaTiO3 (left side) and PDMS material (right side).

The PDMS nanocomposite–based flexible, capacitive, biopotential electrodes are developed as shown in Figure 6.10. The electrodes were circular in shape with an approximate diameter of 2.5 cm. Table 6.2 shows the electrical characterisation of the electrode. Skin-to-electrode resistance and capacitance were measured by placing the electrode on the skin surface. The results show that the average skin-to-electrode resistance of the developed electrode (45 KΩ) was very low compared to cloth-based capacitive electrodes (a few MΩ). A sufficiently high value of coupling capacitance (a few microfarads) was achieved with the proposed electrode in contrast to the cloth-based capacitive electrodes (a few picofarads). The results show that the proposed electrodes improved the skin-electrode interface in overall ECG measurements.

6.4.2   ECG Sensor Electronics

An ECG was observed in the analog as well as digital domain. The observed analog ECG signal using a digital storage oscilloscope is shown in Figure 6.11(a). The ECG data transmitted over Bluetooth was received on an Android-based smartphone. A source-free Android app called 'Bluetooth Data Capture' was used to plot the received ECG data. It captured real-time signals transmitted from the UART channel

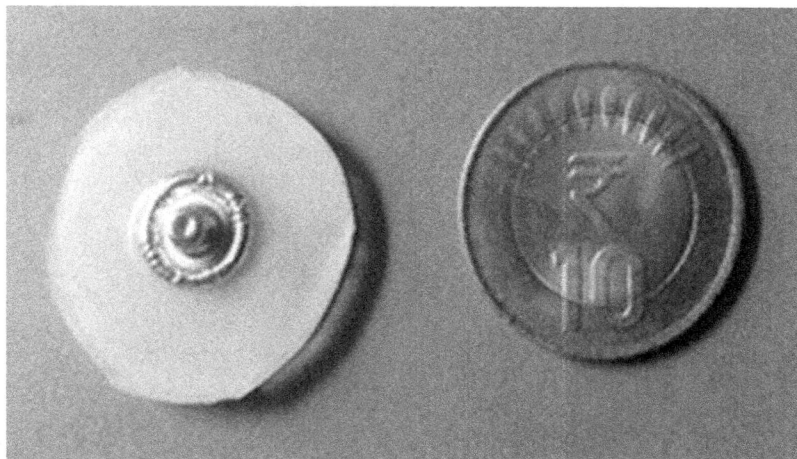

FIGURE 6.10   The developed electrode.

TABLE 6.2
Electrical Characterisation of Electrodes

Subject Number	Subject Particulars	Effective Skin-to-Electrode Resistance (KΩ)	Effective Skin-to-Electrode Capacitance (µF)
1.	27-year-old Male	42	0.05
2.	35-year-old Male	48	0.1
3.	65-year-old Male	45	0.02
4.	28-year-old Female	40	0.2
5.	31-year-old Female	51	0.1
6.	40-year-old Female	45	0.1
Average value		45.17	0.095

over RF Bluetooth to the smartphone. It was possible to store and review the data after the capture. Figure 6.11(b) shows the snapshot of an ECG data plot on the smartphone.

Performance of the sensor electronics was evaluated by measuring various parameters such as gain, CMRR, frequency response, current consumption, battery life, etc., as shown in Table 6.3. Thus, a high value of CMRR was achieved with the proposed prototype. The developed analog front end was capable of sensing small amplitude signals of the order of few microvolts; thus, it was found suitable for measurement

TABLE 6.3
Performance Evaluation of the Proposed System Prototype

Sr. No.	Parameter	Value	Unit
1	Gain	Differential gain = 43.45–75	Unit
		Common mode gain = 0.0497–0.06	
2	CMRR	58.84–61.93	dB
3	Sensitivity	2.38	μV
4	Frequency response	Pass band: 0.5–120	Hz
		Pass band attenuation: 0.5	dB
		Stop band: 50	Hz
		Stop band attenuation: 43	dB
5	Average current	2.95 (PSOC) + 2.98 (BLE) = 5.93	mA
			mA
6	Power consumption	19.404	mW
7	Battery life	253	Hours
	(1500 mAh battery)		

of the physiological parameter. Furthermore, embedded signal processing in part successfully attained the intended frequency response suitable for amplifying frequencies of interest while rejecting others. The average current was measured to find the power consumption of the prototype. It included the average current of the PSOC module and wireless module. The average current of the BLE module was measured with the ammeter connected in series with the supply terminal. High-capacity, small-size batteries were found suitable for the proposed wearable sensors. Power autonomy was achieved with the energy harvester module. Operation of the energy harvesting circuit with a solar module was studied for an indoor environment. The solar module was tested for output voltage and current using a digital multimeter. For indoor illumination the solar module DC output voltage without load was found in the range 2.3 V to 5.2 V and DC current in the range of 1.2 mA to 20 mA with 10 Ω series resistance. It was possible to power the sensor with solar power in the daytime and battery power during the night. A flexible solar module of 5V, 1W rating with a rechargeable lithium-ion polymer battery of 1500 mAH capacity was found appropriate for the proposed sensor. The solar module can be easily integrated into the clothing. The results suggested that a miniature board can be developed for wearable sensor with on-board power management.

6.4.3 Theoretical Implications

The proposed wearable ECG sensor will provide long-term monitoring to assist the cardiac patients and doctors in diagnosis and treatment of CVDs. It will be useful for monitoring an individual at home or in a non-clinical environment. In several clinical applications such as post-intervention monitoring of a heart attack victim,

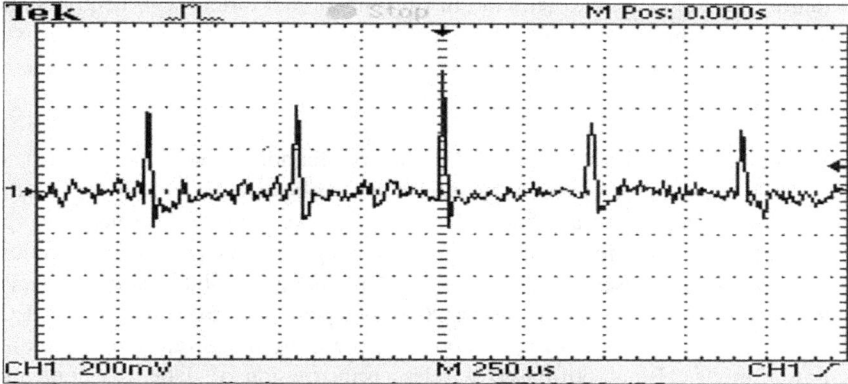

(a)

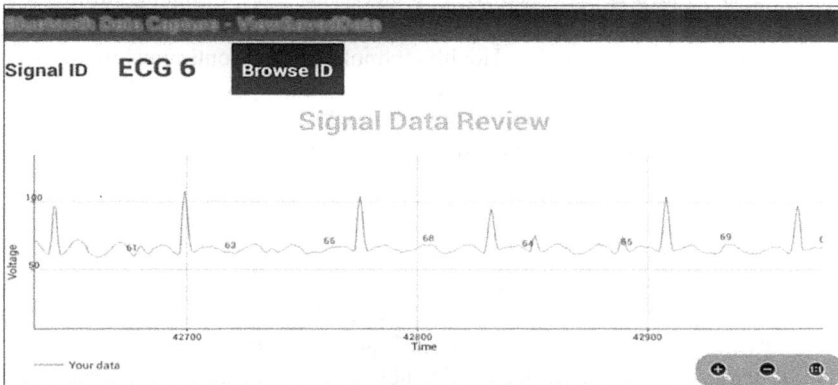

(b)

FIGURE 6.11   The observed ECG signal in (a) analog and (b) digital domain.

the proposed sensor will support little movement and recreation for their physical and mental well-being. It will facilitate continued monitoring of patients as they gradually re-integrate into normal everyday life. Furthermore, wearable monitoring will help overcome the fear of having a further heart attack during rehabilitation, as cardiac patients are encouraged to exercise while in hospital or later on an out-patient basis. Also, it will be useful in assessing the efficacy of on-going treatment and in the planning of subsequent medication. It will enable great ways to reduce healthcare utilisation, decrease the costs, reduce patient visits to doctor, generate research data and increase physician satisfaction. It will be possible to create large ECG datasets suitable for building efficient AI models targeting automated diagnosis and accurate prediction of CVDs. Wearable sensors will improve patient access to healthcare, broadening the scope of telemedicine in rural areas and others who need distance care and monitoring.

6.5 CONCLUSION

The chapter presented broad domain of m-Health technology, wearable devices and AI methods and their integration for intelligent cardiovascular health informatics. A low-power design approach for m-Health-based wearable ECG sensor using a reconfigurable SoC platform was essential for long-term monitoring applications. The key technologies used in the development included high-integration, advanced materials and energy harvesting. A PSOC-based prototype for a single-lead ECG sensor was implemented using a low-power system architecture, components and low-power modes. Bluetooth-based wireless transmission of data was confirmed with storage and display of ECG data on a smartphone. Innovative nanocomposite material–based capacitive-coupled biopotential electrodes were developed and demonstrated with ECG sensor electronics for a robust and wearable solution. The results indicate that PDMS-based flexible electrodes are promising candidates for long-term biopotential recording. The proposed system successfully demonstrated an integration of wearable and m-Health technologies for continuous monitoring of ECG data. The wearable sensor can be used for patient self-monitoring or health provider assessment. It has great potential to transform the overall healthcare system with accurate diagnosis, treatment and post-intervention.

6.6 FUTURE SCOPE

The design of a wearable arrangement such as a chest belt to keep the sensing element and sensor electronics parts intact for long durations was not included in this prototype. Innovations with smart textile materials and suitable wearing arrangements for different age groups of male and female subjects in clinical as well as non-clinical settings can be employed. Despite signal filtering, the prototype suffers from signal noise due to movement, which can be overcome by designing innovative adaptive signal filtering methods along with activity monitoring to improve the accuracy of the measured signal.

There are enormous possibilities of extending the proposed prototype. Other vital body parameter information such as heart rate, respiration rate, blood pressure, etc., can be derived from ECG data with the help of innovative signal processing methods. It can be extended as a multiparameter biosensor node to include other health parameters such as activity monitoring, electroencephalogram (EEG), electromyogram (EMG), body temperature, blood pressure, etc. The proposed system uses separate modules for signal processing, wireless interface and energy management. Integrating all of them, development of a flexible PCB-based small wearable solution, and use of thin film batteries can be explored to improve its performance. The prototype can be extended for an IoT healthcare platform by providing an Internet Protocol (IP) interface to the smartphone-based ECG data for storing it over the IoT cloud. Furthermore, innovative methods may be employed for extracting and classifying the features of ECG signals using deep learning, neural networks, genetic algorithms, etc. The prototype system can further be extended with cloud-based AI methods for intelligent cardiovascular health informatics supporting early detection and prevention of CVDs. A smartphone-based application may be developed to display the measured data and its analysis in suitable form.

6.7 REFERENCES

[1] E. Honeyman, H. Ding, M. Varnfield, and M. Karunanithi, "Mobile Health Applications in Cardiac Care," *Interventional Cardiology*, vol. 6, no. 2, 2014, pp. 227–240.

[2] S. Hong, Y. Zhou, J. Shang, et al., "Opportunities and Challenges of Deep Learning Methods for Electrocardiogram Data: A Systematic Review," *Computers in Biology and Medicine*, vol. 122, 2020.

[3] S. Romiti, M. Vinciguerra, W. Saade, et al., "Artificial Intelligence (AI) and Cardiovascular Diseases: An Unexpected Alliance," *Cardiology Research and Practice*, vol. 2020, 2020.

[4] G.K. Ragesh, and K. Baskaran, "A Survey on Futuristic Health Care System: WBANs," *International Conference on Communication Technology and System Design*, pp. 889–896, 2011.

[5] GSMA/McKinsey & Company, "mHealth: A New Vision for Healthcare," Technical Reports, 2010. https://www.gsma.com/iot/wp-content/uploads/2012/03/gsmamckinsey-mhealthreport.pdf.

[6] Sean Lunde, "The m-Health Case in India," Wipro Council for Industry Research Paper, 2013. https://smartnet.niua.org/sites/default/files/resources/the-mHealth-case-in-India.pdf.

[7] E.N. Schorr, A.D. Gepner, et al., "Harnessing Mobile Health Technology for Secondary Cardiovascular Disease Prevention in Older Adults: A Scientific Statement from the American Heart Association," *Circulation: Cardiovascular Quality and Outcomes*, pp. 659–676, 2021.

[8] World Health Organization, "Towards the Development of an m-Health Strategy: A Literature Review," The Millenium Villages Project Report, 2008. https://toolkits.knowledgesuccess.org/toolkits/mhealth-planning-guide/towards-development-mhealth-strategy-literature-review.

[9] C. Konstantinos, K.C. Siontis, et al., "Artificial Intelligence-Enhanced Electrocardiography in Cardiovascular Disease Management," *Nature Reviews Cardiology*, vol. 18, no. 7, pp. 465–478, 2021.

[10] Z. Ebrahimi, M. Loni, M. Daneshtalab, et al., "A Review on Deep Learning Methods for ECG Arrhythmia Classification," *Expert Systems with Applications: X*, vol. 7, 2020.

[11] Y. He, B. Fu, J. Yu, et al., "Efficient Learning of Healthcare Data from IoT Devices by Edge Convolution Neural Networks," *Applied Sciences*, vol. 10, no. 24, 2020.

[12] Grand View Research, "Wearable Medical Device Market," Technical Reports, 2021. www.grandviewresearch.com/industry-analysis/wearable-medical-devices-market.

[13] Sumant Ugalmugale and Rupali Swain, "Wearable Cardiac Devices Market," Technical Reports, 2020. www.gminsights.com/industry-analysis/wearable-cardiac-devices-market.

[14] Marie Chana, et al., "Smart Wearable Systems: Current Status and Future Challenges," *Artificial Intelligence in Medicine*, vol. 56, pp. 137–156, 2012.

[15] Ali Alzaidi, et al., "Smart Textiles Based Wireless ECG System," *IEEE Systems, Applications and Technology Conference (LISAT)*, pp. 1–5, 2012.

[16] C. Gilsoo, et al., "Performance Evaluation of Textile-Based Electrodes and Motion Sensors for Smart Clothing," *IEEE Sensors*, vol. 11, no. 12, pp. 3183–3193, 2011.

[17] Rita Salvado, et al., "Textile Materials for the Design of Wearable Antennas: A Survey," *Sensors*, vol. 12, pp. 15841–15857, 2012.

]18] David Manuel, et al., "A Novel Dry Active Biosignal Electrode Based on an Hybrid Organic-Inorganic Interface Material," *IEEE Sensors*, vol. 11, no. 10, pp. 2241–2245, 2011.

]19] Prashanth Shyamkumar, et al., "Wearable Wireless Cardiovascular Monitoring Using Textile-Based Nanosensor and Nanomaterial Systems," *MDPI Electronics*, vol. 3, pp. 504–520, 2014.

[20] Z. Stamenkovic, G. Panic, and G. Schoof, "A System-On-Chip for Wireless Body Area Sensor Network," *11th IEEE Workshop on Design and Diagnostics of Electronic Circuits and Systems*, pp. 1–4, 2008.

[21] Yindar Chuo, Marcin Marzencki, Benny Hung, et al., "Mechanically Flexible Wireless Multisensor Platform for Human Physical Activity and Vitals Monitoring," *IEEE Transactions on Biomedical Circuits and Systems*, vol. 4, no. 5, pp. 281–294, 2010.

22. Bertrand Massot, Claudine Gehin, Ronald Nocua, et al., "A Wearable, Low-Power, Health-Monitoring Instrumentation Based on a Programmable System-on-Chip™," *Annual International Conference of the IEEE Engineering in Medicine and Biology Society*, pp. 4852–4855, 2009.

[23] A.C.W. Wong, et al., "A Multi-Parameter Signal-Acquisition SoC for Connected Personal Health Applications," *IEEE International Solid-State Circuits Conference*, pp. 306–310, 2014.

[24] Mozziyar Etemadi, et al., "A Wearable Patch to Enable Long-Term Monitoring of Environmental, Activity and Hemodynamics Variables," *IEEE Transactions on Biomedical Circuits and Systems*, vol. 10, no. 2, pp. 280–288, 2016.

[25] Ya-Li Zheng, et al., "Unobtrusive Sensing and Wearable Devices for Health Informatics," *IEEE Transactions on Biomedical Engineering*, vol. 61, no. 5, pp. 1538–1554, 2014.

[26] Somayeh Imani, et al., "Wearable Chemical Sensors: Opportunities and Challenges," IEEE *International Symposium on Circuits and Systems*, pp. 1122–1125, 2016.

[27] Seulki Lee, et al., "Planar Fashionable Circuit Board Technology and Its Applications," *Journal of Semiconductor Technology And Science*, vol. 9, no. 3, pp. 174–180, 2009.

[28] I. Szendiuch, "Development in Electronic Packaging – Moving to 3D System Configuration," *Radio Engineering*, vol. 20, no. 1, 2011.

[29] Dr Xiaoxi He, "Flexible, Printed and Thin Film Batteries 2016–2026: Technologies, Markets, Players," IDTechEx Energy Storage Report, 2016. https://zh.booksc.eu/book/72583858/4f26d0.

[30] Leslie Mertz, "Convergence Revolution Comes to Wearables," *IEEE Pulse*, vol. 7, 2016.

[31] Xing Li, Chi-Ying Tsui, and Wing-Hung Ki, "UHF Energy Harvesting System Using Reconfigurable Rectifier for Wireless Sensor Network," *IEEE International Symposium on Circuits and Systems*, pp. 93–96, 2015.

[32] Moeen Hassanalieragh, et al., "Health Monitoring and Management Using Internet-of-Things (IoT) Sensing with Cloud-Based Processing: Opportunities and Challenges," *IEEE International Conference on Services Computing*, pp. 285–292, 2015.

[33] PWC, "Health Wearables: Early Days," Technical Reports, 2014. https://www.modern healthcare.com/assets/pdf/CH969211021.PDF.

[34] Francis Morris, William J. Brady, and John Camm, *ABC of Clinical Electrocardiography*. New York: Blackwell Publishing Ltd., 2008.

[35] Yu Mike Chi, et al., "Dry-Contact and Noncontact Biopotential Electrodes: Methodological Review," *IEEE Reviews In Biomedical Engineering*, vol. 3, pp. 106–119, 2010.

[36] J. Devasena, et al., "Development of Non-Contact Capacitive Coupled Electrodes for Bio-Potential Signal Acquisition," *International Conference on Electrical, Electronics, Computer Science & Mechanical Engg*, pp. 1–6, 2014.

[37] Haibo Mao, et al., "One-Dimensional Silver Nanowires Synthesized by Self-Seeding Polyol Process," *Journal of Nanoparticle Research*, vol. 14, 2012.

[38] Mohd Rafie Johan, et al., "Synthesis and Growth Mechanism of Silver Nanowires Through Different Mediated Agents (CuCl2 and NaCl) Polyol Process," *Journal of Nanomaterials*, vol. 17, 2014.

[39] Suryakanta Nayak, et al., "Development of Poly(dimethylsiloxane)/BaTiO3 Nanocomposites as Dielectric Material," *Advanced Materials Research*, vol. 622–623, pp. 897–900, 2012.

[40] Cypress Semiconductor, "PSoC® 5LP Architecture," Technical Reference Manual, 2013. https://usermanual.wiki/Document/Cypress2020PSoC5LP2020Technical 20Reference20Manual.580376874/html.

[41] David Prutchi, and Michael Norris, *Design and Development of Medical Electronic Instrumentation*. Hoboken, NJ: John Wiley & Sons Inc Publication, 2005.

[42] Willis J. Tompkins, *Biomedical Digital Signal Processing*. Upper Saddle River, NJ: Prentice Hall, 1993.

[43] Cypress, "S6AE102A and S6AE103A Evaluation Kit Guide," Technical Reports. www.cypress.com/documentation/development-kitsboards/cyalkit-e04-s6ae102a-and-s6ae103a-evaluation-kit.

7 Recent Trends in Wearable Technologies, Challenges and Opportunities

S. Kannadhasan[1] *and R. Nagarajan*[2]
[1] Cheran College of Engineering, India
[2] Gnanamani College of Technology, India

CONTENTS

7.1 INTRODUCTION

Smart textiles are intelligent textiles that are divided into three categories: Smart textiles that can just detect the environment or the user are known as passive smart textiles. Smart textiles with an actuator and a sensor device that can perceive and respond to stimuli in the environment are known as active smart textiles. Smart textiles that can sense, respond, and alter their qualities to changing environmental circumstances are known as very/ultra-smart textiles. The presence of sensors in a passive smart material is critical because sensors offer a mechanism for detecting signals. Actuators, together with sensors, are the basic ingredient for active smart materials. They respond on detected signals either from a central control unit or autonomously. They're formed of yarn-like strands and filaments that are knitted, woven or non-woven combined with knitted, woven or non-woven structures. Collaboration between the fields of textile design and electronics is critical in the development of smart materials capable of performing a broad variety of tasks found in both flexible and stiff electrical goods. Within the biomedical and safety communities, fabrics-based sensing has been a large field of research. Fabric sensors for electroencephalography (EEG), electrocardiogram (ECG) and electromyography (EMG) may be employed, as well as textiles with intrinsic thermocouples for temperature monitoring. Specific environmental or biological properties, such as oxygen, salinity, moisture or toxins, may be detected using carbon electrodes embedded into textiles. Active features that might be integrated in smart fabric include human interface components, radio frequency (RF) functionality or assistive technology, power production and storage. Human interface components are divided into two categories: display or annunciation devices and input devices. A shape-sensitive fabric capable of recording flexing or motion, pressure, compression or stretching or capacitive patches acting as pushbuttons are examples of input devices, while display or annunciation devices include electroluminescent yarns, fabric speakers or arrays of organic light-emitting diodes (OLEDs) processed into yarns. In smart textiles, simple features that vibrate or offer bio-feedback might be added. The fabric-based antenna is an example of a smart fabrics application [1–5].

These antennas are basically non-conducting materials with precise lengths of conductive yarn weaved or sewn into them. Smart textiles have played an important role in medicine and healthcare, the military, sports and aerospace, to name a few. This article focuses on the fabrication processes used in the creation of smart materials, as well as the applications or products that have been or might be created utilising these processes. For thousands of years, textiles have been an essential component of human existence. Humans utilised textiles primarily as protective garments in the past, although their usage has increasingly expanded. Humans today wear clothing at all times and are surrounded by different types of textiles in almost every location. In recent years, the inclusion of multifunctional qualities in such a common material has been a hot topic. Fabrics, fibres, yarns and a variety of other materials with extra functions have been created for a variety of uses. Textile materials and production processes have become a key source of high-tech breakthroughs. Smart fabrics is a multidisciplinary study topic with roots in chemistry, computer science and engineering, textile design and technology, material science and physics. Wearable technological innovations have revolutionised the learning and teaching process, allowing students to approach their studies in a more constructive, active and self-directed manner. Students may learn more rapidly and access knowledge with fewer mental input and activities thanks to wearable technology. It's vital to remember that using wearable technology in education differs significantly from conventional learning techniques, which require students to attend courses at a set time and place. Educators, on the other hand, must learn how to use wearable computing successfully in the classroom. The possibility of employing four various wearable gadgets recommended by the researchers in their lectures, however, did not excite the participants. Importantly, participants gave a much lower feasibility rating than utility for the four use cases that were thought to be most valuable on average. Remote students may view and listen to lectures at the university without having to be physically there, for example, students in the medical area may watch a surgeon professor do surgery in real time. Students may also use Google Glass to get text messages and alerts on other elements of their education, such as assessment deadlines and instructor notifications. It also provides quantifiable statistics on attention and concentration and answers/translates foreign language questions.

This wearable gadget also keeps instructors and students linked to an interactive environment, allowing instructors to use the face recognition feature to create a 'Student Information System' and record attendance [6–10]. Teachers will be able to access their records, which include information on their academic and non-academic performance, as well as their attendance rate, simply by looking at individual pupils. Students' reports, class times and timetables may all be generated using this information. Virtual reality headsets, such as the Oculus Rift, have had other notable educational effects. It enables students to have a distinct learning experience without taking any risks. It gives students real-world experiences by transporting them to regions that are difficult or impossible to reach in real life, such as space studies, archaeology courses, medical education, chemical engineering and aviation training. In contrast to the passive approach of reading/ watching courses in a regular classroom, the use of virtual reality wearables in education allows students to participate hands-on, engaged and interactively in their learning process.

The Oculus Rift is a wearable head-mounted display (HMD) that is a comfortable, light-weighted, stereoscopic display with an extremely wide field of vision (100 degrees) that provides the immersion required for virtual reality. It is also available at a reasonable cost. Another virtual reality wearable gadget used in teaching is Google Expeditions. It allows instructors to join their students on guided virtual field excursions, creating a unique educational experience. The gadget allows students to participate in more than 200 different journeys to places like museums, the ocean and outer space, where they may immerse themselves in a 360-degree experience that allows them to visit some great destinations. Virtual reality (VR) expeditions are collections of connected VR content and accompanying resources that may be utilised in conjunction with current curriculum. Both 'Augmented Reality' and 'Virtual Reality' have compelling applications in higher education, since their gadgets are meant to transport learners to 'any imagined place in the known universe, altering knowledge delivery and allowing students to participate in deep learning'. The GoPro camera is a wearable gadget that is used to capture a lecture or pupils' performance on an assignment. This gadget assists lecturers in observing the learning environment and evaluating students' performance, as well as documenting their observations [11–17]. 'The GoPro camera is a wearable digital camera that can collect embodied, sensory, kinesthetic, and emotional knowledge and abilities by recording action experiences'.

7.2   WEARABLE GADGETS

In the current day, wearable gadgets are most widely utilised in the healthcare industry. Individuals have employed activity monitoring bracelets and smart watches for health-management goals, and these are typical instances. Recently, a growing number of commercial applications have emerged, allowing organisations to recoup investment expenses more rapidly. Insurers, for example, provide subscribers rewards based on their physical activity measured by such devices, and corporate health insurance groups distribute them for staff health management. Another example is the use of such devices by construction firms to monitor the health of employees on the job. Rehabilitation equipment produced by mediVR employing VR technology is one of the most recent instances of wearable technologies used in healthcare. This technology not only helps medical institutions enhance productivity, but it also helps users regain motor skills while having fun with game-like workouts. The next rehabilitation programme will be offered based on each patient's progress, and rehabilitation evaluation may be measured. It is also feasible to standardise rehabilitative know-how so that it may be shared more readily throughout medical facilities. Patients will be able to complete rehabilitation programmes at home in the future, with medical experts controlling the equipment through remote control, thanks to the technology, which enables one physical therapist to train numerous patients at once. Other Wearable, which include wearable devices for industrial purposes, have consistently risen as a consequence of long-term R&D efforts, and their market size is larger than that of fitness wearable and smart watches, which are both primarily for consumers. In the meanwhile, though, the market for smart glasses and HMD/cameras is still modest, it is growing at the quickest pace of any group. Industrial applications, which will be added to the current market for wearable devices for corporate usage, will likely drive development in such goods when virtual reality/augmented reality (VR/AR) technologies are integrated. As a result, the wearable device market for commercial applications is likely to grow.

Wearable technologies make use of body-worn electronics. Wearable gadgets have been around for around two decades, but their popularity is growing as technology advances, costs fall and more Internet service is accessible. Head-mounted gadgets, smart watches and health-monitoring wristbands are among the most popular wearable gadgets, but the number and variety of gadgets is quickly growing. The Vandrico Wearable Technologies database has 436 gadgets as of 21 June 2016, from a variety of industries, including fitness, medical, entertainment, industrial, gaming and lifestyle. Fitbit, Nike+, Misfit and Jawbone wristbands, Apple and Garmin watches, Oculus Rift, Google Glasses and Google Cardboard headsets, as well as newcomers like Xiaomi bands, Samsung Gear, Epson Moverio, Microsoft HoloLens, Magic Leap's light-weight AR, AMD Sulon and Meta One are examples of already popular wearable devices. Mind reading technologies, hearables, wearable toys, smart clothes, smart coaching, lifesaving and even pet monitoring and GPS mapping are likely to increase the wearables market.

While there is a lot of study into the creation and usage of wearable technology in disciplines other than education, there isn't as much study on the usage of wearable technology in education. The scant research on wearable technologies for learning and teaching suggests that wearable technology's potential in higher education is yet unknown. One explanation for this might be because instructors are unfamiliar with the capabilities of wearable technology. Another explanation might be that the technology is so new that no study into in-form applications has yet been done. There are few instructional paradigms or frameworks that might inspire and guide their work. In the literature, there are just a few empirical instances of the employment of wearable devices in education, as shown in Figure 7.1. There is a current surge of excitement and conceptual development from firms and universities throughout the globe that want to make wearable technology more accessible to people. Using virtual and augmented reality to experience Earth as it was a hundred million years ago; overlaying visual information of the Mars landscape for training purposes; and seeing inside the opportunities for disabilities, impairments and the provision of care or rehabilitation services are just a few examples.

The Internet of Things (IoT) is a vast network of networked devices, sensors, automobiles, embedded software and other items. Wired and wireless connection media are used to link these devices in a seamless manner. Each of these devices/sensors/things is viewed as a separate node that may be set independently. This worldwide linked network of things/nodes operates on a dynamic architecture that is highly supported by communication technologies like as GSM, Wi-Fi, RFID, GPRS and others. The notion of ubiquitous computing is rather popular these days, and the IoT allows and supports it. Global connection, real-time processing and a limited storage space are all characteristics of the IoT. There are certain difficulties with IoT, such as data privacy, security and dependability. Cloud computing and IoT

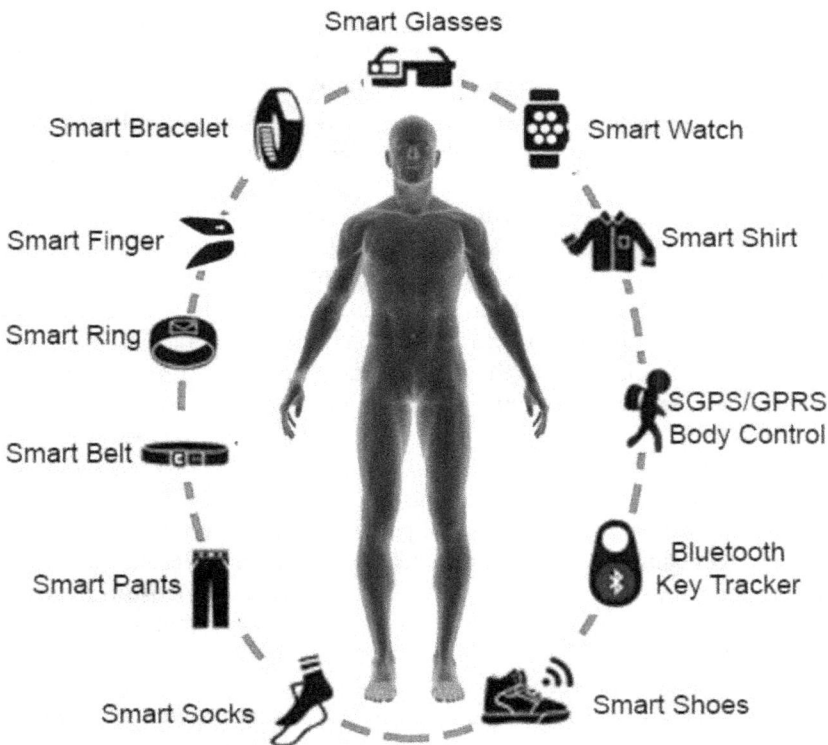

FIGURE 7.1 Wearable technologies.

may be compared and contrasted. In comparison to IoT, the cloud is more developed. However, they have a same goal, which is pervasive computing. In terms of storage space and computing power, the cloud's potential is limitless. IoT seems to be a collection of interconnected gadgets that are linked over the internet. Real-time processing is the result of a continuous stream of data flowing to and from linked devices. The cloud enables IoT processing in real time. Both IoT and the cloud may be said to function in tandem. Every day, the Internet becomes more valuable. Internet access is no longer restricted to PCs and laptops; it now extends to a broad variety of devices, including mobile phones and tablets. The main goal of the IoT is to connect anything that can be connected and to give services to turn everything into smart functioning, such as smart cities, home automation, smart learning, e-healthcare, wearables and so on. Small devices serve as connection points for IoT applications, including a microcontroller and interface to interact, as well as a power source and sensors.

These sensors are used to communicate with the environment. These sensors are mostly used to gather data. The IoT brings a slew of new smart gadgets that businesses may use for real-time business and analytics. Almost all sectors and people are being impacted by the IoT, which is creating new sources of operational savings and income as well as new business models. Computers and other interfaces must be everywhere due to our reliance on them. This need has paved the way for the creation of wearable technology, or computers that can support professionals in personal activities by supplementing and assisting daily living in the tech-savvy world. Wearable technology combined with IoT and cloud computing opens up a plethora of possibilities that pique the interest and creativity of people from all walks of life. Wearable products such as smart watches, eyewear, fitness trackers, health monitoring gadgets and others are on display on the market. Wearables for kids and adults are widely accessible, and their primary purpose is to monitor numerous health concerns in children and adults, such as sleep patterns, growth rates, blood pressure and heart rate. Patients may wear these wearables and have their health progress tracked. After the IoT, which may be defined as a network of things (i.e. 'smart devices' having wireless communication capabilities), the use of wearable technology has skyrocketed. The open-source Wearable Reference Platform (WaRP) based on ARM architecture was announced by Freescale. Due to its powerful signal processing capability, the ARM Cortex – M–based CPU is highly popular in the wearables sector. FreeScale worked with a number of firms, including Circuitco, Kynetics and others. ARM is the global leader in creating sophisticated technologies for mobile and wearable devices, including a wide variety of processors, SoCs (system-on-chip), GPUs (graphics processing units) and intellectual property (IP). Because ARM-based devices can handle a large number of users, developers are urged to utilise them. The IoT is poised to fully use the network's capabilities. It is prepared to apply its technology to a variety of cutting-edge applications, including smart cities, smart homes, building automation and medical/healthcare services. In most IoT applications, the user interacts with their smart environment, which provides them with information and adjusts to their needs and preferences, with or without the user's knowledge. IoT applications use the standard application format, which includes a microcontroller, power supply unit, communication interface and data collection sensors. Activity trackers like Fitbit and Up by Jawbone, as well as more complex gadgets like Google

Glass and Samsung Smart Gear, are examples of wearable computing. These gadgets are constantly linked to the internet. Wearable devices may communicate with other IoT devices to share data and information based on the application's requirements. In the healthcare industry, a wide number of wearable gadgets are employed.

Fitness sensors and other apps aid in the collection of a range of health-related data from users, such as heart rate, sleeping hours, temperature, blood pressure and so on, which may be continuously monitored by healthcare experts in order to give better healthcare services. Although wearables have seen the most progress in the realm of health and fitness, there are other types of wearables on the market today. Apart from their widespread use in the medical field, wearables are also utilised to enhance the lives of end users in a variety of ways. Wearables will undoubtedly alter our way of life by automating every area of our existence, including our homes, automobiles, businesses, health care and entertainment, among others. There are a wide range of health and fitness-related wearables on the market. All of these technologies assist end users in keeping track of their health and staying in shape. Besides end users, doctors may utilise such gadgets for surgery even if they are at a distant place. For instance, activity tracking, weight loss, virtual doctor consultations and hydration tools are just a few examples. Wearables make our lives simpler by simplifying and making everyday chores simpler to do. Wearables have an influence on every aspect of life, from auto tracking to home hunting and home management, a hands-free device to interact with the surroundings, or automotive monitoring. Wearables have infiltrated every aspect of our life. Wearable gadgets may now be used to purchase meals from an online menu. The mobile application of a Canadian restaurant business has been expanded to the wearable Apple Watch. It also has a function that allows you to customise your menu. The wireless mobile's usefulness is hampered by power and networking issues. The wireless network's total performance is measured in bits per second per watt. The open standards that permit interoperability across various services are a key challenge with wireless technology. Typically, one language radio is required to deliver telephone, text messaging, GPS and other services. Communication off body for wearable computers – to the fixed network by various ways, on the body among devices and near the body with things around the user – is what networking is all about, as shown in Figure 7.1. The difficulty with mobile devices is that they are often out of range of the network. Different design considerations are required for each of the three kinds of networks. The designers have a significant difficulty in catering to three different kinds of networks. They must evaluate the possibility of network interference.

Every mobile device's most limiting element is its power consumption. Instead of high-quality electrical circuits, mobile gadgets are rated mostly on their power backup. Researchers should concentrate on the problem of wearable computers' power consumption. Wearable computers are similar to clothing and may take the shape of Google Glasses, a belt buckle or a keyboard incorporated into a garment. Because these gadgets will be worn by people, the power distribution mechanism in them is highly intricate. Because wearable computers are mobile in nature, they need a substantial battery backup, and the end user will get disappointed if the battery backup is inadequate. Strong batteries are necessary to meet the needs of wearable computers' power needs. A klong-lasting power supply, such as plutonium-238, may be utilised in wearable computers and endure for decades. Another option is to utilise batteries with a 16-hour backup time that can be charged while the user is sleeping or eating. The heat produced by the human body ranges from 80 to 10,000 watts. Humans can live in the Sahara Desert and Antarctica for long periods of time and yet maintain a body temperature of 37 degrees Celsius. The human body may be thought of as an effective heat regulator. Wearable computers must be able to match/regulate such circumstances and deal with heat-related difficulties. In order to address these difficulties, wearable computers must be lightweight, modest in size and ergonomic, and they must often function in damp and filthy settings for applications such as marines. The battery pack provides power to wearable gadgets; therefore, power consumption should be kept to a minimum. As a result, power-hungry cooling technologies such as thermoelectric modules aren't the ideal option. Because conductions are the preferred mechanism of heat transmission for wearable computers, it has been proposed that embedding electronics in a polymer-filler composite substrate might assist in the design of wearable computers in various ways. The wearables designers have a significant difficulty. Such gadgets don't put a lot of emphasis on the user interface.

There are a few gadgets that don't utilise displays at all, instead relying on pressure, gestures or touch for interaction. Easy communication utilising light-emitting diode (LED)–based messages and simple visual feedback is their main emphasis. With the increasing demand for these gadgets, designers must modernise them and add new functions. Designers must mature and take a comprehensive approach to designing user interfaces for wearable devices.

7.3   APPLICATIONS OF WEARABLE TECHNOLOGIES

Wearable technologies will transform contemporary life, and in the not-too-distant future, wearables will undoubtedly dominate the development of mobile smart gadgets. Wearable device development is still in its early stages, with the primary functions of these gadgets focusing on performing calculations, navigation, remote image taking and other related services. Cisco's prediction that 50 billion devices would be connected by 2020 is creating greater opportunities for wearable computing and

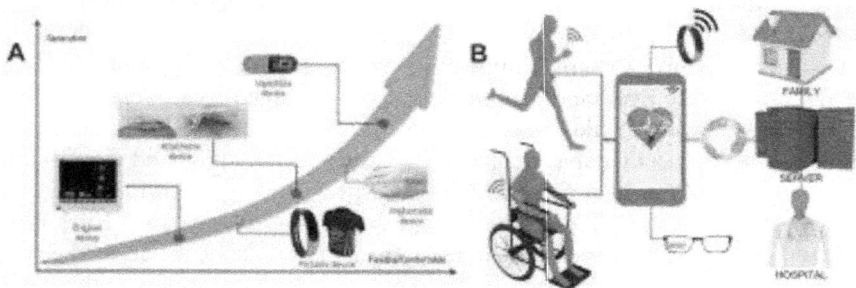

FIGURE 7.2   Various applications of wearable technologies.

gadgets. Wearable gadgets are increasingly touching every aspect of our lives, including health, business, leisure and many more. Healthcare wearable gadgets become attached to a person's body over time, allowing him to monitor changes in his or her body at all times of the day. The user's physical response can be continuously monitored, including what changes will occur if he or she continues to perform certain actions, what changes will occur if he or she continues to perform certain actions, when the most and least movement occurs in the body for a week, and when the heart rate changes significantly. We can observe our bodily changes in real time and at a reasonable cost with the aid of healthcare wearable gadgets. The more information you have, the more correctly you can exercise, prescribe and diagnose your health. As a result, healthcare wearable devices offer a competitive advantage in terms of assisting a healthy living by continually monitoring and assessing bodily changes. Depending on the user's use area, wearable devices may be used in a variety of sectors, including fitness and wellness, healthcare and medical, infotainment, military/industrial and medical applications.

Because the success of technology and the success of the market are measured at separate levels, goods that ignore consumer attributes are more likely to fail in the market. To address customers' different demands, researchers must first determine how they interpret external stimuli, as well as the personal qualities and environmental variables that influence product selection and purchase. We will look at several aspects that influence the continuous usage of IoT-based healthcare devices from a user-centric rather than a technology-centric standpoint in this chapter. In the end, the competitive advantage in the wearable device market is meant to imply that it may be stacked when it focuses on the device's services and user values or advantages. The introduction of wireless communication, for example, has been credited with the creation of inexpensive and portable sensor nodes. These nodes have the capacity to perceive, analyse and convey various indications, making them ideal for health monitoring. Wearable technologies, such as wearable gadgets, electronics and computers, have resulted because of this. Electronic instruments that are incorporated into devices that may be implanted into the body are referred to as health wearable technology (HWT). They are computer devices that take and process inputs and are application-enabled. These technological instruments may be attached to clothes, adhered to the skin using patches, incorporated into accessories such as watches and eyewear and surgically implanted within a patient's body, as shown in Figure 7.2. The HWT's key feature is that they include a hands-free mode that allows users to check their personal health data while conducting regular duties. Accessibility, wearability, comfortability, portability, multifunctionality utility, dependability and practicability are some of the other attributes.

Some of these devices, such as insulin monitors and cardiac event monitors, are approved by the Food and Drug Administration (FDA). Fitness trackers, insulin pumps, cardioverter defibrillators and vital signs monitors are all examples of HWTs. HWTs offer the extra benefit of tracking and monitoring physical activity (PA) and vital signs, which are connected to medical and fitness and wellbeing, thanks to the use of accelerometers and micro-electro-mechanical systems (MEMS). Heart rate, blood pressure, pulse rate, muscular activity, glucose level, sleeping pattern, ECG, core temperature, oxygen saturation, stress levels and eating habits are some of the quantifiable markers. Each of these roles necessitates the use of a certain kind of sensor at a particular location on the human body. These devices have three main components: 1. sensing and data collecting hardware, 2. communication devices that send data to a distant centre and 3. data processing tools or methodologies for retrieving and analysing vital health data for health and wellness purposes.

HWTs are meant to automatically gather data and evaluate it in real time. The Fitbit fitness band, for example, is a technology that demonstrates the value of HWTs in data collection. It tracks data including step count, speed, pace, calories burned, distance walked, skin temperature, heart rate, sweat level, food information and sleeping hours. Fitness and sports HWTs are mostly utilised by athletes and fitness enthusiasts, but they might also be used to motivate obese and diabetic patients to exercise and track their daily food consumption. Trainers or nutritionists may use the data acquired to have a better knowledge of the client's health state and design methods to enhance their health. These multiparameter physiological sensing devices may be used to identify and quantify vital signs to help in medical treatment, in addition to personal health and fitness. A patient discharged after surgery or prone to heart attack, for example, is at a greater risk, therefore remote monitoring of their vital signs using HWTs is crucial. Special HWTs that incorporate adjustable electrical and wave pulses altered according to their requirements aid disabled, paralysed, deaf, blind and patients whose memory has been affected. By recording and monitoring data, HWTs may be used as a preventive healthcare tool and telemedicine. Furthermore, HWTs are extensively employed in the area of research, as shown in Figure 7.2.

They've been used by scientists to better understand the physiology of rare disorders. For example, one research study looked at the potential of a wearable sensor to determine walking quality and balance rate in individuals with frailty syndrome, a condition marked by physical weakness. Researchers were able to discern three stages of frailty using wearable sensors and in-home monitoring. Another research looked at the sensors' capacity to anticipate people with dementia's falling rhythm. When working with patients in distant places, multiparameter physiological sensing devices may help practitioners. In China, a project named 'wireless heart health programme' used wireless health to treat 11,000 patients in remote rural locations. Smartphones with heart-rate sensors were used, and they were linked to the 96-digit phone numbers of local physicians, who could text and contact them, as well as evaluate and offer comments. Following that, doctors reported that the 11,000 individuals in the experimental group who had their health sensors evaluated had major cardiovascular issues, prompting them to seek additional treatment at the clinic. The automated medicine infusion pump is another important use of wearable technology. It regulates the volume and duration of medications or nutrients injected into a patient's body. These pumps have been extensively utilised to treat a variety of chronic conditions, including diabetes (insulin pump) and infections (antibiotic pump). Transdermal drug delivery (TDD) devices or patches, meanwhile, represent a step forward in wearable technology. Heat, electric current and sound waves are used in the devices to enhance medicine administration into the systemic circulation. TDD is currently in the early phases of development, but it intends to improve patient comfort and quality of life. To address the demand for this integration, HWTs will need to have specific characteristics in the future. System interoperability is one of these qualities. Several commercial businesses have produced HWTs utilising a variety of computational methods with a variety of characteristics and features, making it difficult for the electronic medical records (EMRs) to be compatible with them all. It will be easier to integrate HWTs into the EMR if they have a single and consistent computational approach. Furthermore, both computer and data scientists should be involved in the development of these computational techniques.

The goal is to work together with professionals to correctly improve various health issues. Furthermore, in order to improve their operations, data reliability and other usability concerns highlighted by HWTs must be addressed. Another potential idea is to improve the interaction of HWTs. HWTs might be connected with existing interactive computing systems, such as Google Now and Microsoft Cortana, which are currently available in smartphones. Similarly, HWT's interactive interface will create an instructional environment in which physicians may deliver patient alerts and instructive messages. Currently, most HWTs, particularly medical HWTs, are designed and constructed to function as a single-point solution. HWTs in the future should be able to manage a variety of quantifiable data. This will cut down on the amount of HWTs the patient will need to cover, trace and monitor data. Cardiac patients, for example, must have their blood pressure, cortisol levels and cholesterol levels constantly monitored. Multiple-point HWTs exacerbate the previously mentioned problems of prices, weight and discomfort. As a result, they must be cleverly constructed with these factors in mind. Insurance companies will be influenced to embrace these technologies and pay for wearable technologies used in clinical practice if complete, accurate and controllable HWTs are developed. There will be additional FDA rules and standards to oversee and ensure the safe and correct usage of HWTs in the future.

Wearable sensors have become more popular in recent years, and numerous gadgets for personal health care and activity awareness are now commercially accessible. A modern healthcare system should provide superior healthcare services to individuals at any time and in any location, at a cost that is both cheap and patient-friendly. Doctors have always played a vital role. They must go to the doctor for the appropriate diagnostic and advice. There are two drawbacks to this strategy. The IOT has evolved into one of the most influential communication platforms of the twenty-first century. Because of their connection and computational capabilities, all items in our everyday lives become part of the internet in the IOT ecosystem. One of the most basic physiological constraints is heart rate, which is critical for patient monitoring and diagnosis.

7.4   CONCLUSION

Wearable technology is described as any small device, such as a body sensor or HMS, that offers information to users and enables them to interact with them via voice commands or physical input. The goal of this wearable physical gadget is to provide easy, portable and hands-free access to computers, so making ordinary chores easier or more enjoyable. IOT is a commonly utilised technology today. However, in India, wearable gadget technology is not widely utilised or, to put it another way, not fully developed. It is more widely used in other nations. In today's age, wearable technology is defined as having a microprocessor and an internet connection. This article explains how wearable technology works and how it may benefit today's current age. We have described a wearable smart shoe technology utilising IOT in this study. This wearable gadget technology also counts steps, exercises and displays a person's fitness level. With the number of functions built in it, the wearable gadget smart-shoe technology is in increased demand by the consumer market. Embedded characteristics of the proposed system include 1. piezoelectric devices, 2. the Arduino microcontroller and 3. the GPRS (Global Positioning System) gadget (sends alert messages when tapped by foot when in danger). In this work, we show how fitness data may be generated and then communicated from a hardware component to an Android smartphone in the form of graphical and numeric data. Extending multifunctional smart-shoe-related applications may be developed in the future.

7.5　REFERENCES

[1] V. Uma Maheswari, S. Shoba Rani, D. Divakara Reddy and B. Lakshmi, E-Bazaar Innovation Using Iot Device in Cloud Subscription Management, *International Journal of Civil Engineering and Technology*, 8(8), year 2017, pp. 1155–1158.

[2] B. Durga Sri, K. Nirosha, P. Priyanka and B. Dhanalaxmi, GSM Based Fish Monitoring System Using IOT, *International Journal of Mechanical Engineering and Technology*, 8(7), year 2017, pp. 1094–1101.

[3] Hariharr C. Punjabi, Sanket Agarwal, Vivek Khithani, Venkatesh Muddaliar and Mrugendra Vasmatkar, Smart Farming Using IoT, *International Journal of Electronics and Communication Engineering and Technology*, 8(1), year 2017, pp. 58–66.

[4] S. Nithya, Lalitha Shree, R. Kiruthika and B.D. Krishnaveni, Solar Based Smart Garbage Monitoring System Using IOT, *International Journal of Electronics and Communication Engineering and Technology*, 8(2), year 2017, pp. 75–80.

[5] J. Dunn, R. Runge and M. Snyder, Wearables and the Medical Revolution, *Personalized Medicine*, 15(5), year 2018 Sept, pp. 429–448.

[6] C.Y. Jin, A Review of AI Technologies for Wearable Devices, *InIOP Conference Series: Materials Science and Engineering*, 688(4), year 2019 Nov, p. 044072. IOP Publishing.

[7] R. Wright and L. Keith, Wearable Technology: If the Tech Fits, Wear It, *Journal of Electronic Resources in Medical Libraries*, 11(4), year 2014 Oct 2, pp. 204–216.

[8] K.H. Yu, A.L. Beam and I.S. Kohane, Artificial Intelligence in Healthcare, *Nature Biomedical Engineering*, 2(10), year 2018 Oct, pp. 719–731.

[9] E. Bayro-Kaiser, D. Soliño-Fernández, A. Ding and E.L. Ding, Willingness to Adopt Wearable Devices with Behavioral and Economic Incentives by Health Insurance Wellness Programs: Results of a US Cross-Sectional Survey with Multiple Consumer Health Vignettes, *BMC Public Health*, 19(1).

[10] S. Neubert, *Automation Requires Process Information Technologies* [Internet]. Rostock: Center for Life Science Automation (celisca); c2016 [cited at 2017 Jan 25]. Available from: http://139.30.204.254/celisca/index.php?id=987.

[11] Indiegogo, *Hicon Smartwristband with Social Network Icons* [Internet]. San Francisco, CA: Indiegogo; 2015 [cited at 2017 Jan 25]. Available from: www.indiegogo.com/projects/hicon-smartwristband-with-socialnetwork-icons#/.

[12] U. Anliker, J.A. Ward, P. Lukowicz, G. Troster, F. Dolveck, M. Baer, et al., AMON: A Wearable Multiparameter Medical Monitoring and Alert System, *IEEE Trans Inf Technol Biomed*, 8(4), year 2004, pp. 415–427.

[13] S. Kannadhasan, G. Karthikeyan and V. Sethupathi, *A Graph Theory Based Energy Efficient Clustering Techniques in Wireless Sensor Networks*, Information and Communication Technologies Organised by Noorul Islam University (ICT 2013), Nagercoil, 2013, Apr 11–12, Published for Conference Proceedings by IEEE Explore Digital Library 978-1-4673-5758-6/13.

[14] Gas Sensor Developer Kit [Internet]. Newark, CA: Spec Sensors; [cited at 2017 Jan 25]. Available from: www.spec-sensors.com/product-category/gassensor- developer-kits/.

[15] G. To and M.R. Mahfouz, Modular Wireless Inertial Trackers for Biomedical Applications, *Proceedings of 2013 IEEE Topical Conference on Power Amplifiers for Wireless and Radio Applications (PAWR)*, year 2013 Jan 20–23, p. 172–174; Austin, TX.

[16] G. Srividhya, R. Nagarajan and S. Kannadhasan, Enhancement of Clustering Techniques Efficiency for WSN Using LEACH Algorithm, International Conference on Advances in Smart Sensor, Signal Processing, and Communication Technology (ICASSCT 2021), Goa University, Goa, *IOP Journal of Physics: Conference Series*, 1921, year 2021, Mar 19–20. doi:10.1088/1742-6596/1921/1/012013.

[17] P.H. Veltink and H.B. Boom, 3D Movement Analysis Using Accelerometry Theoretical Concepts, in: A. Pedotti, M. Ferrarin, J. Quintern and R. Reiner, editors. *Neuroprosthetics: From Basic Research to Clinical Applications*. Berlin: Springer; 1996. p. 317–326.

8 Intelligent Depression Detection System Using Effective Hyper-Scanning Techniques

Minakshee Patil[1], Vijay M. Wadhai[2],
Dhanashri H. Gawali[3] and Akshita S. Chanchlani[3]
[1] Sinhgad Academy of Engineering, Pune, India
[2] D.Y. Patil College of Engineering, Pune, India
[3] Sant Gadge Baba Amravati University, Amravati, India

CONTENTS

8.1 INTRODUCTION

Depression not only lowers the happiness index of individuals but also reduces mindfulness. The increase in the prevalence of clinical depression has been linked to a range of serious outcomes, particularly an increase in the number of suicide attempts and deaths, making it a public health concern [1]. This underlines the need of an intelligent depression detection system which is able to automatically classify the individual as healthy or depressed. Selection of effective biomarkers plays a vital role in the design of an intelligent depression detection system.

DOI: 10.1201/9781003217107-8

Mental health refers to cognitive, behavioural and emotional well-being. Being a fundamental component of health, good mental health enables individual to cope with the challenges in life, recognise his or her potential, work effectively and contribute to his or her own surroundings. According to ICD-10 (the International Statistical Classification of Diseases and Related Health Problems, Tenth revision), depression, bipolar affective disorder, schizophrenia, anxiety disorders, dementia, substance use disorders and autism are the major mental disorders that cause a high burden of disease worldwide [2]. The study estimates that 10.7% of the global population, i.e. 792 million people, suffered with a mental disorder in 2017 from which 3.4% of the population was affected only by depression showing its prevalence on 264 million people [2].

Depression, which is frequently referred as clinical depression or major depression disorder (MDD) is characterised by persistently low mood or loss of interest in activities, causing significant impairment in daily life. Considering the effect of its severity, depression can be classified as mild, moderate and severe (also called major). Mild depression may cause anger, hopelessness, feeling of guilt and despair, daytime sleepiness and fatigue, whereas moderates depression may lead to excessive worrying, increases sensitivities, problem with self-esteem and reduced productivity. Along with these symptoms, major depression shows severe symptoms as delusions, hallucinations and suicidal thoughts and behaviours [3].

8.2 MOTIVATION

According to the World Health Organization (WHO) key facts, globally, more than 264 million people of all ages suffer from depression [1]. Depression is a leading cause of disability worldwide and is a major contributor to the overall global burden of disease. Today, depression already is the second cause of disability adjusted life years (DALYs) in the age category 15–44 years [3]. Depression alone accounts for 4.3% of the global burden of disease and is among the largest single causes of disability worldwide (11% of all years lived with disability globally). People with mental disorders experience disproportionately higher rates of disability and mortality. For example, persons with major depression and schizophrenia have a 40% to 60% greater chance of dying prematurely than the general population [2].

Figure 8.1 shows the global prevalence by mental and substance use disorder in 2017. It clearly indicates that depression affected 3.44% of the world population [4].

Figure 8.2 indicates the share of the population with depression, which ranges mostly between 2% and 6%, around the world today [4].

Mental Health Action Plan 2013–2020 summarised that health systems have not yet adequately responded to the burden of mental disorders; as a consequence, the gap between the need for treatment and its provision is large all over the world [5]. Between 76% and 85% of people with severe mental disorders receive no treatment for their disorder in low-income and middle-income countries; the corresponding range for high-income countries is also high: between 35% and 50%. The number of specialised and general health workers dealing with mental health in low-income and middle-income countries is grossly insufficient. Almost half the world's population lives in countries where, on average, there is one psychiatrist to serve 200,000 or more people.

Prevalence by mental and substance use disorder, World, 2017

Share of the total population with a given mental health or substance use disorder. Figures attempt to provide a true estimate (going beyond reported diagnosis) of disorder prevalence based on medical, epidemiological data, surveys and meta-regression modelling.

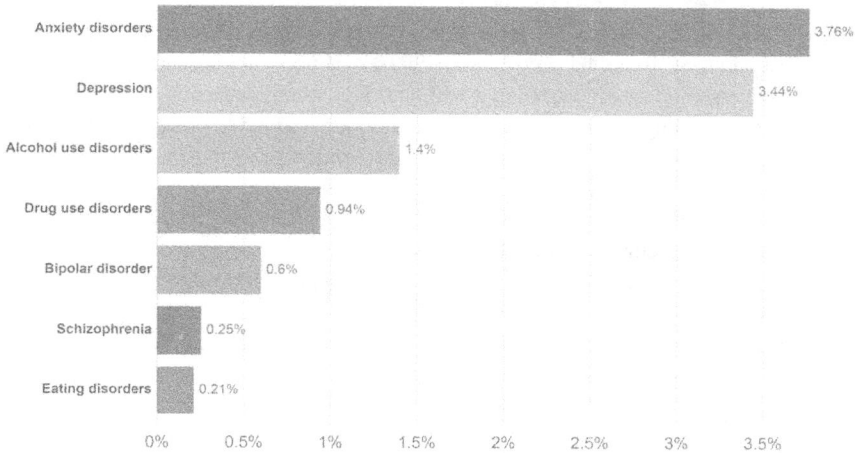

Anxiety disorders	3.76%
Depression	3.44%
Alcohol use disorders	1.4%
Drug use disorders	0.94%
Bipolar disorder	0.6%
Schizophrenia	0.25%
Eating disorders	0.21%

0%   0.5%   1%   1.5%   2%   2.5%   3%   3.5%

FIGURE 8.1   Prevalence by mental and substance use disorder.

Share of the population with depression, 2017

Prevalence of depressive disorders in a given population. This is measured as the age-standardized prevalence, which assumes a constant age structure to compare between countries and through time. Figures attempt to provide a true estimate (going beyond reported diagnosis) of depression prevalence based on medical, epidemiological data, surveys and meta-regression modelling.

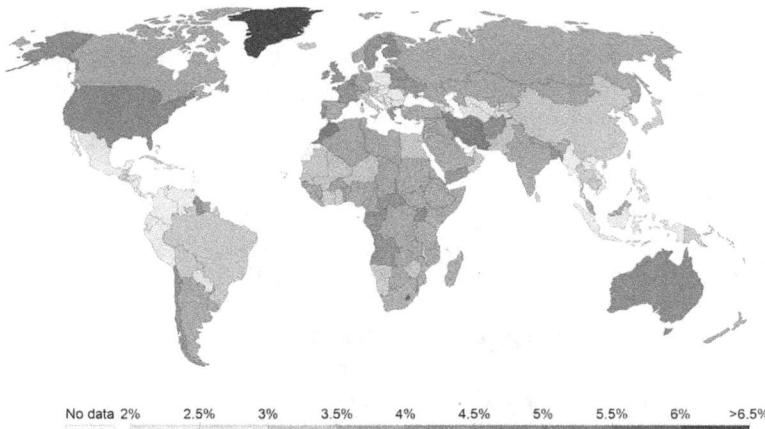

No data 2%   2.5%   3%   3.5%   4%   4.5%   5%   5.5%   6%   >6.5%

FIGURE 8.2   Share of world population with depression.

8.3 CURRENT DIAGNOSTIC SYSTEMS

There are effective treatments for moderate and severe depression. Healthcare providers offer psychological treatments such as behavioural activation, cognitive behavioral therapy (CBT) and interpersonal psychotherapy (IPT) or antidepressant medication such as selective serotonin reuptake inhibitors (SSRIs) and tricyclic antidepressants (TCAs). However, adverse effects are associated with antidepressant medication, so it should not be used for treating depression in children and are not the first line of treatment in adolescents. The majority of mental health services and treatments rely increasingly on accurate diagnosis to decide the path of their treatment. Unfortunately, within the mental health field, clinical diagnoses have been historically unreliable. The current methodologies and tools used to detect depression mostly rely on the patient's response and his communication with clinicians while one is already going through a miserable mental condition. Most of the screening methods used for depression detection are based on questionnaire prepared for the structured assessment [6]. With the help of patient's response to this structured form and face-to-face session with him, clinicians decide the severity of depression and hence the treatment. As this method is subjective, accuracy of diagnosis is largely affected due to the occurrence of 'false positive' and 'false negative' cases.

To avoid or at least to minimise the subjective bias in depression detection, many researchers are working to design automated depression detection system. One of the important steps involved in designing an intelligent depression detection system is selection of effective biomarkers. The evidence to date suggests that biomarkers reflecting the activity of inflammatory, neurotransmitter, neurotrophic, neuroendocrine and metabolic systems may be able to predict mental and physical health outcomes in currently depressed individuals [7–13, 14].

8.4 LITERATURE REVIEW

Although psychiatric disorders have largely been accepted by the medical community as diseases with biochemical dysfunction, researchers are still searching for biomarkers – quantitative indicators that can objectively measure the change in severity of these disorders, much like blood pressure or cholesterol concentrations are biomarkers for cardiovascular disease. In the present work, we have investigated how potentially speech can be used as biomarker to detect depression in adolescents. The ability to speak is closely related to psychomotor function, thinking and concentration and the speed of information processing, all of which are frequently impaired in psychiatric disorders such as clinical depression [8, 13–15]. While the content of speech is consciously controlled, characteristics such as speed, pause and energy and pitch variation in speech are not. Thus, vocal-acoustic data can provide an indirect but objective measurement of clinical depression [7, 9].

Speech energy is one of the widely used features for depression detection. Lower voice energy in a patient can be considered as the indication of clinical depression [10–11]. Pitch, in speech, the relative highness or lowness of a tone as perceived by the ear, depends on the number of vibrations per second produced by vocal cords. It is a widely investigated feature and indicates lower range in the depressed patient when compared with healthy ones [12]. Jitter and shimmer are the two important features and when used in combination have been proven good indicators in depression detection [8, 13, 16].

Jitter is a measure of frequency instability, while shimmer is a measure of amplitude variation in voice. A normal voice has lower jitter while shimmer will have moderate to high range. However in depressed patients, jitter shows higher range while shimmer is very low. Classification using the Markov Transition Matrix method has been investigated in [13]. In this approach, speech samples are labelled in three different states as voiced, unvoiced and silence and then variations in transition probabilities are estimated using discrete time Markov process. Though this method gives good result for unvoiced feature for male and female speakers, further study is required to analyse the effect of classification method and combinations of features on the result. Power spectrum density (PSD) is also one of the significant features investigated in [10, 12, 14] for depression detection. The PSD of the speech signal is nothing but power present in speech as a function of frequency, per unit frequency. PSD showed better classification result, especially with the combination of band 1:3, for both male and female speakers.

For accurate detection of depression, the role of the classifier is equally important as that of the biomarker. After investigating various classifiers for emotion recognition, support vector machine (SVM) has been proven a better classifier due to its better predictability and accuracy [17, 18]. SVM is one of the popular classifiers since it is able to handle smaller datasets, which generally is the case in such studies.

In the present work, we have mainly focused on the effect of spontaneous speech and read speech on depression detection of adolescents. Spontaneous speech samples are collected while interviewing adolescents by the trained interviewer, whereas read speech data is collected while the subject reads out predefined emotional sentences. Also we have investigated the performance parameter of speech features like mel frequency cepstral coefficients (MFCC), pitch, jitter, shimmer and energy. With the present study we have focused only on detecting presence of depression in the subject and not on severity and score rating prediction.

8.5   METHODOLOGY FOR DATASET FORMATION

Acoustic features show remarkably high accuracy in depression detection. Audio data samples used for this study include speech samples of both depressed and healthy individuals, which are labelled as depressed and healthy in the text database. A few entries are described in Table 8.1, where every row gives details of each individual. The labels are assigned based on diagnosis done by the experienced clinician using Patient Health Questionnaire (PHQ-9) and Beck Depression Inventory (BDI) scale.

TABLE 8.1
Sample Entries of Labelled Dataset

File Name	Gender	Age	BDI Scale	PHQ 9 Scale	File Label
Sub23	M	17	6	2	Healthy
Sub24	M	14	22	14	Depressed
Sub25	F	11	9	3	Healthy
Sub26	M	16	4	1	Healthy
Sub27	M	18	19	11	Depressed

While selecting volunteers for this study, 1) only adolescents' speech is recorded, 2) speech samples of siblings are discarded and 3) volunteers with a past history of any type of mental illness are avoided. After careful selection of the volunteers, audio signals are recorded in controlled laboratory environment. To collect read-data audio samples, every volunteer is given the same text which includes sentences (which were arranged in specific paragraphs) that evokes different emotions while reading. The average time of read-data samples is 6 min per individual. Spontaneous data is collected during interview conducted by the trained interviewer using pre-defined open ended questions. In response to these questions, individuals have shared their opinions, different experiences and their life incidents. Average recorded time of these sessions is 11 min per individual. Thus dataset includes audio samples of 54 depressed and 75 healthy individuals. All audio samples are recorded using Sony ICDUX560BLK voice recorder having frequency range 50Hz to 20 kHz.

8.6 SYSTEM DESCRIPTION

The intelligent depression detection (Figure 8.3) system described in the chapter is a step towards saving the lives of depressed patients. The aim of the study is to develop an integrated diagnostic system that will characterise depression symptoms with the help of hyper-scanning methods in ecological and natural conditions.

8.6.1 PRE-PROCESSING

The Sound Forge 5.0 is used to manually extract voiced and unvoiced part of recorded audio data. Along with comparing the role of spontaneous and read speech in depression detection, one of the focus of this study is to decide the effect of duration of speech signal on the accuracy of classification. Read audio data collected for every volunteer during reading sessions is manually arranged as 1) All paragraphs: In this approach, complete speech duration for every volunteer is collected. Average voice

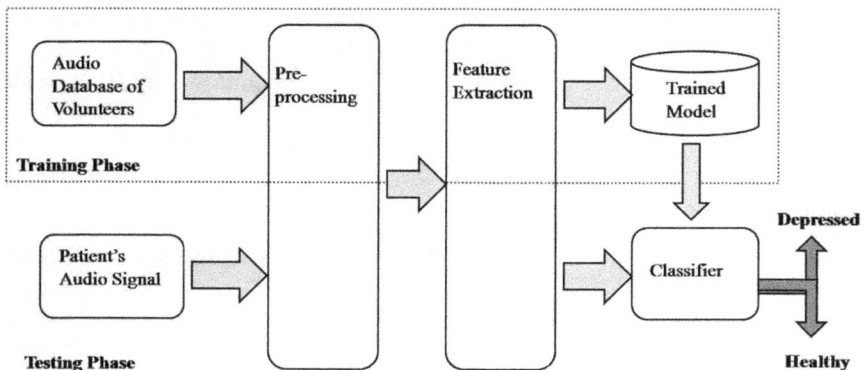

FIGURE 8.3 Intelligent depression detection system using acoustic features.

duration collected is 5 min per volunteer. 2) Initial part of every paragraph: Every paragraph is designed to evoke different feelings while reading. In this approach the initial 10-sec duration from every paragraph is collected and all such chunks are concatenated to form a sample file for every volunteer. 3) End part of every paragraph: In this approach, the last 10-sec duration from every paragraph is collected and concatenated to form a sample file. Similarly, spontaneous data, which has been collected during interview sessions conducted by the trained interviewer, is manually prepared and labelled in three categories: 1) Response for all questions: initially, it was planned to consider complete duration of interview, but the average duration for spontaneous data was 11 min and that for read data was 6 min. So to have comparable durations, the initial 5 min of audio data for every volunteer is extracted. 2) Initial part of every question: as every question is open ended, it demands a subjective response from the volunteer based on his experiences, feelings and approach. So, in this approach, the initial 5 sec from every question is collected and is concatenated to prepare a sample file for every volunteer. 3) End part of every question: in this approach, a sample file is prepared by extracting the last 5-sec duration from every question followed by concatenation.

8.6.2 FEATURES EXTRACTION

Depression affects muscles in the human voice production system [8, 19]. This clearly indicates that depression affects acoustic features prominently. In the present work, acoustic features like jitter, shimmer, log energy, pitch and MFCC (12 coefficients) have been investigated for both spontaneous and read data.

Acoustic feature of the speech is nothing but physical characteristics of speech sounds such as loudness, amplitude and frequency, which varies among individuals depending upon their speech production system with the help of vocal tract and air flow through the voice-box [20, 21]. Some acoustic features are robust in nature and so can be used for experimental purpose for various speech applications. Jitter can be defined as a change in pitch. It is figured utilising the fundamental frequency of each cycle, subtracting from a past estimation of f0 and then afterward partitioning by f0 takes place. Shimmer is calculation of the period-to-period variability of the signal's peak to peak amplitude (Ai). Thus jitter is cycle-to-cycle fluctuations in the fundamental frequency of speech, whereas shimmer is the fluctuations in peak-to-peak amplitude. MFCC computation is a replication of the human hearing system intending to artificially implement the ear's working principle with the assumption that the human ear is a reliable speech recogniser. MFCC features are rooted in the recognised discrepancy of the human ear's critical bandwidths with frequency filters spaced linearly at low frequencies and logarithmically at high frequencies have been used to retain the phonetically vital properties of the speech signal. Speech signals commonly contain tones of varying frequencies, each tone with an actual frequency, f (Hz), and the subjective pitch is computed on the mel scale. The mel-frequency scale has linear frequency spacing below 1000 Hz and logarithmic spacing above 1000 Hz. Pitch of 1 kHz tone and 40 dB above the perceptual audible threshold is defined as 1000 mels and used as a reference point.

During preprocessing, audio data is arranged in different files containing either the complete part or a small chunk of the speech, as explained in Section 6.1. Acoustic features are extracted with the help of Praat 6.0 which is open source and widely used software for speech analysis. Features are extracted frame to frame and are normalised for the same subject. The frame size is selected as 25 msec having 50% overlapping with a hamming window.

Extracted features are arranged in a tabular form as shown in Table 8.2, where each column represented all the features extracted for a particular volunteer and is labelled as '0' for a healthy or '1'for a depressed volunteer.

8.6.3   CLASSIFICATION

Speech data is classified into two classes, namely depressed and healthy, using SVM with hyper-plane. SVM is a very effective machine learning algorithm and has proven its significance as a classifier even for smaller datasets. The SVM algorithm is implemented in the system using a kernel. A kernel transforms an input data space into the required form. SVM uses a technique called the kernel trick. In this technique, the kernel takes a low-dimensional input space and transforms it into a higher dimensional space. In other words, we can say that it converts non-separable problem to separable problems by adding more dimensions to it. It is most useful in non-linear separation problems. The kernel trick helps us to build a more accurate classifier.

To design a trained model, training data can be selected using selection criteria like 1) Equal test train: where the same data is used for training as well as for testing; 2) Leave one out: where only one sample is used for testing and all the remaining samples are used for training the classification model; and 3) Cross validation: in this

TABLE 8.2
Extracted Features for a Few Subjects

Subject – >	47	48	51	52
Feature1	−0.150	−0.253	−0.197	−0.225
Feature2	0.123	−0.751	0.245	0.823
Feature3	−0.210	−0.268	−0.123	−0.811
Feature4	0.245	0.796	0.976	0.628
Feature5	−0.341	−0.242	0.271	−0.102
Feature6	−0.144	−0.656	−0.673	−0.297
Feature7	−0.949	−0.209	−0.262	−0.112
Feature8	−0.136	0.211	−0.223	0.111
Feature9	−0.266	−0.333	−0.519	−0.177
Feature10	−0.416	−0.322	0.155	−0.100
Feature11	0.594	−0.330	−0.200	−0.645
Feature12	−0.242	0.653	−0.167	0.714
Feature13	−0.170	−0.506	−0.718	−0.219
Label	0	0	1	1

approach dataset is separated into desired proportions of training and testing data. We have used the cross validation method to select training and testing data (80% training and 20% testing data). Training data has been fed to the SVM classifier to generate a trained model. The result is obtained by feeding testing samples to the trained model.

8.7   RESULT AND DISCUSSIONS

Our work mainly focuses on the binary decision system to classify adolescents as healthy or depressed. Among linguistic and acoustic features of speech, the latter is selected for classification, as family and social background, culture, age and educational status have a major impact on linguistic features of the subject. After investigating many acoustic features, those features having insignificant impact on classification, possibly due to voice box development observed during adolescent age, particularly in male subjects, have been discarded.

The main objective of the experiments is to correctly classify the volunteers as either depressed or healthy. In the study, the correct classification of depressed and healthy adolescents in measured in terms of overall accuracy along with sensitivity and specificity. The accuracy is defined using the following terms:

True Positive (TP): Number of depressed volunteers classified as depressed
False Negative (FN): Number of depressed volunteers classified as healthy
True Negative (TN): Number of healthy volunteers classified as healthy
False Positive (FP): Number of healthy volunteers classified as depressed

$$\%\text{Accuracy} = \frac{TP + TN}{(TP + FN + TN + FP)}$$

Table 8.3 shows the result in terms of percentage accuracy for both spontaneous and read data with different subsets of speech. In spite of using a smaller dataset, (which problem is stated in similar research work), the overall accuracy of classification is above 65%, which clearly indicates that speech can be used as a promising biomarker for depression detection. Accuracy obtained with spontaneous speech is remarkably higher than that with read speech for almost all subsets of speech. This emphasises the role of spontaneous speech in depression detection for adolescents.

Among all, performance of MFCC is better (above 81%) followed by jitter (above 80%). When the results for the initial-part-dataset are compared with the end-part-dataset for both read and spontaneous speech, it is observed that the initial part gave better accuracy. This emphasises that the initial response of a volunteer gives better result before he or she engaged in the task. The hypothesis that the voice of a depressed person is monotonous is supported with the result obtained with shimmer and pitch. The accuracy for pitch (76.1%) and shimmer (76.2%) being nearly equal underlines the fact that the monotonous voice quality of depressed adolescents can easily classify them from healthy ones.

When experiments are carried out with different datasets of both read and spontaneous speech to decide how much portion of speech is adequate for classification, it is observed that the initial part gives better accuracy instead of the entire speech. This observation will be helpful while working with bigger datasets where the overall

TABLE 8.3

Depression Detection Results (in %) Using Different Parts of Speech

Acoustic Features	All Read Sentences	Read Speech		Spontaneous Speech		
		Initial Part of Each Paragraph	End Part of Each Paragraph	Response for All Questions	Initial Part of Each Question	End Part of Each Question
Jitter	75.1	79.6	73.8	80.4	84.1	81.2
Shimmer	65.8	66.1	66.9	76.2	77.2	77.7
Log Energy	67.4	69.3	67.7	79	85.5	79.8
MFCC	74.5	75.2	74.1	81.3	83.7	82.5
Pitch	67.2	66.4	66.9	76.1	79.3	78.6

speed of the system might be affected due to larger training period required for the whole part of the speech.

8.8 CONCLUSION

The work in this study shows that speech can be used as effective biomarker. Acoustic features can be used as an indicator for depression in adolescents. When compared with the experimental results, accuracy obtained with spontaneous speech is significantly more than that with read speech data. Overall accuracy obtained with MFCC and jitter is higher than other acoustic features for almost all datasets, which underlines the contribution of these acoustic features in binary classification of adolescents as depressed or as healthy. One more significant finding of the experimental study is related to effect of duration of speech samples on the accuracy. The results clearly indicate that initial part of speech gives better accuracy than the entire portion of speech sample. This finding is very useful in saving training-phase duration for the larger datasets. The intelligent depression detection system will assist psychologists in effective diagnosis and ongoing monitoring during the treatment. Furthermore, it will help in reducing productivity losses and improve human performance. Early detection leads to overcome the restrictions on specialist, drug and psychotherapeutic care. In addition, the early detection, intervention and appropriate treatment can significantly improve the quality of human life.

8.9 FUTURE SCOPE

In this chapter, we have studied and experimented capability of acoustic features to detect the depression in the adolescents. The system has adopted binary classification technique to categorise the individual either as depressed or as healthy. Thus, system is able to detect the presence of depression in adolescents with very good accuracy. But it is not able to detect the severity of depression. In general, severity of depression is considered in three categories as mild, moderate and severe (which also called major depression). In our further research, we will work to design an automated depression detection system which will classify the depressed individual according to the severity of depression.

In the current study, while investigating the contribution of acoustic features in depression detection, we have examined them on individual basis. There is need to investigate effect of fusion of features on the accuracy and sensitivity of the classification. To improve the accuracy we can use more than one classifier simultaneously for the detection. The decision weight can be allocated to every classifier depending upon their individual performance and the resultant group decision can be used to predict the classification.

8.10   REFERENCES

[1] NMH Communications, *Mental and Neurological Disorders*. Fact Sheet: The World Health Report 2014. Geneva, Switzerland: World Health Organization, 2014.

[2] GBD 2017 Disease and Injury Incidence and Prevalence Collaborators, Global, Regional, and National Incidence, Prevalence, and Years Lived with Disability for 354 Diseases and Injuries for 195 Countries and Territories, 1990–2017: A Systematic Analysis for the Global Burden of Disease Study 2017, *The Lancet*, 392, 2018.

[3] A.D. Lopez, C.D. Mathers, M. Ezzati, D.T. Jamison and C.J. Murray, *Global Burden of Disease and Risk Factors*. Washington: The World Bank, 2006.

[4] Hannah Ritchie and Max Roser, *Mental Health*, 2018. OurWorldInData.org, https://ourworldindata.org/mental-health.

[5] World Health Organization, *Mental Health Action Plan 2013–2020*. World Health Organization, 2013. https://apps.who.int/iris/handle/10665/89966.

[6] A.T. Beck, R.A. Steer, R. Ball and W.F.Ranieri, Comparison of Beck Depression Inventories-IA and-II in Psychiatric Outpatients, *Journal of Personality Assessment*, 67(3), pp. 588–597, Dec. 1996; P. Tavel, *Modeling and Simulation Design*. Natick, MA: AK Peters Ltd., 2007.

[7] N.S. Melissa, L. Margaret, J.S. Shannon and B.A. Nicholas, Detection of Adolescent Depression from Speech Using Optimised Spectral Roll-Off Parameters, *Biomedical Journal of Scientific & Technical Research*, 5(1), 2018. doi:10.26717/BJSTR.2018.05.001156.

[8] S. Marmor, K.J. Horvath, K.O. Lim and S. Misono, Voice Problems and Depression Among Adults in the United States, *The Laryngoscope*, 126(8), 1859–1864, 2016, Dec. doi:10.1002/lary.25819.

[9] James C. Mundt, Peter J. Snyder, Michael S. Cannizzaro, Kara Chappie and Dayna S. Geralts, Voice Acoustic Measures of Depression Severity and Treatment Response Collected Via Interactive Voice Response Technology, *Journal of Neurolinguistics*, 20(1), 50–64, 2007.

[10] M.N. Stolar, M. Lech and N.B. Allen, Detection of Depression in Adolescents Based on Statistical Modeling of Emotional Influences in Parent-Adolescent Conversations, *Acoustics, Speech and Signal Processing (ICASSP)*, 2015. https://pages.uoregon.edu/psi/CVs/AllenCV%206-2016.pdf.

[11] Lu-Shih Alex Low, Namunu C. Maddage, Margaret Lech, Lisa B. Sheeber and Nicholas B. Allen, Detection of Clinical Depression in Adolescents' Speech During Family Interactions, *IEEE Transactions on Biomedical Engineering*, 58(3), 574–586, Mar 2011.

[12] Sharifa Alghowinem, Roland Goecke, Michael Wagner, Julien Epps, Tom Gedeon, Michael Breakspear and Gordon Parker, Comparative Study of Different Classifiers for Detecting Depression from Spontaneous Speech, *IEEE International Conference on Acoustics, Speech and Signal Processing (ICASSP)*, 8022–8026, 2013.

[13] Kuan Ee Brian Ooi, Margaret Lech, Nicholas Allen, Multichannel Weighted Speech Classification System for Prediction of Major Depression in Adolescents, *IEEE Transactions on Biomedical Engineering*, 60(2), 497–506, Feb 2013.

[14] H. Azam et al., *Classifications of Clinical Depression Detection Using Acoustic Measures in Malay Speakers*, 2016 IEEE EMBS Conference on Biomedical Engineering and Sciences (IECBES), Kuala Lumpur, pp. 606–610, Dec 2016. doi:10.1109/IECBES.2016.7843521.

[15] J. Cavenar, H. Keith, H. Brodie and R. Weiner, *Signs and Symptoms in Psychiatry*. Philadelphia: Lippincott Williams & Wilkins, 1983.

[16] National Institute of Mental Health, *Depression*, 2016. Retrieved March 1, 2016, from www.nimh.nih.gov/health/topics/depression/index.shtml.

[17] T. Seehapoch and S. Wongthanavasu, *Speech Emotion Recognition Using Support Vector Machines*, 2013 5th International Conference on Knowledge and Smart Technology (KST), Chonburi, Thailand, pp. 86–91, May 2013. doi:10.1109/KST.2013.6512793.

[18] R. Kessler, P. Berglund, O. Demler, R. Jin, K. Merikangas and E. Walters, Lifetime Prevalence and Age of Onset Distributions of DSM-IV Disorders in the National Comorbidity Survey Replication, *Archives of General Psychiatry*, 62(6), 593–602, June 2005.

[19] Rutter, M., Relationships Between Mental Disorders in Childhood and Adulthood, *Acta Psychiatrica Scandinavica*, 91(2), 73–85, Feb 1995.

[20] C. Qin and M.A. Carreira-Perpnan, *An Empirical Investigation of the Non Uniqueness in the Acoustic-to-Articulatory Mapping*, Eurospeech, London, 2007.

[21] K. Richmond, *Estimating Articulatory Parameters from Acoustic Speech Signals*, Ph.D. thesis, University of Edinburgh, Edinburgh, 2001.

9 Design of an Intelligent System for Diabetes Prediction by Integrating Rough Set Theory and Genetic Algorithm

Shampa Sengupta[1], *Kumud Ranjan Pal*[2]
and Vivek Garg[3]
[1] MCKV Institute of Engineering, India
[2] Seharabazar C.K. Institution, India
[3] University of Greenwich, United Kingdom

CONTENTS

9.1   INTRODUCTION

Diabetes is a non-communicable disease. A research report of World Health Organization [1] presented about how the impacts of diabetes of any person affect physically, financially, economically on his or her families too. According to a report, this uncontrolled health issue leads to 1.2 million deaths.

Diabetes [2] can occur if the body cannot generate insulin or is unable to use produced insulin properly. Our daily food is broken down into glucose and enters into our bloodstream. Insulin hormone has an important role in our body to metabolise glucose. Today many people are suffering from diabetes mellitus. The causes behind this are lifestyle, age, bad diet, obesity, high blood pressure, etc. Diabetic people have a risk of diseases like vision loss, heart disease, stroke, nerve damage and kidney disease. General symptoms of diabetes are weight loss, increased hunger, extreme fatigue, blurry vision, frequent urination, etc. Diabetes is of three types: type 1 diabetes [3], type 2 diabetes [4] and type 3 diabetes [5], which is called gestational diabetes. Each type of diabetes is caused for different reasons. Non-production of insulin is the main cause behind type 1 diabetes. Type 1 diabetes patients require insulin to inject and are referred as insulin-dependent diabetes mellitus (IDDM) patients. Genetics and lifestyle factors causing extra weight are the reasons behind type 2 diabetes, also referred to as non-insulin-dependent diabetes mellitus (NIDDM) patients. In type 2 diabetes the patient's cells are unable to use insulin properly. Hormonal changes during pregnancy can cause gestational diabetes. Hormones, which are produced by the placenta, make a pregnant woman's cells almost insensitive to the effects of insulin.

There is a need to handle electronic health records from the healthcare industry. The modern healthcare system requires proper information technology solutions to process this medical data to prevent the disease by warning people whether they are prone to diabetes or not, that is to save the people from this deadly disease.

In this chapter, a working model of the prediction of diabetes disease is proposed. The method uses the popular soft computing techniques rough set theory [6] (RST) and genetic algorithm (GA) [7]. The method actually consists of two important stages wherein the first stage, selection of important disease features from the diabetic dataset is done, and after that, classification algorithms are applied on the reduced dataset to predict the disease in the second stage. The algorithm handles medical data effectively for an optimised solution. We have used a few heuristics in the method. The details of the heuristics and their importance are specified later in the chapter. The method provides a good accuracy in predicting the diabetes disease. The proposed method has been modelled in Figure 9.1.

The primary contribution of the work is:

- Efficient processing of medical disease data in the healthcare domain for a better prediction result.
- Optimal feature subset selection from the original feature set using RST-based GA method.
- Development of an efficient disease prediction system using machine learning techniques in an integrated environment.

In this chapter the recent development of artificial intelligence (AI) in the prediction of diabetes is presented in Section 2. Section 3 demonstrates the proposed method for developing the prediction model. Section 4 illustrates the results of the conducted experiment. Section 5 discusses the important characteristics of the working model and provides a conclusion.

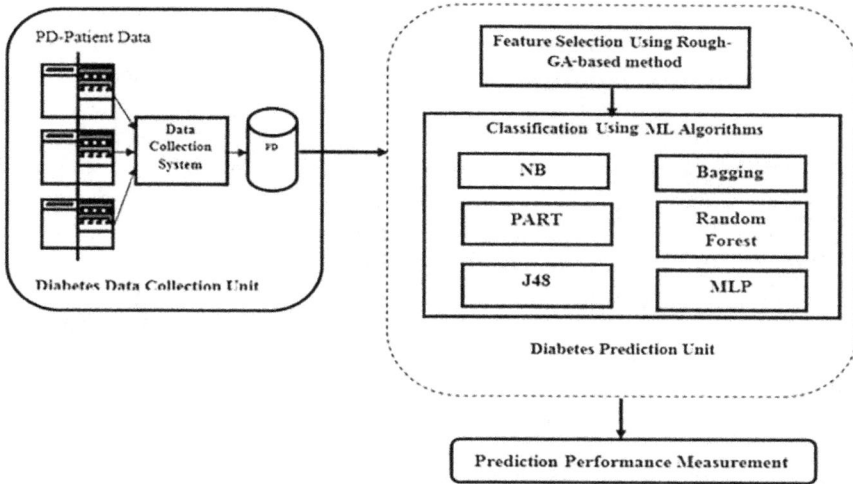

FIGURE 9.1 Proposed model of intelligent diabetes prediction system.

9.2 ARTIFICIAL INTELLIGENCE IN DIABETES PREDICTION

The technical challenges that current AI solutions provide to clinicians to predict the diabetes disease are discussed in this section. To manage the healthcare data efficiently for data mining and pattern recognition [8–10] purposes, its dimensionality needs to be reduced. With feature selection [11] and reduct computation [6, 12–14], RST [6] is frequently used as a pre-processing step for knowledge discovery [12–14]. Important and relevant features are selected from the feature space based on certain evaluation criterion, which actually increases the efficiency of the data analysis tasks like clustering [15] and classification [16–17].

9.2.1 DIMENSION REDUCTION TECHNIQUES

Nowadays a large amount of structured and unstructured data is being generated in the healthcare field through patient data and medical test reports. Rows and columns can represent this structured data, such as in a spreadsheet, where each row indicates the individual patient object and columns are treated as the patient's disease features/symptoms. So, features are known as a set of input variables or attributes that represent the health status of a patient. More input features are often producing poor performance of various classification algorithms [16–17]. The study of dimensionality reduction [18–19] is concerned with reducing the number of input features and maximising the accuracy of learning algorithms [16–17].

There are two broader-level dimensionality reduction techniques [18–19] known as feature selection [11] and feature extraction [20]. Feature selection [11] is the method of selecting the important subset of features from the feature pool without compromising the system accuracy as represented by the original features. The objects with its conditional features and the decision feature most often represent a decision system. A conditional feature is important or significant if it contributes much to take the prediction on a decision feature accurately. This process is playing an important role to enhance the performance of the model by reducing the computational cost in terms of space and time. Feature selection is of three types (based on the evaluation process) such as a *filter* approach [11], *wrapper* approach [11] and *embedded* method [11]. If the feature selection job is performed independent of any learning algorithm, then it is the *filter* approach [11], whereas in case of the *wrapper* approach the feature selection method is integrated with the learning algorithm where accuracy of the induction algorithm is considered as the measure of suitability of the subset.

Wrapper methods produces better results but are costly to run as evaluation of subsets depends on the learning algorithms, which may suffer from problems with the bigger datasets. An *embedded* method [11] takes advantage of its own variable selection method and performs feature selection and classification at the same time. The tree algorithms like random forest [21], extra tree, etc., are the most common embedded techniques. Jain et al. [22] and Bishop [23], found that the feature selection identifies significant features from a set of candidates, while feature extraction [20] is concerned with transformations of features in order to generate useful and novel features from the original ones.

9.2.2 ROUGH SET THEORY

RST is a soft computing tool proposed by Z. Pawlak [6] to handle ambiguous, vague, inconsistent and uncertain data. RST (Pawlak, 1991; Polkowski, 2002) is used as a dimension reduction tool by the researchers to solve different real-world problems. In the real world, everything is treated as an object and every object is described by its attributes. To identify the object, detection of important attributes are very much necessary. RST can be used to find out the most informative attribute/feature subset from the original feature set by removing the irrelevant attributes with minimal information loss. To get the insight from the data using RST, only the data itself is sufficient; no additional parameters are needed – that's why RST is such a popular research tool used nowadays. RST is used for the dimension reduction [6, 11] and the classification purpose by keeping the informative features to predict the class label of the data [16–17]. Here two terms, namely attributes and features, have been used in this chapter synonymously.

There exist many RST-based attribute reduction or feature selection algorithms [6, 12–14], which were developed for providing the solutions of different kinds of real-life problems. However, determining the minimal set of attributes, called reduct, is an NP-complete [24–26] problem, and for a particular dataset there is more than one reduct for most of the cases. Research works are going on for the selection of the particular reduct for better model. To find the reduct by the exhaustive method is quite infeasible and so heuristic methods are also applied. In reality, the possibility of multiple reducts exists in a decision system, but the best reduct is generally used for the developing the classifiers.

Let us consider a decision system $DS = (U, F, C, D)$, where U is the universe of discourse and F is the total number of features, including conditional features (C) and decision feature (D), so that $F = C \cup D$. Suppose, universe $U = \{O_1, O_2 \ldots O_n\}$, so considering any feature subset $A \subseteq F$, A-indiscernibility relation $IND(A)$ is defined by equation (9.1).

$$IND(A) = \{(x, y) \in U^2 \mid \forall f \in F, f(x) = f(y)\} \tag{9.1}$$

If $(x, y) \in IND(A)$, then x and y are indiscernible with respect to feature set A where class of objects are denoted by $[x]_A$.

The lower approximation of a target set X with respect to A is the set of all objects, which certainly belongs to X, as defined by equation (9.2).

$$\underline{AX} = \{x \mid [x]_F \subseteq X\} \tag{9.2}$$

The positive region $POS_A(D)$ is calculated by taking the union of the lower approximations AX under A for all target set $X \in U/D$, given in equation (9.3).

$$POS_A(D) = \cup_{X \in U/D} \underline{AX} \tag{9.3}$$

The upper approximation of the target set X with respect to A is the set of all objects, which can possibly belong to X, as defined by equation (9.4).

$$\overline{AX} = \{x \mid [x]_F \cap X \neq \varnothing\} \tag{9.4}$$

Finding the dependency between the features is very much necessary to understand the correlation between the features for any kind of data analysis purpose. RST describes the concept of data dependency in a simplified manner. Consider two (disjointed) sets of features, M and N, and finding out the degree of dependency between these two sets is discussed here. As we know, each attribute set induces an (indiscernibility) equivalence class structure, so in this case, the equivalence classes induced by M is $[x]_M$, and N is $[x]_N$. Then, the dependency of feature set N on feature set M is denoted by $\gamma_M(N)$ and is given by equation (9.5).

$$\gamma_M(N) = \frac{\sum_{i=1}^{N} |FX_i|}{|U|} \tag{9.5}$$

Where, N_i is a class of objects in $[x]_N$; $\forall i = 1, 2, \ldots, N$.

In RST, a reduct is the necessary set of attributes or features to tell about the category structure and the decision system as well. That is, the equivalence class structure obtained by the reduct will be same as considering the whole attribute set of the decision system. R is a reduct of a decision system if the dependency of decision attribute D on R is equal to the dependency of D on the full attribute set F.

$$\gamma_R(D) = \gamma_F(D) \tag{9.6}$$

It is not true that only one reduct can exist for a decision system. There may be multiple reducts or many subset of features, which can preserve the knowledge property of the decision system.

9.2.3 Evolutionary Algorithms

To find the best or optimal solution of a problem, the use of an optimisation principle or technique is needed. It selects the best element based on some criteria from some set of available alternatives. Optimisation technique is used in data mining for optimal feature subset selection as well as for optimal classification rule generation. Evolutionary algorithms (EAs) [7] use randomness and genetic inspired operations like selection, recombination and random variation, etc., to develop the evolutionary computational models to get the optimal solution of a problem. GA [7] is an evolutionary algorithm that simulates the process of natural evolution.

9.2.3.1 Genetic Algorithm (GA)

GA is a nature-inspired evolutionary algorithm which is often used to get the optimum solution of a given problem with basic tasks such as selection, crossover and mutation. In GA [7], a chromosome is defined as a simple string, which defines a proposed solution to the problem. Generally, chromosome representations are redefined according to the problem. A gene is a part of chromosome and contains a part of the solution. Fitness is a central idea in evolutionary theory. Fitness value describes the quality of the individual solution, which actually helps to search for the optimal x by maximising/minimising the objective function $f(x)$ over a given space X.

9.2.3.2 Steps of GA

1. *Start*: Generate random population.
2. *Evaluation*: Calculate the fitness of each chromosome in the population.
3. *Variation*: Repeat the following steps:
   a) *Selection*: Select two parents according to their fitness.
   b) *Crossover*: Perform crossover according to crossover probability.
   c) *Mutation*: Mutate each offspring according to mutation probability.
   d) *Acceptance*: Add offspring to new population.
4. If the termination condition is not satisfied, go to step 2.
5. Stop.

9.2.4 Learning Algorithms

Learning algorithms [16–17] play a significant role in the design of an automated and intelligent disease prediction system. Machine learning automates analytical model building through a data analysis method. Machine learning algorithms are traditionally divided into three categories: supervised learning [16], unsupervised learning [17] and reinforcement learning [17]. Predictive models are developed using supervised learning algorithms. This type of learning algorithm builds a realistic model using set of input and output training data to make the predictions for the response to new data. Supervised learning algorithms include artificial neural network (ANN) [16],

Bayesian method [27], decision tree [28], ensemble method [29], etc. Unsupervised learning algorithms are used to develop descriptive models. This type of algorithm uses a known set of input data to analyse and discover a pattern within but othe utput is known. Two important examples are clustering and dimension reduction. K-means clustering [15] and k-median clustering [15] are the two important unsupervised algorithms. Semi-supervised learning [16–17] falls between supervised learning and unsupervised learning. This type of learning method uses labelled and unlabelled data on a training dataset. Classification and regression techniques [16–17] are similar to semi-supervised learning.

Classification [16–17] is a major research area in the field of data mining [8–9] for the static as well as dynamic environment. Correct classification analysis serves a better understanding of the underlying data. Recently the structure of the different dataset is so difficult to understand directly, so it is necessary to apply many machine learning tools for classification of the dataset [16–17]. These methods include the k-nearest neighbours (KNN) [16], Bayesian approaches [27], support vector machines [30], ANN [16] and decision trees [28]. Prediction of a single classifier depends on the training capability of the classifier on the data itself. Ensemble classification [16–17] is an efficient and combined approach of the decision of the base classifiers for the classification job in machine learning [31].

9.2.5 PREVIOUS WORKS ON DIABETES PREDICTION

Many researchers are working in this healthcare analytics domain for predicting diabetes to save people from this deadly disease.

In [32], the authors made predictions in the field of medical diagnosis by using different data mining algorithms on the same dataset and analysed their efficiency. Three algorithms such as naive Bayes (NB), ANN [16] and KNN [16] are implemented to design their own prediction model. Author found that ANN is performed best with 96% accuracy compared to NB with 95% accuracy and KNN with 91% accuracy. In [33], the authors used a logistics regression (LR) model to identify the risk factor for diabetes on p-value (p <0.005) and odds ratio (OR). They used NB, decision tree, Adaboost (AB) and LR classifiers for feature selection. In their proposed model, they compared four classifiers for three K2, K5 and K10 partition protocols to calculate the classification accuracy and reached 94.25% of accuracy for the K10 protocol.

In [34], the authors designed a framework for analyzing risk for diabetes mellitus type 2 by applying six classification methods through a questionnaire significant to diabetes, and the same was applied on a Pima Indian diabetes database (PIMA). The results compared with different statistical models also. In both cases, random forest produces the best accuracy of 94.10%, which is the highest among the rest. In [35], the authors build a prediction model using learning techniques to handle different complicacies related to retinopathy, nephropathy and neuropathy. They have considered seven features for their prediction model, which are age, gender, body mass index (BMI), blood glucose level, blood pressure, family history of diabetes and duration of diabetes. The method used for feature selection techniques also validated different subset of features, and finally NB and C4.5 classification techniques for the generation of classification rules, and predicted the risk factor for retinopathy and nephropathy as well. The method achieves 68% overall accuracy. In [36], the authors proposed a methodology to classify and detection of diabetes mellitus by F-score feature selection and fuzzy-SVM with a promising accuracy result. F-score is used to identify the important features of dataset, and fuzzy SVM is used to generate the fuzzy rules. They have applied their methodology on a Pima Indian diabetes dataset and achieved good accuracy in predicting the diabetes patients. In [37], the authors proposed a hybrid intelligent system combined by self-organizing map (SOM), neural network (NN) and principal component analysis (PCA) for diabetes classification using machine learning techniques. They used SOM clustering algorithms to cluster the dataset and NN for classification of diabetes types. They also used PCA for multivariate analysis as a dimension reduction technique to retain the desired information in the easiest way. PCA eliminates the redundant information from the diagnosis system. The combination of clustering, PCA and NN provides better classification accuracy. Several diagnosis systems have been developed to improve the decision making to reduce the time consumption in diagnosing a disease. In [38], authors proposed a diagnosis system using RST and results prove that the RST-based system produces better results than the rule-based system.

In our work, we are proposing a novel integrated RST-GA based method for the development of an intelligent, automated diabetic prediction model, a better approach to the developed method [38] with better classification results.

9.3   DEVELOPMENT OF THE DIABETES PREDICTION MODEL

In the proposed work, an intelligent diabetes prediction model has been developed to predict diabetes through important diabetes feature selection using RST [6] and GA [7]. There are a few number of research proposals [11–14] which tell about novel optimised approaches for feature selection from the diabetes data to predict the disease to help te mankind. In the proposed method, a novel Rough-GA–based feature selection technique is devised to select the important features (reduct) from the dataset, and after that, classification algorithms are applied on the reduced dataset to predict the disease. The fitness function of GA [7] is defined using the RST concepts only. As we know, designing the suitable or the appropriate fitness function is very important to get the good results. The proposed intelligent method can select the important feature subset R from the decision system S. The method starts with generating a random population of size P with the length of each binary chromosome is $|F| = N$. Consider $F = \{F_1, F_2, F_3 \ldots F_N\}$ and j-th bit of a chromosome chr corresponds to feature Fj. All '1' in chromosome chr corresponds a feature subset say, $F_1 \subseteq F$. To check if F_1 is the target feature subset of the system S, fitness value of chromosome chr is calculated. Here a heuristic is used to define the fitness function where a positive region overlapping value [39] between the Feature subset F_1 and the whole feature set F in S is considered and at the same time, the length of the feature subset F_1 is also taken care of. The positive region of S considering the whole feature set F and feature subset F_1 are $POS_F(D)$ and, $POS_{F_1}(D)$ respectively. Overlapping positive region $P_F(D) = POS_F(D) \cap POS_{F_1}(D)$ [39] actually depicts the number of objects in S correctly classified by both F and F_1. Here, importance is given to maximise the fitness value for getting the reduct or important feature subset. Fitness function $f(chr)$ for a chromosome chr is defined in equation (9.7) to compute the feature subset R of the system S.

$$f(chr) = \left(\left(\frac{P_F(D)}{|U|} \right) / F_1 \right) \qquad (9.7)$$

The overall procedure is summarised as follows:

Inputs: Decision system $DS = (U, F, D)$
Outputs: Feature subset R of S
Step I: Calculate the positive region $POS_F(D)$ of S with the feature set F.
Step II: Initialise the population of GA with population size = N. The chromosome length (N) is equal to the number of features in F.
Step III: Compute the fitness value of each chromosome chr in the population using $f(chr)$ defined in equation (9.7).
Step IV: Considering fitness value, the genes are chosen for the mating pool using the rank selection technique.
Step V: The chromosomes in the mating pool are operated using the uniform crossover operator and the mutation operator, having crossover probability cr_p and mutation rate, m_p.
Step VI: The chromosomes for the next generation are chosen with some percentage of replacement of the parent population.
Step VII: Step III to step VI are repeated until the GA converges.
Step VIII: The best chromosome of the GA, after it has terminated, forms the feature subset R of the entire system S.

9.4   EXPERIMENTAL RESULTS

To measure the performance of the proposed method, a benchmark diabetes dataset with 768 instances with eight numeric features were collected from UC Irvine machine learning repository (UCI) [40]. The proposed model is developed using the Python programming language.

The results achieved from the proposed feature selection technique are compared with some standard feature selection methods such as 'Correlated Feature Subset Evaluator'(CFS) [41], 'Consistency Subset Evaluator'(CON) [42], and 'Relief-F' [43] from the Weka tool [44]. Later, comparative analysis is also done based on the classification accuracies achieved on the reduced datasets. We considered standard classifiers such as NB [27], partial decision tree algorithm (PART) [45], random forest [21], bagging [46], tree-based classifier (J48) [28] and multi-layer perceptron (MLP) [47].

Experiments were carried out to measure the performance of the algorithm, where the proposed method is compared with the benchmark feature selection techniques. The main goal of the experiments were on major issues like number of features, classification accuracy and execution efficiency. Experiments are performed using the k-folds cross validation method [48].Here we have taken the k value as 10.

TABLE 9.1

Prediction Results Obtained for Diabetes Dataset

Dataset (#original Features)	Methods (#features)	Classifiers (%)					
		NB	Bagging	PART	Random Forest	J48	MLP
PIDD (8)	Whole Data (8)	76.30	75.65	74.47	73.43	73.82	75.13
	CFS (4)	77.40	75.10	72.08	70.31	74.28	75.16
	CON (4)	76.77	76.07	71.82	72.87	72.32	75.07
	Relief-F (5)	76.19	75.24	72.07	72.81	72.01	73.21
	Proposed Method (4)	**77.47**	**75.13**	**72.13**	**73.30**	**74.86**	**75.26**

After certain values are tested experimentally, GA parameter values have been fixed as follows: population size (N) = 200, crossover probability (cr_p) = 0.9 and mutation rate (m_p) = 0.001.

The original number of features, number of features after applying the proposed and existing feature selection methods and the classification accuracies (%) on the reduced data are computed and listed in Table 9.1. The detail accuracy and other statistical parameter values of the classifiers [49] of the proposed method are also given later after the table.

After applying the proposed method on the Primary Immuno Deficiency Disease (PIDD) data [40], the following important features are selected: 'Plasma glucose concentration', 'BMI', 'Diabetes pedigree function' and 'Age in years' to predict the diabetes disease. Now classification accuracies obtained by proposed and existing methods are given in Table 9.1.

The detail classification results of the proposed method through the Weka tool [44] are given in Table 9.2. As we know, accuracy [49] is not only the single parameter to describe the goodness of the classifier, so other measures like precision [49], recall [49], F-measure [49] and Fall_out [49] have been evaluated for each of the classes, and finally the average of these measures are given for the proposed method.

Results achieved from the diabetes dataset prove that the proposed method generates better or similar prediction results as compared to the standard feature selection and classification methods. Hence, we can say that the proposed method selects the most important features with better classification performance.

Other benchmark datasets collected from the UCI repository [40] prove the effectiveness of the method. Table 9.3 provides the results of the experiment and shows that the proposed method is better compared to other standard methods in terms of selecting the feature subset as well as the classification accuracies.

Table 9.4 describes the results of the detail statistical parameters of the considered classifiers. Detail results prove that the proposed model is good in terms of selecting the important features to give not only the high classification accuracy, but all

TABLE 9.2
Detail Statistical Results Obtained for Diabetes Dataset

Dataset	Classification Methods	Classifier Parameters			
		Precision	Recall	F-Measure	Fall_out
PIDD (8)	NB	0.770	0.775	0.769	0.298
	Bagging	0.746	0.751	0.747	0.311
	PART	0.726	0.721	0.723	0.321
	Random Forest	0.736	0.733	0.734	0.306
	J48	0.742	0.749	0.743	0.315
	MLP	0.749	0.753	0.75	0.308

TABLE 9.3
Prediction Results Obtained for Other Datasets

Dataset (#original features)	Feature Selection Methods (#features)	Classifier Accuracy (%)					
		NB	Bagging	PART	Random Forest	J48	MLP
Breast Cancer (9)	CFS (4)	95.71	94.85	94.34	94.42	94.56	94.13
	CON (5)	95.99	94.70	94.50	94.70	93.56	94.56
	Relief-F (5)	95.93	94.82	93.46	94.01	93.75	94.27
	Proposed Method (3)	**95.72**	**94.87**	**94.98**	**95.33**	**93.89**	**95.32**
Dermatology (33)	CFS (9)	98.76	98.06	98.10	98.64	98.07	98.62
	CON (9)	98.52	98.25	98.21	98.73	98.86	98.67
	Relief-F (11)	98.72	98.45	98.50	98.48	98.76	98.46
	Proposed Method (9)	**99.85**	**98.85**	**98.76**	**98.90**	**98.90**	**99.31**
Mushroom (21)	CFS (4)	97.52	96.01	97.01	97.19	97.01	97.01
	CON (5)	98.52	98.85	98.67	99.01	99.05	98.16
	Relief-F (5)	97.04	98.03	98.12	98.22	98.10	98.10
	Proposed Method (3)	**99.86**	**99.84**	**98.80**	**99.03**	**99.00**	**98.26**

other measures are also providing very promising results in terms of evaluating the classifier.

9.5 CONCLUSION

A novel rough-GA–based expert healthcare system has been developed to predict diabetes by selecting the important disease features to improve the rate of classification.

TABLE 9.4

Detail Statistical Results for the Other Dataset

Dataset with Selected Number of Features Generated by the Proposed Method	Classification Methods	Classifier Parameters			
		Recall	Fall_out	Precision	F-Measure
Dermatology (9)	NB	0.98	0.01	0.98	0.98
	PART	0.99	0.01	0.99	0.98
	Bagging	0.99	0.02	0.98	0.98
	J48	0.98	0.02	0.97	0.98
	MLP	0.99	0.01	0.98	0.97
	Random Forest	0.98	0.02	0.98	0.99
Mushroom (3)	NB	0.99	0.01	0.98	0.98
	PART	0.99	0.01	0.98	0.99
	Bagging	0.99	0.01	0.98	0.98
	J48	0.97	0.03	0.97	0.97
	MLP	0.99	0.01	0.96	0.97
	Random Forest	0.99	0.01	0.98	0.99
Breast Cancer (3)	NB	0.96	0.04	0.96	0.96
	PART	0.95	0.05	0.96	0.96
	Bagging	0.95	0.05	0.95	0.95
	J48	0.94	0.06	0.94	0.94
	MLP	0.95	0.05	0.94	0.95
	Random Forest	0.95	0.05	0.95	0.94

The method gives very good classification results through optimal feature selection process efficiently. The advantages of our proposed method is that it can select a more compact and optimal feature subset with good classification accuracy. The method is a generalised one and can be used for the prediction of other diseases too. In spite of these benefits, some more experiments need to be conducted for the bigger datasets with more samples with big data approaches.

9.6 REFERENCES

[1] World Health Organization, *Diabetes Statistics Reports for the World*, March, 2021. www.who.int/diabetes/en/.

[2] V.V. Vijayan and C. Anjali, "Prediction and Diagnosis of Diabetes Mellitus – A Machine Learning Approach," IEEE Recent Advances in Intelligent Computational Systems (RAICS), 2015.

[3] P. Indoria and Y.K. Rathore, "A Survey: Detection and Prediction of Diabetes Using Machine Learning Techniques," *International Journal of Engineering Research &Technology (IJERT)*, vol. 7, issue 3, 2018, ISSN: 2278-0181.

[4] D. Brown, A. Aldea, R. Harrison, C. Martin and I. Bayley, "Temporal Case-Based Reasoning for Type 1 Diabetes Mellitusbolus Insulin Decision Support," *Artificial Intelligence in Medicine, Science Direct*, vol. 85, pp. 28–42, 2018.

[5] P. Sonar and K.J. Malini, "Diabetes Prediction Using Different Machine Learning Approaches," IEEE Third International Conference on Computing Methodologies and Communication (ICCMC), 2019.

[6] Z. Pawlak, "Rough Set Theory and Its Applications to Data Analysis," *Cybernetics and Systems*, vol. 29, pp. 661–688, 1998.

[7] J. Li, J. Chen and H.Q. Min, "A Classification Method Based on Immune Genetic Algorithm," International Conference on Machine Learning and Cybernetics, 2012.

[8] Y. Anzai, *Pattern Recognition and Machine Learning*. Elsevier, Chapter 4, 2012.

[9] M. Fatima and M. Pasha, "Survey of Machine Learning Algorithms for Disease Diagnostic," *Journal of Intelligent Learning Systems and Applications*, vol. 9, issue, 1, 2017.

[10] P.A. Devijver and J. Kittler, *Pattern Recognition: A Statistical Approach*. Prentice Hall, 1982.

[11] S. Mishra, P.K. Mallick, H.K. Tripathy, A.K. Bhoi and A. González-Briones, "Performance Evaluation of a Proposed Machine Learning Model for Chronic Disease Datasets Using an Integrated Attribute Evaluator and an Improved Decision Tree Classifier," *Applied Sciences*, vol. 10, 2020.

[12] A.K. Das, S. Sengupta and S. Chakrabarty, "Reduct Generation by Formation of Directed Minimal Spanning Tree using Rough Set Theory," *Advances in Intelligent and Soft Computing*, Springer, vol. 132, pp.127–135, 2012.

[13] S. Sengupta and A.K. Das, "Single Reduct Generation by Attribute Similarity Measurement Based on Relative Indiscernibility," *Second International Conference, Part II. Springer LNICST Series*, vol. 85, pp. 476–487, 2012.

[14] J. Liang, F. Wang, C. Dang and Y. Qian, "A Group Incremental Approach to Feature Selection Applying Rough Set Technique," *IEEE Trans Knowl Data Eng*, vol. 26, issue 2, pp. 294–308, 2014.

[15] W. Chen, S. Chen, H. Zhang and T. Wu, "A Hybrid Prediction Model for Type 2 Diabetes Using K-Means and Decision Tree," IEEE International Conference on Software Engineering and Service Science (ICSESS), 2017.

[16] F.Y. Osisanwo, J.E.T. Akinsola, O. Awodele, J.O. Hinmikaiye, O. Olakanmi and J. Akinjobi, "Supervised Machine Learning Algorithms: Classification and Comparison," *International Journal of Computer Trends and Technology (IJCTT)*,vol. 48, issue 3, pp. 128–138, 2017.

[17] N. Dogan and Z. Tanrikulu, "A Comparative Analysis of Classification Algorithms in Data Mining for Accuracy, Speed and Robustness," *Information Technology and Management*, vol. 14, pp. 105–124, 2013.

[18] V. Arunasakthi and L. Kamatchi-Priya, "A Review on Linear and Non-Linear Dimentionality Reduction Techniques," *Machine Learning and Applications: An International Journal (MLAIJ)*, vol. 1, issue 1, pp. 65–76, 2014.

[19] A.K. Das and J. Sil, "Dimensionality Reduction and Optimum Feature Selection inDesigning Efficient Classifiers," Springer Verlag Lecture Notes, International Conference on Swarm Evolutionary and Memetic Computing, 2010.

[20] R. Aminah and A.H. Saputro,"Diabetes Prediction System Based on Iridology Using Machine Learning," IEEE 6th International Conference on Information Technology, Computer and Electrical Engineering (ICITACEE), 2019.

[21] W. Xu, J. Zhang, Q. Zhang and X. Wei, "Risk Prediction of Type II Diabetes Based on Random Forest Model," Third International Conference on Advances in Electrical, Electronics, Information, Communication and Bio-Informatics (AEEICB), 2017.

[22] A. Jain and D. Zongker, "Feature Selection: Evaluation, Application, and Small Sample Performance," IEEE Transactions on Pattern Analysis and Machine Intelligence, 1997, https://doi.org/10.1109/34.574797.

[23] C.M. Bishop, Ed., "Neural Networks and Machine Learning, NATO ASI Series," Series F: Computer and Systems Sciences, 168, Springer-Verlag, 1998.

[24] K. Thangavel and A. Pethalakshmi, "Dimensionality Reduction Based on Rough Set Theory: A Review," *Applied Soft Computing*, vol. 9, issue 1, pp. 1–12, 2009.

[25] R. Jensen and Q. Shen, "Rough Set-Based Feature Selection: A Review," *Rough Computing: Theories, Technologies and Applications*, 2007, doi:10.4018/978-1-59904-552-8.ch003.

[26] N. Hoque, H.A. Ahmed and D.K. Bhattacharyya, "A Fuzzy Mutual Information-Based Feature Selection Method for Classification," *Fuzzy Information and Engineering*, Elsevier, vol. 8, pp. 355–384, 2016.

[27] V. Roth and T. Lange, "Bayesian Class Discovery in Microarray Dataset," *IEEE Transaction on Biomed Eng*, vol. 51, issue 5, pp. 707–718, 2004.

[28] S. Teli and P. Kanikar, "A Survey on Decision Tree Based Approaches in Data Mining," *International Journal of Advanced Research in Computer Science and Software Engineering*, vol. 5, issue 4, pp. 613–617, 2015.

[29] S. Al-Azani and E.S.M. El-Alfy, "Using Word Embedding and Ensemble Learning for Highly Imbalanced Data Sentiment Analysis in Short Arabic Text," *International Conference on Ambient Systems, Elsevier Networks and Technologies*, vol. 109C, pp. 359–366, 2017.

[30] A.K. Das, A. Paul and J. Sil, "Generation and Analysis of Classifiers Using Reducts and Support Vector Machines," *International Conference on Intelligent Systems and Networks*, pp. 159–164, India, 2009.

[31] D. Sisodiaa and D.S. Sisodia, "Prediction of Diabetes Using Classification Algorithms," *Internatio*nal Conference on Computational Intelligence and Data Science (ICCIDS), 2018.

[32] A. Sarwar and V. Sharma, *Comparative Analysis of Machine Learning Techniques in Prognosis of Type II Diabetes*, AI & Society, Springer, vol. 29, pp. 123–129, 2014.

[33] M. Maniruzzaman, M.J. Rahman, B. Ahammed and M.M. Abedin, *Classification and Prediction of Diabetes Diseaseusing Machine Learning Paradigm*, Health Information Science and Systems, Springer Nature Switzerland AG, 2020.

[34] N.P. Tigga and S. Garg, "Prediction of Type 2 Diabetes using Machine Learning Classification Methods," International Conference on Computational Intelligence and Data Science (ICCIDS), 2019.

[35] C. Fiarni, E.M. Sipayung and S. Maemunah, "Analysis and Prediction of Diabetes Complication Disease Using Data Mining Algorithm," The Fifth Information Systems International Conference, 2019.

[36] R.B. Lukmantoa, Suharjitoa, A. Nugrohoa and H. Akbara, "Early Detection of Diabetes Mellitus Using Feature Selection and Fuzzy Support Vector Machine," 4th International Conference on Computer Science and Computational Intelligence (ICCSCI), 2019.

[37] M. Nilashi, O. Ibrahim, M. Dalvi, H. Ahmadi and L.Shahmoradi, "Accuracy Improvement for Diabetes Disease Classification: A Case on a Public Medical Dataset," *Fuzzy Information and Engineering*, vol. 9, pp. 345–357, 2017.

[38] S. Anouncia, S. Margret, J. Clara, P. Jeevitha and T. Nandhini, "Design of a Diabetic Diagnosis System Using Rough Sets," *Cybernetics and Information Technologies*, vol. 13, 2013, doi:10.2478/cait-2013-0030.

[39] A. Das, S. Sengupta and S. Bhattacharyya, "A Group Incremental Feature Selection for Classification Using Rough Set Theory Based Genetic Algorithm," *Applied Soft Computing*, vol. 65, 2018, doi:10.1016/j.asoc.2018.01.040.

[40] P. Murphy and W. Aha, *UCI Repository of Machine Learning Databases*, 1996, www.ics.uci.edu/mlearn/MLRepository.html.

[41] M.A. Hall, "Correlation-Based Feature Selection for Machine Learning," PhD thesis, Dept. of Computer Science, University of Waikato, Hamilton, 1998.

[42] H. Liu and R. Setiono, "A Probabilistic Approach to Feature Selection: A Filter Solution," Proc.13th Int'l Conf. Machine Learning, pp. 319–327, 1996.

[43] Y. Zhao, L. Fang, L. Cui and L. Bai, "Application of Data Mining for Predicting Hemodynamics Instability During Pheochromocytoma Surgery," *BMC Medical Informatics and Decision Making*, Article number 20, vol. 165, 2020.

[44] WEKA, *Machine Learning Software*, www.cs.waikato.ac.nz/.

[45] C. Bishop, *Pattern Recognition and Machine Learning*, 1st ed., Springer, 2010.

[46] S.K. Somasundaram and P. Alli, "A Machine Learning Ensemble Classifier for Early Prediction of Diabetic Retinopathy," *Journal of Medical Systems, Springer Link*, vol. 41, Article number: 201, 2017.

[47] M. Jahangir, M. Ahmed, H. Afzal and K. Khurshid, "An Expert System for Diabetes Prediction Using Auto Tuned Multi-Layer Perceptron," IEEE Intelligent Systems Conference, 2017.

[48] M.K. Hasan, M.A. Alam, D. Das, E. Hossain and M.Hasan, "Diabetes Prediction Using Ensembling of Different Machine Learning Classifiers," *IEEE Access*, vol. 8, pp. 76516–76531, 2020.

[49] E. Alpaydin, *Introduction to Machine Learning*, 2nd edition. PHI, 2010.

10 Blockchain for the Healthcare Sector
Application and Challenges

Richi Chhabra[1], Mohammad Shahnawaz Nasir[2],
Khalid Ali Qidwai[2] and Mohammad Shabbir Alam[2]
[1] Deenbadhu Chotu Ram University of
Science and Technology, India
[2] Jazan University, Saudi Arabia

CONTENTS

DOI: 10.1201/9781003217107-10

10.1 INTRODUCTION

10.1.1 BACKGROUND AND WORKING OF BLOCKCHAIN

The blockchain technology and architecture were developed in 2008 and launched in 2009 [1]. Blockchain came up as a technology that empowered bitcoin (a cryptocurrency) by Satoshi Nakamoto with his white paper in 2009 [2]. It aims at recording and tracking valuable information through the collection and maintenance of segregated ledgers. Blockchain stores information in batches called blocks, and these blocks are connected to each other in a sequence to form a line or a string of blocks. These blocks are distributed among various members associated with that specific network. These are easily accessible and are called open ledger chains, as all the participants have access to the information.

Every time a user wants to share data with another user using a network, they get into a transaction. Each transaction is represented by a block. Also, to add a new block in existing chain, it needs verification from all the hubs in the network [3]. Once verified, the block is added to the chain and is assigned a unique code called a hash. Information about the hash of the previous block is also added in the block, i.e. each block has its own hash and the hash of the previous block in the chain [4]. After being added to the block chain, the block is accessible to all the participants in the chain.

Blockchain operates by storing data in ledger records. The information is distributed among various blocks, and these blocks together make up a blockchain. The key characteristics that make the blockchain technology desirable are non-centralisation, privacy, verifiability and persistency [1]. These benefits not only help reducing cost but also increases efficiency.

A blockchain design works in a peer-to-peer circulated network providing two essential benefits: more noteworthy registering power than a centralised engineering, since the processing force of all hubs is consolidated together, and network trustworthiness, in light of the fact that there is a single failure. Blockchain can likewise accomplish and keep up with information trustworthiness in conveyed frameworks because of the great degree of safety carried out in blockchain innovation [5].

Blockchain as a distributed ledger system allows autonomous operators to work together in the ecosystem in a way that ensures clarity and time-stamped recording of the data to bring improvement in handling speed, economic benefits and security, while reducing risk and cost [6]. In contrast to conventional ways of storing the data at a central location, the blockchain is based on peer-to-peer (P2P) network, wherein numerous duplicates of the information are stored in distinct devices. A peer permits a set of computing assets to be utilised by other members without the requirement for focal coordination by servers. Such hubs can take various jobs inside the organisation while guaranteeing protection, coordination and security of business information trades [7].

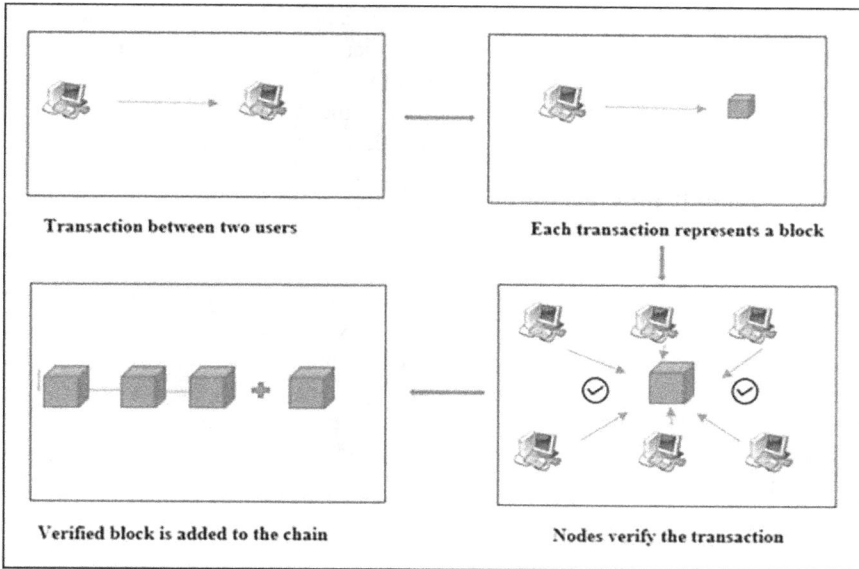

FIGURE 10.1 Process of blockchain.

In light of shared organisations, one of the advantages of utilising blockchain is it refreshes constantly, leaving no space for mediators and related expenses [7]. Being impervious to changes, blockchain offers a straightforward climate where medical experts and patients alike can get to their records without added costs [7]. It additionally builds security into the framework by lessening the probability of lost records.

The security of the blockchain is executed utilising cryptographic keys, a conveyed network and an organisation overhauling convention by recording data in a block. When data (for example, a financial transaction) is approved, meta-information is recorded in a block and cannot be questioned, eliminated or adjusted without the information and consent of the people who made the record, such as the organisation.

Monetary usage of blockchain applications should be referenced initially on the basis of Bitcoin, which is as of now the principal application case for this innovation. Bitcoin is an advanced form of money, dependent on shared systems administration innovation and public key (a huge mathematical worth which is utilised to scramble information) cryptography. Complete exchanges are unknown and irreversible as shown in Figure 10.1. Also the utilisation of a distributed conveyed record makes it essential for all gatherings to affirm the exchanges. The origination of Bitcoin was traced back to 2008 when Satoshi Nakamoto conceptualised a hypothetical idea, and since then this terminology has seen a quick ascent being developed, reception and general use as a digital exchange currency.

10.2 LITERATURE REVIEW

10.2.1 KEY CHARACTERISTICS OF BLOCKCHAIN

10.2.1.1 Decentralisation

Centralised networks can be defined as networks in which communication, information and data enter into and leave through a central hub, which are in form of private servers. Decentralised capacity is a significant component of the blockchain innovation, and the reason for the upgraded security and validation of the information stored in the system. Decentralisation helps in sharing data among various users without any central authority [5]. The decentralisation process is one of the most common ways of segregating the files from one significant server to multiple servers through blockchain's record.

10.2.1.2 Immutability

Information stored in a blockchain is immutable; it cannot be changed or modified easily. For it to be changed it is required to have a consensus of a minimum 51% of peers participating in the blockchain [8]. Blockchain is not dependent on any central authority; rather there are multiple nodes, all the hubs which are part of the chain and have a replica of the digital ledger. To add an exchange transaction, each hub needs to actually look at its legitimacy. If the majority of hubs reach the consensus, a new block is added to the chain. This adds to transparency and makes it safe from any fraudulent attacks. Once the new block is added to the network, no user can alter it or delete it.

10.2.1.3 Enhanced Security

Blockchain offers enhanced security, as there is no controlling central authority, and all the transactions are to be verified by the hubs; thus no one can make alterations in the chain without consensus. All the information in the blockchain is based on cryptography. All the text is encrypted and stored in form of a hash. Each block in the chain stores its hash and the hash of the previous block. If any information is to be updated even in one of the blocks, the hash of subsequent blocks will also change, which would not need large computing power, thus enhancing security.

10.2.1.4 Consensus

A blockchain is supported by multiple hubs, and transactions without a prior trust relationship are associated with a peer-to-peer network. For the blockchain to be helpful, there should be some technique by which the hubs can commonly concur upon adding the next legitimate block in the chain.

The two most broadly used techniques for building up such an appropriated consensus are summed up as follows:

- Proof-of-work is a consensus algorithm for block approval where hubs compete with each other to create the following block by using computational work to solve a difficult numerical issue. The hub solves the problem first, and showing proof of its work, acquires and adds the next block in the chain. This algorithm requires extensive computing capabilities to complete the mathematical problems.
- Proof-of-stake avoids the calculation of the computational test, as a randomly chosen node is selected and is given the chance to create each block. The likelihood of choice is weighted by each node's degree of existing stake in the framework. The higher the investment in the blockchain, the greater the chances of being selected for adding up a new block in the framework. Ray et al., 2021 suggested proof of stake is more suitable than proof of work for the e-healthcare framework [9].

10.3 TYPES OF BLOCKCHAIN

Currently blockchain technology is categorised into two parts: public and private blockchain. Public blockchain gives access of transaction and information to all the participants to participate in a consensus-creating process. The agreement systems like Bitcoin's proof of work in open blockchains requires all the nodes in the network to arrive at the agreement on the condition of exchanges. Public blockchains likewise have less data security because of their intrinsic nature. The public blockchains depends upon information process prompting permanent information storage. Further, in open blockchains the whole hub should concur on any change as it records similar data. Accordingly, any change ought to be recorded in all succeeding blocks [10]. On the other hand, in a private blockchain framework all the nodes in the network are a part of the same organisation. The number of participants authorised are limited in number, thus it has a strong data privacy in the network. In order to make any change, all the nodes can come to a consensus and the necessary changes can be made [10]. Public blockchains require no outsider confirmation, thus private blockchain might be more important for being utilised in medical care. With completely private blockchains, consents are permitted uniquely to all the stakeholders of an association, yet read authorisations can in any case be public or limited to a few or all members of the organisation, thus giving a more noteworthy degree of security. Along these lines, keeping patients' clinical records, adjusting balances, returning exchanges and changing the blockchain rules would all be able to be effectively accomplished by an organisation or a wellbeing association running their private blockchain.

There are likewise other blockchains which share some common ground with both public and private blockchains. These are called semi-private blockchains, and they are controlled by a solitary organisation or association. However, they award admittance to clients, mainly to associations, that satisfy specific pre-set accreditations or measures [7]. Such frameworks also try to figure out how an organisation deals with their private applications and its utilisation; examples might include storage of files by government authorities, possession records, public records, medical services expenses and repayment information. Later on, these semi-private blockchains could fundamentally affect medical services strategy [11].

10.4 SMART CONTRACTS

Smart contracts are certain codes and protocols which are followed by all the parties entering the agreement. They are an essential part of the applications that are based on blockchain technology [12]. They are different from the traditional contracts, as traditional contracts are executed by a third party, which adds to the cost and time. Smart contracts are self-executing programs [13] that automatically execute themselves after the terms of the contract have been fulfilled. Smart contracts are stored and copied in the blockchain network [14].

With the healthcare sector going through a digital revolution and using blockchain technology in its operations, it is important to ensure security to all the patients regarding their data. The healthcare sector empowers various stakeholders to work cooperatively and proficiently for better and upgraded clinical benefits. Thus, formalising suitable guidelines while framing smart medical care contracts, incorporating timely concerns and providing approvals of concerned stakeholders can truly enhance the acceptance of such agreements. Therefore, blockchain applications in medical care should sync the information provided by patients and associated organisation partners. The acknowledgement and approval of this healthcare information is a perquisite condition for the formation and fostering of smart healthcare contracts [12]. The purpose of this whole process is to segregate the information and channelising its accessibility only to the concerned parties.

10.5   BLOCKCHAIN AND HEALTHCARE

Blockchain technology has been popular in areas of finance, banking, real estate and healthcare. The finance part of the blockchain has been popular and has been researched thoroughly. However, application of blockchain in healthcare (Figure 10.2) and the medical sector is getting popular among researchers [15], since it one of the most regulated industries, and blockchain can positively impact the healthcare sector. The attributes of the blockchain, which are its decentralised nature, receptiveness and autonomy, may offer a remarkable answer for medical services. More extensive pertinence of the innovation clears its direction into various parts of medical care, including wearables and progress of the clinical examination. The medical care area has developing requests for blockchain improvements, and a new review by Deloitte shows that the conventional business is effectively investigating new roads for the utilisation of the blockchain to address its basic necessities [6].

Blockchain is a decentralised dispersed record of all the proceedings executed among various stakeholders. This virtual record is repeated and composed of cooperatively using cryptographic codes and dispersed approval of all peers. The business rationale is inserted in the record and is regularly executed along with exchanges utilising appropriated applications. The innovation empowers anonymous exchanges that are difficult to alter, eradicate or debate. Exchanges are considered irreversible with no unified authority controlling the transactions, and in the healthcare area, specifically, sharing of patients' health data is managed electronically among different stakeholders in the area [16]. All the parties engaged with the assortment, storage and handling of clinical data will approach a private and straightforward circulated record that can likewise further develop healthcare research. The innovation tries to build up a base limit within which the authority and responsibility can be delegated to the healthcare specialist. Blockchain innovations likewise can follow up on clinical information sharing, either through putting away the actual information or providing guidelines on who can get to that information (possibly through savvy contracts), getting patient and supplier identification and accreditations, enhancing the management of the medical supply chain, information sharing and assent for research and clinical preliminaries (counting information adaptation) and protection and settlement of insurance claims and decrease of false practices. Patients connect with a number of medical care suppliers during various stages of life, leaving information dispersed throughout.

10.5.1   HEALTHCARE DATA COLLECTION

Technology for monitoring health includes wearables, which creates a huge amount of personal data. Appropriate administration and safe extraction of this data are significant for information-driven choices in the medical care framework. Additional healthcare data is also generated by day-to-day administration services and operating activities performed by healthcare providers. Healthcare data is not only huge in size but also diverse and dynamic. It is non-uniform and dependent on various factors. Since individuals meet a huge number of healthcare providers throughout their lives, and the data is often is dispersed and fragmented, making it difficult to access, use and share.

10.6 APPLICATIONS OF BLOCKCHAIN IN HEALTHCARE

10.6.1 MEDICAL RECORDS MANAGEMENT

Healthcare information is a data-sensitive sector, as a huge amount of data is generated, dispersed and circulated on a regular basis. It is essential that the data is stored and circulated with care due to its sensitive nature and security and privacy concerns [17]. In the healthcare sector it is important that the data shared is safe, secure and scalable, as it is not only used for diagnosis but also for decision making. Doctors and healthcare professionals ought to be capable to share the clinical information of their patients in a way that the privacy of the patient is maintained and data is shared in timely manner to guarantee that the concerned doctors are well aware of the patient's ailments. Patients are the medium of possessing and controlling admittance to their medical care information. This eliminates all deterrents to patients gaining duplicates of their medical care records or moving them to another medical services provider. Blockchain might ensure clinical information can't be changed by anyone, including doctors and patients. Also the data stored in blockchain is encrypted, which makes it safe, as it cannot be read by a malicious party. Blockchain also reduces the danger of patient recordkeeping because information is put away on a decentralised organisation; there is no single organisation or authority that can be ransacked or hacked to get an enormous number of patient records.

10.6.2 MEDICAL EDUCATION

Medical education is one of the areas where use of blockchain can prove to be more useful. Blockchain can be used to keep the academic records of medical professionals even before they graduate from medical school. It can also be used to keep a record of understudy accomplishments all through the educational program and archive skills obtained through a scope of contrast clinical settings and strengths, consequently going about as an advanced record framework for each stakeholder. Also, in light of the fact that clinical training is a course of long-lasting learning, information on this digital ledger could keep on developing, adding conferences attended, each article composed and all successful procedures performed. Clinical experts could then choose if they might want to share this data and, along these lines, confirmed certificates could be given all the more effectively, with the cycle additionally being more feasible and secure. Specialist versatility would increment incredibly, while superfluous desk work and endorsements would be limited [11].

10.6.3 DRUG SUPPLY MANAGEMENT

The importance of blockchain has been realised by drug manufacturers. As per the World Health Organization, 10% of medications are counterfeit around the world; in developing nations the number ascends up to 30%. Such malpractices in the pharmaceutical industry not only affect the lifestyle products but have severe impact on drugs related to cardiovascular diseases, pain relievers, contraceptives, antibiotics and other prescribed drugs. This can have a severe effect on the human life. Some drug-manufacturing organisations have effectively begun carrying out blockchain in the drug supply chain management system, since fake medications are a significant threat to the health industry and a risk for the wellbeing of patients, especially in the developing nations [18]. Pham et al., 2019 suggested a practical framework for application of an anti-counterfeit drug system, so as to avoid circulation of fake drugs in the market [19]. The study suggested application of Ethereum blockchain and Inter Planetary File System (IPFS) networks to give a secure and dependable framework, which can trace the origin of medicines. In sync with the listed advantages, the applications of blockchain must be promoted with concerned populations so that they can verify and validate the authenticity of items through an analysis of their identity numbers and associated tags. This mechanism can be used to track and stop the cross-selling of medicinal and clinical drugs exhaustively to some extent [11].

10.6.4   Implementing Public Health Policies

The outbreak of coronavirus highlighted the importance of public healthcare and the importance of public health data. Health data for the population is a powerful tool for analysing the data for a large group of people. It can be helpful in treating various medical conditions. Researchers have shown that funds can be used judiciously by healthcare stakeholders and insurance agencies for the execution of blockchain technology. Medical data that is encrypted and anonymous could be utilised by the drug organisations to improve and help customise drug development. Resources could be employed at the right place, and healthcare policies can be implemented by using a huge pool of patient data in public healthcare. Additionally, the Centers for Disease Control and Prevention (CDC) is examining the way blockchain can be put to use to share clinical information with various medical associations. Blockchain can possibly keep the information secure and concealed. It can simultaneously permit the medical experts to move the data and offer it as quickly as it is needed. The capability of blockchain innovation can be seen in the fields of medication, genomics, telemedicine, tele-observing, e-health, neuroscience and customised medical care applications by its system of balancing out and getting the informational index with which clients can associate through various kinds of transactions [17].

10.6.5   Health Insurance

Claims handling has been distinguished as an objective for blockchain upgrade, comprehensive of smoothing out process of preauthorisation entries, medical insurance claims settlement and checking for eligibility. A project has been developed by Massachusetts Institute of Technology Media Lab and Beth Israel Deaconess Medical Center called MedRec. It empowers patients to have command over who can get to their information and under what conditions, guaranteeing more smoothed out medical coverage and quicker and safer access for investment in biomedical examination [11]. The blockchain system has investigated claim processing through a decentralised infrastructure for medical care administration utilising non-fungible tokens. Claims settlement and related parts attached to shortening instalment cycles are additionally focused areas for the coordination of smart contracts application to mechanise and speed up.

Blockchain innovation has prompted enormous answers for conventional medical care space issues [20], for example, giving a protected framework and incorporating private wellbeing records. Blockchain can be utilised to give secure correspondence among partners and convey clinical reports productively.

10.6.6 ORGAN TRANSPLANT

Blockchain can revolutionise healthcare in the area of organ transplant. Organ transplant surgeries are subjected to various conditions and are also complicated. Finding a right donor can take several years. Various organs like heart, liver, kidney, lungs, pancreas and intestines can be transplanted. However, they go waste due to inefficiency in the system. Blockchain can be utilised to preserve the data related to

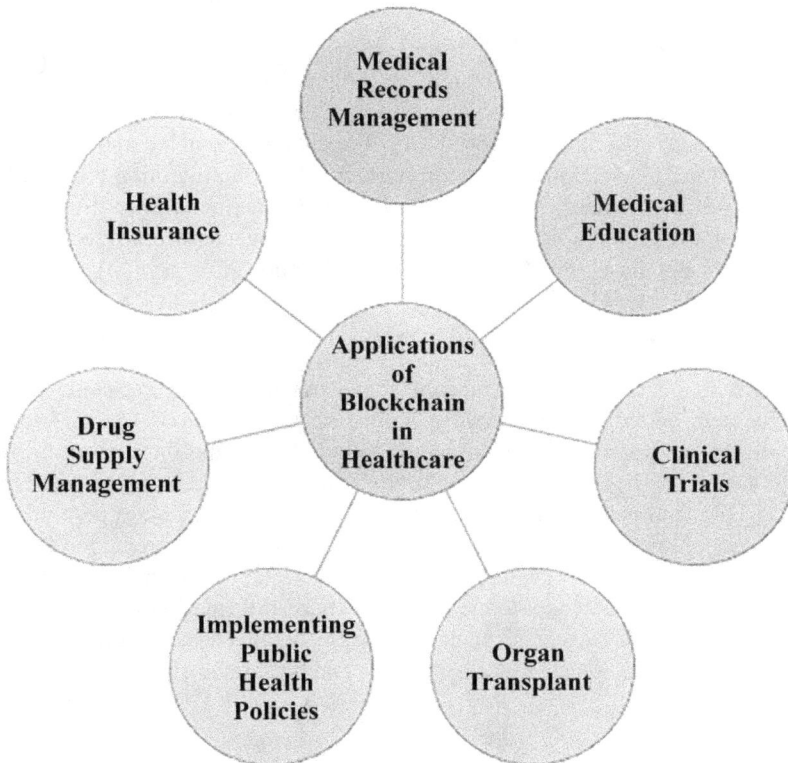

FIGURE 10.2 Application of blockchain in the healthcare sector.

organ donation and should be in sync with the local systems of hospitals so as to store updated information [21]. With the blockchain technology, as the data-related patient would be stored in one place, it would be easier to reach the right place at right time. Organtree is one such non-profit organisation that is bridging the gap between patients, donors and healthcare practitioners [22].

10.6.7 CLINICAL TRIALS

Clinical trial enables the controlled testing and viability of medicinal drugs resulting in the generation of large quantities of data. The interaction is costly, takes a couple of years to finish and without using any unfair means. It is essential to have a straightforward arrangement that allows anybody to audit the clinical reports and guarantee that the consequences of the preliminary testing are not altered. Blockchain can be an extraordinary innovation to work with clinical trials by giving information trustworthiness, and the validity of the archives could be confirmed. The disseminated network guarantees that no information can be changed without approved admittance [23].

10.7 BENEFITS OF USING BLOCKCHAIN TECHNOLOGY IN HEALTHCARE

10.7.1 ACCESS TO ACCURATE DATA

Digital records of the patients are usually not aligned or stored in one place. The data is scattered between the hospitals, clinics and insurance providers. So as to access the accurate data, it becomes important that the data is assembled and is stored in a safe place. Here, blockchain plays an important role by maintaining a record of all patient data at a one place. This empowers medical care experts to give effective, ideal and legitimate therapies to patients. Utilising blockchain innovation, medical care suppliers can have a total image of a patient's clinical history [24].

10.7.2 INTEROPERABILITY OF HEALTH DATA

Interoperability is defined as the ability of systems to use and exchange information. The electronic data generated by healthcare providers exists in different formats with differentiating technical specifications [25]. Thus, it becomes difficult to align and share the data. There might be certain cases wherein electronic health record (EHR) frameworks based on similar platforms are not interoperable on the grounds that they are intended to meet some particular requirements and inclinations of some specific hospital. The absence of standardised information is a significant issue that restricts the capacity to share information electronically for patient consideration. However, blockchain can solve this issue. All the data stored on blockchain is based on standardised codes, and thus are uniform and can be used by hospitals.

10.7.3 SECURITY

the healthcare sector has always been prone to cyber security attacks. Several organisations in this sector are based upon a centralised infrastructure, which stores and manages EHRs of the patients. Such systems are not safe and can become victim to malicious attacks. Hardware failure can also be the reason for loss of data, as the data is centralised. Blockchain networks follow uniform codes and are based upon the concept of decentralisation; thus the chances of loss of data can be reduced by storing all the electronic health data on the blockchain network and can be used by only a medical care facility with access to the network.

10.7.4 OPERATING COSTS

There is a high operating cost involved in the recovery and transfer of patient data. Most of the times, the patient's medical information is distributed across various medical facilities. Gathering this data from electronic sources and hard copies not only involves time but also huge handling cost. Blockchain innovation can help to lessen the operating expenses by reducing the involvement of third parties. Moreover, it can also collect and align data from wearables and other medical devices. Thus, it can help decrease the cost of healthcare facilities, as it helps them get easy access to healthcare data, rather than collecting it from multiple sources [24].

10.7.5 AUDIT OF MEDICAL DATA

The medical industry undergoes audits to check their performance, whether or not they follow specific arrangements, techniques, rules, guidelines and laws enforced by healthcare institutes. The auditing process helps in assessing the adequacy of a medical service through orderly and objective appraisals. Most of the medical data currently exists in traditional formats and needs to be audited manually. This not only hampers the auditing process but also affects its quality. Blockchain technology can work with the medical institute's innovation with medical services organisations to deal with their information in a certain way, so that it can be verified and cannot be meddled by any malicious attack. Auditing the blockchain-based healthcare information can be used to improve patient administration; also it can help in tracking and following all the necessary compliance by the medical organisations.

10.8 CHALLENGES OF APPLICATIONS OF BLOCKCHAIN IN HEALTHCARE

Whenever a new technology is developed and implemented, it involves several challenges. Blockchain technology is no different. Application of blockchain in the healthcare sector involves three categories of challenges: technical challenges, organisational challenges and social challenges (Figure 10.2).

10.8.1 TECHNICAL CHALLENGES

10.8.1.1 Scalability

One challenge commonly found in blockchain is scalability. Healthcare data is generated continuously due to the various wearable devices available. This regularly generated data not only requires storing capacities but also computational capabilities. The network might not be able to process a high number of transactions. Bitcoin

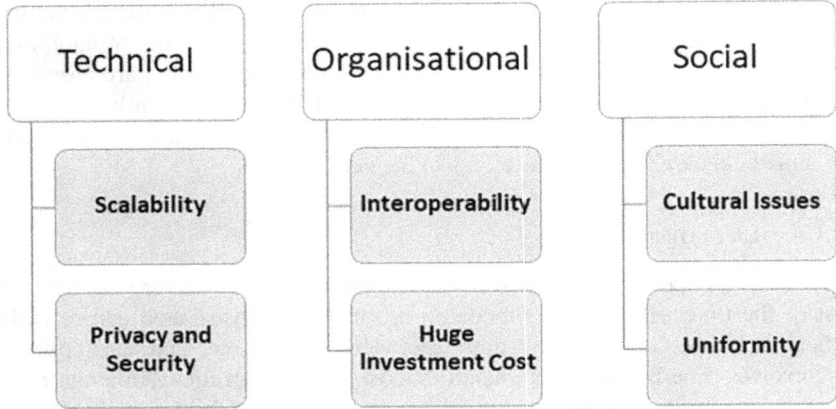

FIGURE 10.3 Challenges of applications of blockchain in healthcare.

can process 2–3 transactions per second, Ethereum can process 20 transactions per second, and VISA processes more than 1600 transaction per second [26]. A trade-off between storing limits and computational skill could restrict the adaptability of such medical care frameworks [12]. In this case, the healthcare service providers are not able to provide enough storing space and computational technology, and the potential for expanded centralisation and delay in information approval and affirmation develops as shown in Fig.10.3 [27].

10.8.1.2 Privacy and Security

In the conventional database management system there is a centralised authority which stores, manages and maintains the data. Contrary to the conventional database, blockchain technology is based upon the concept of decentralisation. There is no trusted third party to manage the data; all the data is accessible to all, which poses many security and privacy threats [17]. Healthcare data is all about confidentiality of the patient – it is given by the patient and is to be used for them. Therefore, it is unsafe to replicate all the information in each hub. Though blockchain provides and follows high-security protocols, the most concerning subject for the existing blockchain technology is keeping a record of personal identified information and electronic health records of patients [28].

10.8.2 Organisational Challenges

10.8.2.1 Huge Investment Cost

The blockchain-based healthcare architecture might involve high infrastructure and operations costs. The authorities and the healthcare sector actually need to identify the various types of development, expansion, operations and complete distribution costs for all the parties involved. Consequently, it is essential to track down the ideal ways of diminishing the general expense and assets for building such frameworks [12]. While the expense of setting up and working such a framework to transition from conventional healthcare data frameworks isn't identified yet, open-source advancements and the decentralisation of blockchain can assist with decreasing it.

10.8.2.2   Interoperability

Interoperability is another challenge that is common with blockchain. Healthcare data exists in multiple formats, and there are numerous blockchain networks available with different consensus models and different codes. Lack of standardisation has led to the challenge of interoperability, which further poses a barrier for seamless data sharing [17]. Certain standard need to be developed and used for the application of blockchain technology so to ensure uniformity and maximum utilisation of data.

10.8.3   SOCIAL CHALLENGES

10.8.3.1   Cultural Issues

A knowledge drift is needed to empower the reception of blockchain innovation in the medical services area. The existing healthcare frameworks is not only prone to data breaches but system failure, since it is operated manually and controlled centrally. Since blockchain and its applications in healthcare industry are fairly new, there is a dire need of skilled professionals who are able to handle the health records. Not only do they need IT know-how but also medical knowledge [29–30]. The existing blockchain network requires the right manpower to manage P2P networks. Since blockchain is a fairly new concept, it will take time for developers to adopt it [24]. Training programs can be developed and staff can undergo training so as to maximise the utilisation of blockchain technology.

10.8.3.2   Standardisation

For the successful arrangement in medical services applications, uniform norms should be characterised by authorised bodies. For instance, on account of medical care data stored on the blockchain, it ought to be clarified what information, size and configuration can be shared and which information is restricted. The lack of standardisation hampers the wide applicability of blockchain in the healthcare sector [15].

10.9   CONCLUSION

In this study, the integration of blockchain technology in the healthcare industry is discussed. The chapter discusses how using blockchain technology can help manage healthcare data. Blockchain, with its features like decentralisation, immutability and security, makes the healthcare data safe when compared to the existing data management system. The benefits and applications of blockchain technologies in healthcare were also explored and highlighted. The chapter also discusses various challenges that are posing barriers to the wide adaptability of blockchain technology in the healthcare sector. Blockchain technology has extensive scope to revolutionise the healthcare industry by providing ease of access of data to healthcare professionals and pharmaceutical companies, which they can use for providing better services to patients, reducing costs, providing data security to patient personally identifying information, and improving the industry overall.

10.10 REFERENCES

[1] Z. Zheng, S. Xie, H. Dai, X. Chen, and H. Wang, "An Overview of Blockchain Technology: Architecture, Consensus, and Future Trends," *Proc. – 2017 IEEE 6th Int. Congr. Big Data, BigData Congr. 2017*, pp. 557–564, 2017.

[2] S. Nakamoto, *Bitcoin: A Peer-to-Peer Electronic Cash System*, 2009. https://www.bibsonomy.org/bibtex/423c2cdff70ba0cd0bca55ebb164d770.

[3] N. Honest, "Blockchain Concept and Its Area of Applications," *Interdiscip. Res. Technol. Manag.*, June, pp. 331–335, 2021.

[4] A. A. Monrat, O. Schelén, and K. Andersson, "A Survey of Blockchain from the Perspectives of Applications, Challenges, and Opportunities," *IEEE Access*, vol. 7, pp. 117134–117151, 2019.

[5] H. D. Zubaydi, Y. W. Chong, K. Ko, S. M. Hanshi, and S. Karuppayah, "A Review on the Role of Blockchain Technology in the Healthcare Domain," *Electron.*, vol. 8, no. 6, pp. 1–29, 2019.

[6] Deloitte, *Breaking Blockchain Open Deloitte's 2018 Global Blockchain Survey*, 2018, https://www2.deloitte.com/lt/en/pages/legal/articles/innovation-blockchain-survey.html.

[7] M. Prokofieva and S. J. Miah, "Blockchain in Healthcare," *Australas. J. Inf. Syst.*, vol. 23, pp. 1–22, 2019.

[8] H. F. Atlam, *Blockchain with Internet of Things : Benefits, Challenges, and Future Directions*, June 2018. https://www.researchgate.net/publication/325486515_Blockchain_with_Internet_of_Things_Benefits_Challenges_and_Future_Directions.

[9] P. P. Ray, Di. Dash, K. Salah, and N. Kumar, "Blockchain for IoT-Based Healthcare: Background, Consensus, Platforms, and Use Cases," *IEEE Syst. J.*, vol. 15, no. 1, pp. 85–94, 2021.

[10] R. Yang *et al.*, "Public and Private Blockchain in Construction Business Process and Information Integration," *Autom. Constr.*, vol. 118, February, p. 103276, 2020.

[11] I. Radanović and R. Likić, "Opportunities for Use of Blockchain Technology in Medicine," *Appl. Health Econ. Health Policy*, vol. 16, 2018.

[12] T. Kumar, V. Ramani, I. Ahmad, A. Braeken, E. Harjula, and M. Ylianttila, *Blockchain Utilization in Healthcare: Key Requirements and Challenges All-IP Application Supernetworking View project Blockchain Utilization in Healthcare: Key Requirements and Challenges*, 2018. https://cris.vtt.fi/en/publications/blockchain-utilization-in-healthcare-key-requirements-and-challen.

[13] R. W. Ahmad, K. Salah, R. Jayaraman, I. Yaqoob, S. Ellahham, and M. Omar, "The Role of Blockchain Technology in Telehealth and Telemedicine," *Int. J. Med. Inform.*, vol. 148, November 2020, p. 104399, 2021.

[14] Z. Zheng *et al.*, "An Overview on Smart Contracts: Challenges, Advances and Platforms," *Futur. Gener. Comput. Syst.*, vol. 105, pp. 475–491, 2020.

[15] T. McGhin, K. K. R. Choo, C. Z. Liu, and D. He, "Blockchain in Healthcare Applications: Research Challenges and Opportunities," *J. Netw. Comput. Appl.*, vol. 135, January, pp. 62–75, 2019.

[16] G. Epiphaniou, H. Daly, and H. Al-Khateeb, "Blockchain and Healthcare," *Adv. Sci. Technol. Secur. Appl.*, pp. 1–29, 2019.

[17] A. A. Siyal, A. Z. Junejo, M. Zawish, K. Ahmed, A. Khalil, and G. Soursou, "Applications of Blockchain Technology in Medicine and Healthcare: Challenges and Future Perspectives," *Cryptography*, vol. 3, no. 1, pp. 1–16, 2019.

[18] I. Radanović and R. Likić, "Opportunities for Use of Blockchain Technology in Medicine," *Appl. Health Econ. Health Policy*, vol. 16, no. 5, pp. 583–590, 2018.

[19] H. L. Pham, T. H. Tran, and Y. Nakashima, "Practical Anti-Counterfeit Medicine Management System Based on Blockchain Technology," *TIMES-iCON 2019–2019 4th Technol. Innov. Manag. Eng. Sci. Int. Conf.*, pp. 1–5, 2019.

[20] T. K. Mackey *et al.*, " 'Fit-for-Purpose?' – Challenges and Opportunities for Applications of Blockchain Technology in the Future of Healthcare," *BMC Med. 2019 171*, vol. 17, no. 1, pp. 1–17, March 2019.

[21] C. A. C. Yahaya, A. Firdaus, Y. Y. Khen, C. Y. Yaakub, and M. F. A. Razak, "An Organ Donation Management System (ODMS) Based on Blockchain Technology for Tracking and Security Purposes," *Proc. – 2021 Int. Conf. Softw. Eng. Comput. Syst. 4th Int. Conf. Comput. Sci. Inf. Manag. ICSECS-ICOCSIM 2021*, pp. 377–382, 2021.

[22] Organtee-The First Free Online Donor Registration I Indiegogo. [Online]. www.indiegogo.com/projects/organtee-the-first-free-online-donor-registration#/. [Accessed: 26 November 2021].

[23] M. Attaran, "Blockchain Technology in Healthcare: Challenges and Opportunities Article in International Journal of Healthcare Management November 2020 Challenges and Opportunities," *Int. J. Healthc. Manag.*, 2020. DOI:10.1080/20479700.2020.1843887.

[24] I. Yaqoob, K. Salah, R. Jayaraman, and Y. Al-Hammadi, "Blockchain for Healthcare Data Management: Opportunities, Challenges, and Future Recommendations," *Neural Comput. Appl.*, vol. 0123456789, 2021.

[25] M. Reisman, "EHRs: The Challenge of Making Electronic Data Usable and Interoperable," *Pharm. Ther.*, vol. 42, no. 9, p. 572, 2017.

[26] D. Mechkaroska, V. Dimitrova, and A. Popovska-Mitrovikj, "Analysis of the Possibilities for Improvement of BlockChain Technology," *2018 26th Telecommun. Forum, TELFOR 2018 – Proc.*, pp. 1–4, 2018.

[27] E. Gökalp, M. Onuralp Gökalp, S. Gökalp, S. Çoban, and P. Erhan Eren, *Analysing Opportunities and Challenges of Integrated Blockchain Technologies in Healthcare Cloud Computing Based Predictive Maintenance Framework for Medical Imaging Devices View Project Cloud Computing Based Predictive Maintenance Framework for Medical Imaging Devices View project Analysing Opportunities and Challenges of Integrated Blockchain Technologies in Healthcare*, 2018. https://www.researchgate.net/publication/327229059_Analysing_Opportunities_and_Challenges_of_Integrated_Blockchain_Technologies_in_Healthcare.

[28] M. M. H. Onik, S. Aich, J. Yang, C.-S. Kim, and H.-C. Kim, *Blockchain in Healthcare: Challenges and Solutions*. Elsevier Inc., 2019.

[29] I. Abu-elezz, A. Hassan, A. Nazeemudeen, M. Househ, and A. Abd-alrazaq, "The Benefits and Threats of Blockchain Technology in Healthcare: A Scoping Review," *Int. J. Med. Inform.*, vol. 142, August, p. 104246, 2020.

[30] J. H. Beinke, C. Fitte, and F. Teuteberg, "Towards a Stakeholder-Oriented Blockchain-Based Architecture for Electronic Health Records: Design Science Research Study," *J. Med. Internet Res.*, vol. 21, no. 10, 2019.

11 Blockchain-Enabled Secured Medical Supply Chain Management

Anuj Tripathi[1], Vivek Garg[2], Binu Kuriakose Vargis[3] and Chaitanya P. Agrawal[4]
[1] Affle (India) Limited, India
[2] University of Greenwich, United Kingdom
[3] Inderprastha Engineering College, Ghaziabad, India
[4] Makhanlal University, Bhopal, India

CONTENTS

11.1 INTRODUCTION

11.1.1 MEDICAL SUPPLY CHAIN MANAGEMENT IN HEALTHCARE FACILITY

Supply chain management is a vital process for the medical industry so that the overall operations can run efficiently [1–3]. For the past two years, the international medical sector has been working to deal with coronavirus, creating a need for the streamlined supply chain management. This has created a demand for adapting to the latest and

DOI: 10.1201/9781003217107-11

sophisticated technology available to work with and ensuring that the products and services are delivered as soon as possible. The technologies used in hospitals and other medical institutions are at their all-time high [4, 5]. In such a situation, every healthcare institution has made efforts to modernise its operations, including the medical supply chain. The significant benefits of having tech ecosystems in place can streamline the flight floor and automate the processes. By simplifying and standardising the practices of the medical supply chain, hospitals could cut their operational costs.

The supply chain practices of the medical industry are more complex and different than other sectors [6]. The primary reason behind the same is that various stakeholders have varying objectives to achieve at every step of the supply chain. While procuring and distributing the equipment and services to reach the patient, the healthcare institution follows many steps. The medical supply chain deals with various issues such as demand for specific inventory, expiration of products, issues in stocking and decrease and increase in order [7–9]. The medical supply chain management capabilities benefit the medical operations and patients by reducing functioning costs [10]. It enables distributors, manufacturers and pharmacies to hold smaller inventories to make substantial enhancements in savings and offer associated products at highly affordable prices. An optimised supply chain system reduces costs and adds to the betterment of the lifecycle of the entire medical supply chain.

The healthcare industry also leverages its medical supply chain for improved access [11]. Shortage of the required drugs and medicines has been a significant issue in both developing economies and developed countries. By providing access to short supply products, the companies can generate high revenue and grab into new opportunities for growth. They can also adopt different strategies to improve savings and reduce costs. Improved access also ensures that the patients and applicable users receive the product they need to maintain a healthy and balanced lifestyle. The medical supplies also benefit the organisation by enhancing safety [12, 13]. In recent times, the rise in security breaches has posed a threat to patients' safety. Due to this, people's trust has considerably reduced in the healthcare system, which can be regained with the optimised operations and supply chain management system.

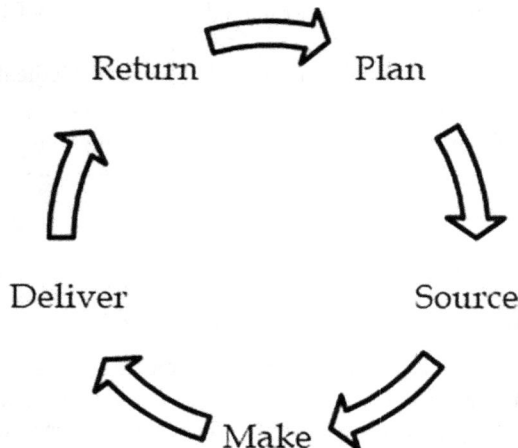

FIGURE 11.1   Components of the medical supply chain.

11.2   COMPONENTS OF THE MEDICAL SUPPLY CHAIN

Figure 11.1 highlights the process of the medical supply chain. This refers to the organisation's stages to fulfill to conduct the functions. The first component of the medical supply chain is planning [14]. It is imperative for controlling manufacturing processes and inventory. Companies try to match their supply with the customers' demand by formulating a course of action based on analytic findings. The company sources the products as per planning to make sure that they consider the factors of development and quality. It is essential to be vigilant regarding the variations and demands along the medical supply chain to avoid the 'Bullwhip Effect'. For example, medical organisations intended to secure the demand of the market by using tools for analysis also plan the required materials by using tools of material planning such as Netsuite, Biz21 and Oracle Cloud ERP. The second stage in the medical supply chain is sourcing [15–17]. It revolves around identifying vendors who will most efficiently and economically source medical products and services to meet the anticipated or current demand.

The suppliers need to set specific standards and fulfill the same to ensure that they can deliver good-quality products for their clients. The items within the sourcing could be perishable or non-perishable. In the case of perishable products, the supplier must have minimum lead time, which would minimise inventory cost. On the contrary, for the non-perishable products, the lead time the supplier promises should be less than the number of days on which the product can last so that there is no loss in revenue [18, 19].

The third stage in the medical supply chain is made, which revolves around production and manufacturing [20]. It has been found that as per the consumer's preference, the organisation will perform all the activities in terms of transforming the raw material into the final product. It will also perform actions such as testing, assembling and packing as a part of medical supply chain management. The make stage is concerned with the production and integrates feedback received from the consumer [21]. It makes sure that a win-win situation is created for both the producer and the customer. As a result, the firm can continuously improve its production operations.

One of the most critical components of medical supply management is to contribute to indirect or direct integration within the consumers [22]. It is accomplished in the delivery stage of the supply chain. This stage has a significant contribution to improving the brand image of the healthcare organisation. When the equipment and services demanded by the customers are launched in the market to meet their expectations through the delivery channel of the business and logistics services, it can secure credibility and reliability from the customers. The business uses various transport methods such as railway, air or road to perform seamless operations. Return is the most crucial aspect of medical supply chain management, as it is a part of the post-delivery customer support process [23]. It is linked with all types of products and devices returned in the medical supply chain. It is also referred to as reverse logistics. One of the critical aspects of supply chain management is that it minimises the potential degradation of business relationships.

The process of 'Return' provides the same course of action for the business organisation towards its suppliers. This involves returning defective, low-quality or expired materials to the suppliers [24]. It ensures that the patients' health is protected and they are not given sub-quality products. The leaders in the healthcare ecosystem reflect upon the components of the medical supply chain while making strategic decisions [25]. All the medical supply chain management elements arere vital for vertical diversification and logistic attainment. Due to recent technological developments in the medical supply chain regarding digital transformation, many initiatives have been taken for making the supply chain lean. This is likely to contribute to the competitive advantage of the business organisation [23].

11.2.1   CURRENT TRENDS IN MEDICAL SUPPLY CHAIN MANAGEMENT

The healthcare industry has changed. Organisations have identified new ways of cutting costs and improving patient care by removing waste. This value directly impacted the biggest suppliers in the world as their perspectives regarding how the supply chain will help provide a healthcare transformation in the coming decade [24]. The medical supply chain is arising as a gold mine for data analysis. The value of accurate and clean data is disputed, but many healthcare organisations have to go a long way to analyse their ultimate potential [25]. Currently, the information coming from the medical supply chain ecosystem is focused on transactional values and leverages the business's capabilities. The medical supply chain would be capable of utilising the gold mine of data with the proper documentation and transactional data to make better decisions for patient care. As more data is collected from patients, every department will gain an unprecedented understanding of patient care [26]. This is so because the data would include information about the current area of improvements across the levels. It could be strengthened to fulfill the ultimate goals of medical care within the healthcare facility.

The medical supply chain is anticipated to be a part of the C-suite and be involved in strategic projects [27]. Due to the increasing focus on the medical supply chain across the healthcare industry, it is projected that the future individuals will have a better position in the C-suite. It would also be a significant component in projects across different areas of the healthcare facility. It is vital to understand that the supply chain was relegated to the basement in the last few years. Instead, it is becoming the pillar of the healthcare organisation.

It has been identified that medical supply chain management has led to the standardisation of care across all stages [28]. One of the most critical ways healthcare could achieve sustainability is by emphasising the standardisation of care. It mainly revolves around maintaining consistency in care from the perspective of the patient. The current supply chain can guide and support this change as it is developed upon valuable data to determine the crucial aspects. This includes the best prices and outcomes, which will help modify inefficient, long-standing and wasteful procedures.

The medical supply chain management modifications need to be in lockstep with healthcare professionals [29]. Patients predict that a clinically integrated supply chain would perform the operations better than the standard medical supply chain. As such, healthcare professionals work closely side by side for delivering the best patient care. [30] explained that physicians had recognised the need to adjust their logistic processes to prioritise the patients' health. They are putting efforts into curating a supply chain that fosters support, guidance and knowledge on price points of the products and their outcomes and alternatives. In turn, the supply chain professionals would gain the trust of healthcare professionals by demonstrating the return on investment of a supply chain optimisation. The composition of the medical ecosystem would collaborate to ensure that continuous improvements are carried out in the medical supply chain.

However, [31] argued that a medical supply chain is predictable. It is vital to note that the data derived from the medical supply chain can be used to make better decisions and act as leverage for predictive analytics. Supply chain professionals use data to predict what is needed to quickly get products to the market. This is because the supplied equipment could lose its speed if it is backordered or discontinued later.

One of the future trends of the medical supply chain would be that it will be long-term and likely to benefit relationships between partners [13]. For multiple years, healthcare trading partners have discussed creating more transparent and communicating relationships with each other. However, only a few have succeeded in building better relationships. The future of a medical supply chain starts with the scope for having ideal relationships when it comes to fruition. Suppliers and providers are likely to achieve the mutual goal of improved patient care and will also find better channels for aligning incentives to succeed.

The medical supply would expand wherever the patient goes [32]. This means that the future of the medical supply chain will no longer revolve around inpatient and outpatient facilities; instead, it would expand to wherever the patient is physically located. This is because of greater collaboration and consolidation among healthcare systems. This includes nursing home partnerships and telemedicine networks. The primary focus of expanding the scope of the medical supply chain is to reduce the readmission rates of the patients, as this has become very critical with the reform of healthcare.

Unlike the present scenario, the medical supply chain of the future would extend its presence beyond the confines of the hospital [8]. The primary motive behind the same is to ensure that the patients are getting the care they deserve wherever they are, even if they cannot return to the hospital. The medical supplies are also adapted to personalised medicine and will lead to more informed consumers [33]. Disruptive technologies such as 3D printers and improved diagnostics have shaped the current medical supply chain. Due to this, it will adapt to new manufacturing and buying processes that revolve around personalised medicine. It will further lead to more connected consumers of the healthcare industry who emphasise identifying the best hospitals and products for them. The future medical supply chain must be prepared to allow the customer to shop for products and services online [27].

11.3 IMPACT OF FORCE MAJEURE ON MEDICAL SUPPLY CHAIN MANAGEMENT

The COVID-19 pandemic triggered force majeure by governments worldwide, which disrupted the medical supply chain [34]. The pandemic did not only threaten the supply of essential medicines and other devices. It had an acute impact and developing countries along with healthy nations. For example, Kenya, along with other African countries, was exposed to a medicine shortage where citizens' lives depended upon the imported medicines to stop the widespread nature of these problems are reflected in the complex presence of a globalised supply chain for healthcare commodities and pharmaceuticals. The channel of medical supply chain management is illustrated in Figure 11.2.

Figure 11.2 explains the channel of the medical supply chain. It starts from manufacturing active pharmaceutical ingredients and ends when the finished product reaches the point of dispensing. The figure also depicts the process of the medical supply chain starting with active pharmaceuticals turned into manufactured products. They are exported and transported overseas. These materials are then exported and then taken into the warehouse. The process highlights the last stage of dispensing.

As the COVID-19 pandemic erupted, the supply of critical materials was severely disrupted because of lack of labour and forced quarantine [36]. It is vital to note that sometimes the link between regional warehouses of a medical supply is not smooth, leading to severe disruption in the allocation of raw materials between the regions. The COVID-19 pandemic led to a shortage of medical resources in the frontline. It forced governments to issue a guideline that only diagnosed patients with severe conditions could be hospitalised [37]. Research organisations worldwide put time into identifying the pathogenic mechanism of the virus, which further prolonged the development of specific drug and treatment for the patients.

Respiratory-support devices such as atomisers, life support machines, oxygen generators and monitors are primary clinical treatment devices [24]. Hence, the need for instruments to measure temperature, life support machines and antiviral medical products drastically increased from diagnosis to cure. To restore the balance between the demand and supply of medical products, an emergency approval procedure was launched by governments for registration application of medical devices that were initially needed for protection and control COVID-19 pandemic [38]. However, as the borders were closed and international trade was disrupted, it led to a shortage of significant materials, which further acted as a further roadblock in the production of medical devices.

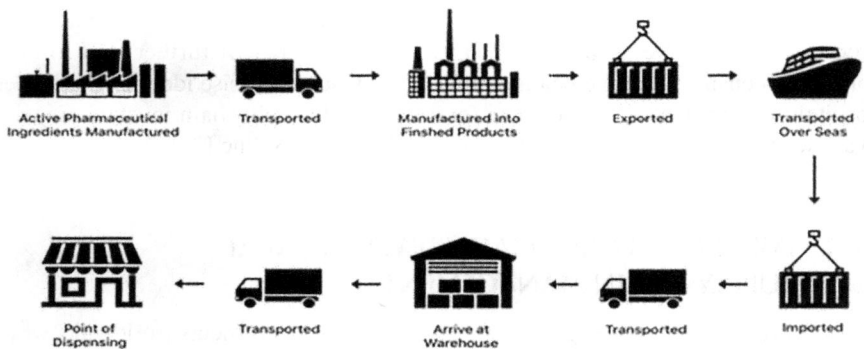

Active Pharmaceutical Ingredients Manufactured → Transported → Manufactured into Finshed Products → Exported → Transported Over Seas

Point of Dispensing ← Transported ← Arrive at Warehouse ← Transported ← Imported

FIGURE 11.2 Channel of medical supply chain management [35].

During the initial stage of the COVID-19 outbreak, a large part of the affected population was frontline workers. This highlighted the difficulty individuals face in maintaining their safety while they treating affected patients [7]. Within these situations, long-term treatment services showed their advantages. Hospitals started using self-disinfection kits and personal protective equipment for frontline workers to continue helping and treating patients with the new coronavirus. It could be stated that high-tech medical devices are expected to play an increasingly important role until COVID-19 is wholly eradicated from the Earth.

11.3.1 LOOPHOLES IN EXISTING MEDICAL SUPPLY CHAIN MANAGEMENT

The healthcare supply chain is unique due to its continuous monitoring nature during the acquisition of products. It is also necessary that a business organisation traces the path of products from the origin to destination, as the supplies could create a difference in life. Medical supply chain management leads to a significant expense for healthcare providers. Even though the collections make a difference in healthcare delivery, overnight shipping is still a challenge in the healthcare industry [13]. Unexpected situations can occur, and it is the responsibility of the hospitals to address them despite the costs. Still, one or two orders that need to be sent overnight do not have a detrimental impact on the supplier's bottom line. Still, as this regularly occurs, there are chances that suppliers would see significant losses in their revenues.

Another challenge that medical suppliers face is that of the hidden cost in every product. Most of the suppliers historically look at the product cost and the shipping cost; however, there are also additional expenses such as that of holding inventory [39]. Suppliers must plan their budget around total supply cost and are aware of the losses they could encourage from expired products and accessories. This means that they need to consider the aspect of product standards and purchase price variance.

Due to the unpredictability of demand in the medical supply chain, drug shortages are also one of the significant challenges [40]. It could create a mess in the supply chain because the deficiency of a drug is causing suppliers to either purchase costly alternatives or maintain a backup inventory of products that are at risk of getting short in supply. If the supplier goes for the second option, then the provider needs to manage the added cost of inventory management and deal with the risk of product expiration. Shortage of data is a significant loophole in the existing capabilities of the medical supply chain [41]. Data and medical supply chains enable businesses to improve their effectiveness and efficiency. It also allows them to see what the industry has been missing in optimising their processes. Since the suppliers have reported a lack of actionable data, this has impacted the executives in hospitals who recognised that their decisions are not sufficiently informed as they do not have access to advanced modelling and real-time reports.

One of the primary reasons behind the lack of actionable data is that the information derived from a supply chain is absolute due to inherent vertical internal structure [42]. This problem needs to be addressed as most IT professionals in the healthcare field believe that the supply chain is the area where the most actionable data lies. This data goes beyond the purchasing activity and instead reflects consumption activity.

The medical supply chain management lacks integration. This is because healthcare facilities and hospitals are becoming more consolidated. As an outcome of this, the health systems are growing, merging and acquiring. Supply chains within these systems are integrated, which means that even though the organisations remain separated, they follow a linked model. It is essential that healthcare suppliers address the inconsistency in supply which could negatively impact the bottom line [43]. Poor workflow design in the medical supply chain is a disruptive loophole. The primary reason behind the same is that throughout the stages of the healthcare supply chain, a lot of processes are unnecessarily duplicated since the entities and systems embedded in the supply chain are not connected [44]. It is necessary that healthcare organisations consider the fact that many of the tasks could be integrated and automated to allow all the participants to share information more easily. The healthcare facility should address the supply chain gaps with appropriate solutions and technology to ensure that it does not impact its capacity and ability to deliver as per the needs of the patients.

11.4 BLOCKCHAIN TECHNOLOGY IN MEDICAL SUPPLY CHAIN MANAGEMENT

Blockchain is a distributed database shared among the nodes of a network that is used for storing information electronically in a digital format [45]. The innovation of blockchain guarantees the security infidelity of a record of data and generates trust by eliminating the need for a third party. This is so because blockchain collects information within groups, also known as blocks, that hold the data. These blocks have considerable storage capacities. They are then filled, closed and linked to the previously served block, creating a chain of data known as the blockchain [46]. All the new information added to the data set in the future is compiled into a fresh new block and then connected to other blocks in the chain. A database is usually structured into tables, whereas the blockchain structures the data into blocks connected. This data structure develops an irreversible timeline of information when applied in a decentralised nature. Whenever a block is filled, it is closed and then it becomes a part of the timeline. It is vital to know that each block within the same ecosystem is given the exact time it was added to the chain [47].

The basic principle of blockchain is decentralisation which makes it very different from the existing data storage technologies. This decentralisation takes place within a public forum [48]. The transactions within the blockchain are peer-to-peer. This eliminates the need for any third party to verify the steps being taken in a particular chain [49]. It has been identified that blockchain provides transparency with the pseudonymise to the participants involved [50]. This means that the details of two entities within a blockchain could be either kept secret or opened to stakeholders based on needs. Blockchain technology is built upon the principle of transparency with specific reference to selective or disguised identity. This includes the transaction of documents between the entities involved, which could be related to logistics and supply chains, among others.

Even though blockchain has considerable flexibility on behalf of the parties involved, it does not enable them to undertake the irreversibility of records [51]. This means that the documents cannot be modified once the blockchain transaction is processed in the database and the accounts have been updated. Various algorithms are developed to make sure that the data required on the blockchain is permanent and segregated in a chronological manner. This makes it easier for the people available on the network to access the data of a specific date or keyword. Even though the irreversibility of records as a principle of blockchain would not seem attractive, it is instrumental in identifying fraud irrespective of the parties involved [52]. Blockchain provides better and reliable transactions between the parties as compared to traditional technologies due to its capability of minimal manual intervention and robust connectivity over the internet.

11.4.1 Need for Blockchain Technology in Medical Supply Chain Management

The medical supply chain needs blockchain to protect personally identifiable information and only allow a limited number of entities to conduct transactions within a particular chain. This provides them with better connectedness while directly improving security and ensuring that they follow the regulatory compliances and help to reduce the long-term operational cost. The presence of blockchain in the supply chain tokenises the transaction related to personal and confidential drug information [2]. It further creates a unique and verifiable identifier for purchase orders, bills of lading and inventory management in the organisation.

By integrating blockchain, every participant within the medical supply chain would have their digital signature, which they would use to sign the tokens as they move through the chain of data [41]. This will enable the business organisation to verify the transactions at every phase when they are recorded. It will also provide them with the clarity of transfers between the stakeholders by providing a built-in audit trail that cannot be tempered by blockchain insurance irreversibility of records. With the extensive need for blockchain in the medical supply chain, e.g. integration of blockchain, the medical records of patients would be easily accessed from any part of the world [53]. The entire medical history could be seen by accessing the information about patient data such as fingerprints, etc. This will further facilitate the urgent needs of the medical situation where the patient shows any deviation with the prescribed precautions, and it would alert the paramedics so that they can respond quickly.

11.4.2 Role of Blockchain Technology in the Medical Industry

Blockchain technology can streamline the functions of the medical industry in various ways. Identifying the research procedures in the medical sector could be facilitated with the help of blockchain technology. In the current times, electronic health records are automatically updated. They could share the medical information of a given patient within the health care facility or a selected network of organisations only. This could be further extended if the organisation was part of a more extensive set of information, the topmost blockchain layer [46]. This revolves around the secure transfer of personally identifiable information (PII). The blockchain would enable other organisations and researchers to access a broad spectrum of communication with the cohort data of hundreds of thousands of patients [45]. This availability of massive amounts of data would also promote better clinical research in the medical industry. It is likely to improve safety measures and streamline the procedures of event reporting and identification within public health. Blockchain technology could also enable seamless switching of doctors and paramedics between patients. This is so because different people could access the same information on the blockchain through a unique identification code which the patient has with himself [1]. In this way, the medical history and other important information related to the patient's health could be easily unlocked and shared with organisations and providers through a private key. This would help the medical industry make better health information technology that streamlines collaboration between different healthcare professionals despite their geographical location.

It has been identified that blockchain could create a single system for informational healthcare that could be embedded in the same so that information could be stored and constantly updated along with rapid and secured retrieval by authorised users. It would also lead to miscommunication between different healthcare professionals who are involved in caring for the same patients. In addition to this, countless mistakes could be prevented, along with the provision of faster interventions and diagnostics [54]. By using blockchain and its secured features, healthcare ecosystems have been able to provide personalised care for each patient.

Apart from this, interoperable electronic health records are also possible now due to the integration of blockchain technology in healthcare logistics. The primary reason behind this is that blockchain provides a single transaction, and therefore organisations could deal with shared data through a single system [55]. It also enables them to store the specific set of standardised data on the chain with private encrypted links for separately complete information such as images for test results. The use of intelligent contracts and uniform authorisation protocols, etc., can be seamless through blockchain technology. It has immensely supported unified connectivity within all the nodes of the medical industry.

In the last decade, millions of data breaches occurred in reference to healthcare records. Blockchain provides security features that could help the organisation protect information about the health of their patients. This could be done by giving everyone a public identifier or a private key to open the health records as and when required [56]. Moreover, as the aspect of hacking is a concern for data security in general.

Along with this, mobile health apps and remote monitoring have also become possible due to the integration of blockchain technology in the medical industry. It is necessary to understand that as the use of smartphones is increasing, mobile health applications are becoming more critical in the current times with advancing technology [57]. In this context, it has become necessary to keep electronic medical records secure only within the blockchain network. It would facilitate sending data to the medical professional rapidly, as well as making it available for self-monitoring. It is necessary to understand that mobile applications are sensitive to malware attacks on the smartphone. If a hacker can enter into the smartphone of the patient, they could gain access to the private key whenever it is embedded, which further exposes the highly secure blockchain to a phishing attack.

Blockchain technology has also streamlined the tracing and sourcing of medical supplies in the industry. It has been found that blockchain can help secure as well as identify the trail of medical and pharmaceutical supplies with complete transparency on behalf of the supplier and the organisation [58]. Due to its expanded capability of openness, as well as a rapid transfer of information, it could also provide real-time monitoring of labour costs and carbon emission, which was involved in the manufacturing of the supplies in the first place. Blockchain has also made it easier for patients to claim their health insurance in the medical industry. It is necessary to understand that blockchain is uniquely adapted to the process of claim because of its ability to present medical events as and when they took place. This is so because each set of information that is embedded in the blockchain is given a particular timestamp which creates a series of blocks in the sequence of time when the information was registered.

Due to this, without the potential for changing the data at a later stage for purposes of fraud from either of the parties, such as the patient on the insurance company, complete transparency could be ensured in the claim process in the concerned industry. It is vital to note that the unique capabilities of blockchain could help organisations track as well as real-time report conditions [5]. This attribute could be beneficial in times of global epidemics such as that of the coronavirus crisis where patterns of the diseases could explode along multiple channels, and the data could be used to identify its origins and parameters of transmission.

In addition to this, blockchain technology could also play an integral role in safeguarding genomics within the medical industry. Many business organisations are bringing the technology of DNA and genome sequencing, which has opened the gates of genomic data theft. The capabilities of blockchain could prevent this, along with providing an online marketplace where scientists could legally buy genomic information of different samples in order to facilitate their research. The capabilities of blockchain could promote safe selling and eliminate expensive intermediaries as far as DNA sequencing and study is concerned [59].

Therefore, it could be said that applications of blockchain in the medical industry are considered at an early stage. Even though there are some examples of blockchain Technology frameworks, they are currently being used at a relatively small scale within the medical industry. With improved systems and security in blockchain, the medical industry would be able to facilitate synchronised transactions along with better management of healthcare data.

11.4.3 Effectiveness of Blockchain Technology in Medical Supply Chain Management

Blockchain ttechnology offers a digital and automated process of storing data which is highly beneficial to the management processes of the supply chain. It has been identified as one of the keys lags that invoice in the supply chain contain inaccurate information sometimes. These inaccuracies may lead to miscommunication and have been found to do with the potential sources of conflict [60]. Blockchain is used to log in the product activities throughout the supply chain automatically. It enhances the effectiveness of the supply chain processes by integrating automation which decreases the potential for human error. Automation and a reduced number of mistakes could also increase the delivery speed of products in the medical supply chain. When the delivery speed is enhanced, it could lead to a better customer service experience and increased rates of retention.

Blockchain technology also improves collaboration within supply chain management. As there are numerous logistics organisations that work at differentiating technology levels, the complexity within the entire supply chain has considerably increased. This is so because the availability of a lot of information has led to transparency and difference in non-standardised processes.

Blockchain has increased the effectiveness of this by combating collaboration issues through increased data transparency. The essential central point within the logistics aspect of supply chain management is the need for intermediaries. It is vital to note that the need for intermediaries arises while working with different third-party entities, which could be alternative suppliers in partners. Blockchain has helped the supply chain to eliminate the requirements of intermediaries, which saves both money and time to the business along with improving relationships [61]. Blockchain could be used throughout the logistics industry for decreasing errors and miscommunication and increasing the effectiveness of supply chain operations. It also enables the business to partner with the different suppliers within the global supply chain so that they can work together efficiently.

Within supply chain management, blockchain also improves the transparency and traceability of products. It has done the same by creating a traceable digital record for each product that has entered the supply chain. If any issues occur throughout the operations of the supply chain ecosystem, it has become much easier to identify the aspect where the mistake was committed and could be further rectified. Tractability and traceability are specific attributes when medical safety issues arise in the supply chain [62]. For instance, cold chain tracking technology uses sensors to confirm that the products which are currently in the logistics are being maintained at an appropriate temperature throughout the life cycle, which makes sure that the highest and safest quality is provided to the customers.

Blockchain technology can combine increased supplies and transparency with innovative contract technology. It offers businesses distributed ledger and enhanced compatibility of the management systems. Blockchain technology has also made the supply chains more effective by helping both consumers and companies to be more aware and knowledgeable about the products which are purchased [63]. For example, healthcare businesses use blockchain technology for confirming that the materials were disbursed from a specific location, which further decreases the probability of fraudulent purchases and invoices. From the perspective of the customers, blockchain could provide the necessary information about reservation techniques and the ethical knowledge of the raw materials which have been procured. It has become essential because, in recent times, consumers are becoming more concerned about ethical production and sourcing, which has been solved through the effectiveness of blockchain solutions in the supply chain.

Blockchain technology also optimises the aspect of security within the supply chain in which further improves effectiveness. It is necessary to note that security is always a top priority of the business [64]. Blockchain helps logistic professionals to keep the data about the same secure throughout the entire healthcare ecosystem without any flaws. This is because blocks within the blockchain are tough to falsify, which reduces the probability of forgery or fraudulent activity [65]. Security embedded within blockchain provides businesses with an opportunity of improving their reputation and enhance the credibility of operations. Malpractice within the supply chain is greatly minimised with the help of blockchain technology which decreases the likelihood of damaging Public Relations or other cost implications on behalf of the business entity.

11.4.4 Working of Blockchain-Enabled Medical Supply Chain Management

Blockchain involves the time stamp series of data records that are managed by a network of computers. These systems are not under the entitlement of any single organisation or entity [66]. The blocks of data involve the blocks that are connected by using cryptographic principles. This further leads to the development of a chain. Public blockchain ledgers are autonomous on a primary basis and are used in peer-to-peer networks for exchanging data between a group of parties that are connected with each other. As the nature of blocks is independent itself, there is no need for an administrator to monitor the operation set. The users collaborate through a collective administrator. Another form of blockchain within supply chain management is known as the permission or private blockchain [67]. It is usually developed by an organisation for creating as well as monitoring transactional networks which could be used by partners. This enables the business organisations to share data internally and with each other.

It is necessary to note that every blockchain transaction within the supply chain goes to the same stepper regardless of the industry with which it is being used. For instance, within the medical supply process, blockchain performs numerous functions, as stated earlier, which includes the protection of data maintenance of health records and sharing information across geographical borders [68]. However, the basic working of blockchain with a supply chain could be broken down into four contiguous and distinct steps. Figure 11.3 highlights the process of a blockchain-enabled supply chain. It includes nodes and stages, which explain the whole process.

Record of Every Transaction: Whenever data is embedded within a blockchain, it becomes a record. This record, which contains specific details of people who were making the transaction along with the data embedded in the same, is authenticated by utilising the digital signature [70]. Each record is given a timestamp which cannot be altered later, which protects the sanctity of the data and ensures security.

Verification: It is highly essential to verify the data which is being embedded in the supply chain. This is so because if data is being entered by a party that is not given access to the blockchain, it could interfere with the security of the information which is already present. The verification process is completed by the computers which are connected to the network. Within this, the laptop independently checks to make sure that the transaction made within the blockchain and the new information

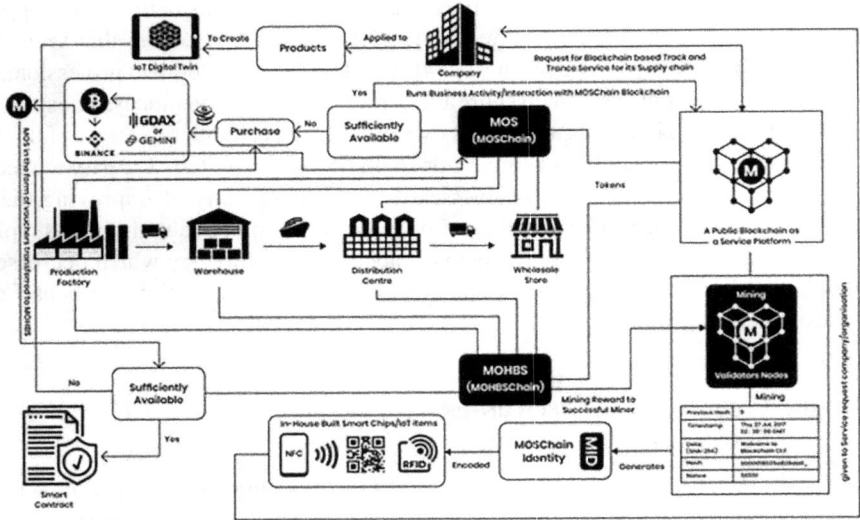

FIGURE 11.3   Working of a blockchain-enabled supply chain [69].

which has been added is legitimate in nature [71]. It is necessary to note that as blockchain is a decentralised process, it means that every node which is being entered or retracted from the changing needs to agree with the codes before the process can be completed as a supply chain management.

Transaction Is Added to the Block: After the transaction is verified, it is then added to the block. Blocks are basically a group of transaction records, but it is necessary to understand that each of the blocks and its information is unique in nature. Each block carries a unique code known as a hash digestive or hash value. It is used for uniquely identifying the block and registering its position within the blockchain [68]. The hash also ensures that the sanctity of information and data is maintained and has not been changed as it was embedded in the block.

Block Is Added to the Supply Chain: Once the hash value is given to the information and the block is closed, it is then added to the end of the blockchain. This marks the end of the blockchain and process of verification in supply chain management. Once a single block is completed and into the supply chain, another block follows the same procedure again.

11.4.5   USE CASES OF BLOCKCHAIN-ENABLED SECURED MEDICAL SUPPLY CHAIN

Nebula Genomics: The piece of genome sequence single has a free fold since the first Human Genome Project was completed. The white paper which was written on Nebula Genomics highlighted that the opportunities around personal genome sequencing would soon lead to the creation of a genome data market that will be worth billions of dollars. The team behind Nebula Genomics believes that this market would have similar opportunities and challenges as any other market where data is involved [72]. The organisation has adopted blockchain technology to solve data security issues and to make sure that the data can be sold directly from the patient to the end user without any intermediary. Blockchain technology has been used for enhancing genomic data protection. It has also enabled the customers to efficiently acquire genome data and resolve the challenges of big data.

Doc.AI: This was founded by Walter and Sam in 2016. Physical education is focused on visualising the future, which is blockchain-based, consumer-controlled and powered by artificial intelligence (AI). The data offered by the company is centred around all kinds of biological data, which includes microbiome and genome. The platform is used in natural language processing along with computer vision for securing data through blockchain technology. It then uses the data for generating insights from medical data [72]. Any entity could launch the data trial, which involves a collection of health data on the platform for a particular cause or when the data scientists are given the task of connecting dots and making predictive data models. As an outcome of this, the entity involved gets insights about their own data, which they bring to the doctor. This organisation presents a great example of how the power of community could be enhanced with the use of blockchain and artificial intelligence for the decision of medicines in a more efficient manner.

Iryo: This Slovakia-based enterprise has a participatory and global healthcare ecosystem. It was established two years ago and built an open-source electronic health record (EHR) platform with a zero-knowledge data repository [72]. Being a zero-knowledge data repository, it makes sure that the sensitive medical data will remain secure and impervious to breaches of cyber security, which includes phishing attacks sponsored by the state. The overall business objective of Iryo is to build an appropriate platform for keeping all the health records unified in a single blockchain. The problem currently being solved is that all kinds of medical data, which is collected from various providers, are stored in different formats and are usually scattered across systems. The solution offered by the organisation promises to keep data in a secure manner, which enables patients to share their medical history anywhere in the world through secured channels.

Patientory: This Atlanta-based company has developed a blockchain platform for securing healthcare data for providers, patients and medical institutions. It is an advanced healthcare application enables the user to create a patient profile and embed the information of which they could keep track of throughout their health history. The software provides the patient with an easy way of tracking the wizards of the doctor, personal medical information, medical bills, pharmacy medications, immunisation information and health insurance details [72]. The start-up had urged the United Kingdom government to get behind a blockchain-enabled National Health system. It also requested the government to remove legal obstacles which are currently standing in the way of blockchain technology within the movement of data among concerned entities and providers.

Chronicled: This San Francisco–based tech leader has been applying blockchain technology combined with Internet of Things (IoT) systems within the medical supply chains. The purpose of integrating blockchain within supply chains is to improve accountability and the traceability of data. It is highly crucial in the pharmaceutical industry that deals in susceptible commodities [72]. For instance, healthcare products are highly temperature-sensitive such as vaccines which need to be safely delivered in a certain time frame. Integration of blockchain solutions within the supply chain has helped the clients of Chronicled to speed up the process of logistics, undertake potential cost savings and minimise the discrepancies from an already streamlined process. Organisations helped medical institutions to improve the product visibility and add the component of transparency as their products travelled through the medical supply chain.

11.5 RESEARCH IMPLICATIONS

Theoretical Implications: This research significantly contributes to the existing literature related to blockchain-enabled medical supply chain management. It would also act as a foundation for other researchers who are looking forward to studying and researching about the blockchain and supply chain constructs in reference to the medical industry. The chapter has also highlighted the critical analysis e.g. the loopholes of the existing medical supply chain. The research highlighted the current trends in medical supplies management and the role of blockchain technology in healthcare.

Managerial Implications: The healthcare organisations such as medical institutions, suppliers, patients, professionals, etc., would benefit with the research by identifying the in-depth use of the blockchain technology. From this study, they could gain practical knowledge about the ways in which the medical supply chain functions and the role of blockchain for streamlining the process. The supply chains function in a similar way despite the specific industry, such as the medical or retail. The findings of the current study could also act as a baseline for other business organisations looking forward to integrating a blockchain within their business functions. In addition to this, the chapter has also discussed the successful use cases of blockchain-enabled secured medical supply chains at global level. The research highlights the success story of healthcare clients who have adopted blockchain and will motivate other organisations to streamline the processes.

11.6 REFERENCES

[1] Abbas, Khizar, et al. "A blockchain and machine learning-based drug supply chain management and recommendation system for the smart pharmaceutical industry." *Electronics* 9.5 (2020): 852. https://doi.org/10.3390/electronics9050852
[2] Jamil, Faisal, et al. "A novel medical blockchain model for drug supply chain integrity management in a smart hospital." *Electronics* 8.5 (2019): 505. https://doi.org/10.3390/electronics8050505
[3] Dasaklis, Thomas K., Nikolaos Rachaniotis, and Costas Pappis. "Emergency supply chain management for controlling a smallpox outbreak: The case for regional mass vaccination." *International Journal of Systems Science: Operations & Logistics* 4.1 (2017): 27–40. https://doi.org/10.1080/23302674.2015.1126379
[4] Sodhi, ManMohan S., and Christopher S. Tang. "Supply chain management for extreme conditions: Research opportunities." *Journal of Supply Chain Management* 57.1 (2021): 7–16. https://doi.org/10.1111/jscm.12255

[5] Cole, Rosanna, Mark Stevenson, and James Aitken. "Blockchain technology: Implications for operations and supply chain management." *Supply Chain Management: An International Journal* (2019). https://doi.org/10.1108/SCM-09-2018-0309

[6] Lee, Hwee Khei, and Yudi Fernando. "The antecedents and outcomes of the medical tourism supply chain." *Tourism Management* 46 (2015): 148–157. https://doi.org/10.1016/j.tourman.2014.06.014

[7] Kovas, Gyöngyi, and Ioanna Falagara Sigala. "Lessons learned from humanitarian logistics to manage supply chain disruptions." *Journal of Supply Chain Management* 57.1 (2021): 41–49. https://doi.org/10.1111/jscm.12253

[8] Durach, Christian F., Joakim Kembro, and Andreas Wieland. "A new paradigm for systematic literature reviews in supply chain management." *Journal of Supply Chain Management* 53.4 (2017): 67–85. https://doi.org/10.1111/jscm.12145

[9] Abdulsalam, Yousef, Dari Alhuwail, and Eugene S. Schneller. "Adopting identification standards in the medical device supply chain." *International Journal of Information Systems and Supply Chain Management (IJISSCM)* 13.1 (2020): 1–14. https://doi.org/10.4018/IJISSCM.2020010101

[10] Adebanjo, Dotun, Tritos Laosirihongthong, and Premaratne Samaranayake. "Prioritising lean supply chain management initiatives in healthcare service operations: A fuzzy AHP approach." *Production Planning & Control* 27.12 (2016): 953–966. https://doi.org/10.1080/09537287.2016.1164909

[11] Vafaeenezhad, Taha, Reza Tavakkoli-Moghaddam, and Naoufel Cheikhrouhou. "Multi-objective mathematical modeling for sustainable supply chain management in the paper industry." *Computers & Industrial Engineering* 135 (2019): 1092–1102. https://doi.org/10.1016/j.cie.2019.05.027

[12] Chukwu, Otuto Amarauche, Valentine Nnaemeka Ezeanochikwa, and Benedict Ejikeme Eya. "Supply chain management of health commodities for reducing global disease burden." *Research in Social and Administrative Pharmacy* 13.4 (2017): 871–874. https://doi.org/10.1016/j.sapharm.2016.08.008

[13] Moons, Karen, Geert Waeyenbergh, and Liliane Pintelon. "Measuring the logistics performance of internal hospital supply chains – a literature study." *Omega* 82 (2019): 205–217. https://doi.org/10.1016/j.omega.2018.01.007

[14] Hasani, Aliakbar, Seyed Hessameddin Zegordi, and Ehsan Nikbakhsh. "Robust closed-loop global supply chain network design under uncertainty: The case of the medical device industry." *International Journal of Production Research* 53.5 (2015): 1596–1624. https://doi.org/10.1080/00207543.2014.965349

[15] Mathur, Bhavana, et al. "Healthcare supply chain management: Literature review and some issues." *Journal of Advances in Management Research* 15.3 (2018): 265–287. https://doi.org/10.1108/JAMR-09-2017-0090

[16] Govindan, Kannan, Prakash C. Jha, and Kiran Garg. "Product recovery optimisation in closed-loop supply chain to improve sustainability in manufacturing." *International Journal of Production Research* 54.5 (2016): 1463–1486. https://doi.org/10.1080/00207543.2015.1083625

[17] Tripathi, Anuj, Teena Bagga, Sharma Shubham, and S.K. Vishnoi. "Big data-driven marketing enabled business performance: A conceptual framework of information, strategy and customer lifetime value" (Jan. 2021). *Proceedings of the 11th International Conference on Cloud Computing, Data Science & Engineering* (pp. 315–320). IEEE Confluence, 2021. https://doi.org/10.1109/Confluence51648.2021.9377156

[18] Gabriel, Cle-Anne, et al. "How supply chain choices affect the life cycle impacts of medical products." *Journal of Cleaner Production* 182 (2018): 1095–1106. https://doi.org/10.1016/j.jclepro.2018.02.107

[19] Ghadimi, Pezhman, Farshad Ghassemi Toosi, and Cathal Heavey. "A multi-agent systems approach for sustainable supplier selection and order allocation in a partnership supply chain." *European Journal of Operational Research* 269.1 (2018): 286–301. https://doi.org/10.1016/j.ejor.2017.07.014

[20] Khatter, Kiran. "Non-functional requirements for blockchain enabled medical supply chain." *International Journal of System Assurance Engineering and Management* (2021): 1–13. https://doi.org/10.1007/s13198-021-01418-y

[21] Alizadeh, Mehdi, Ahmad Makui, and Mohammad Mahdi Paydar. "Forward and reverse supply chain network design for consumer medical supplies considering biological risk." *Computers & Industrial Engineering* 140 (2020): 106229. https://doi.org/10.1016/j.cie.2019.106229

[22] Montecchi, Matteo, Kirk Plangger, and Michael Etter. "It's real, trust me! Establishing supply chain provenance using blockchain." *Business Horizons* 62.3 (2019): 283–293. https://doi.org/10.1016/j.bushor.2019.01.008

[23] Alotaibi, Shoayee, Rashid Mehmood, and Iyad Katib. "The role of big data and twitter data analytics in healthcare supply chain management." *Smart Infrastructure and Applications*. Springer, Cham (2020): 267–279. https://doi.org/10.1007/978-3-030-13705-2_11

[24] Golan, Maureen S., Laura H. Jernegan, and Igor Linkov. "Trends and applications of resilience analytics in supply chain modeling: Systematic literature review in the context of the COVID-19 pandemic." *Environment Systems and Decisions* 40 (2020): 222–243. https://doi.org/10.1007/s10669-020-09777-w

[25] Schniederjans, Dara G., Carla Curado, and Mehrnaz Khalajhedayati. "Supply chain digitisation trends: An integration of knowledge management." *International Journal of Production Economics* 220 (2020): 107439. https://doi.org/10.1016/j.ijpe.2019.07.012

[26] Lamba, Kuldeep, and Surya Prakash Singh. "Big data in operations and supply chain management: Current trends and future perspectives." *Production Planning & Control* 28.11–12 (2017): 877–890. https://doi.org/10.1080/09537287.2017.1336787

[27] Xu, Song, et al. "Disruption risks in supply chain management: A literature review based on bibliometric analysis." *International Journal of Production Research* 58.11 (2020): 3508–3526. https://doi.org/10.1080/00207543.2020.1717011

[28] Behl, Abhishek, and Pankaj Dutta. "Humanitarian supply chain management: A thematic literature review and future directions of research." *Annals of Operations Research* 283.1 (2019): 1001–1044. https://doi.org/10.1007/s10479-018-2806-2

[29] Rowan, Neil J., and John G. Laffey. "Challenges and solutions for addressing critical shortage of supply chain for personal and protective equipment (PPE) arising from Coronavirus disease (COVID19) pandemic – Case study from the Republic of Ireland." *Science of the Total Environment* 725 (2020): 138532. https://doi.org/10.1016/j.scitotenv.2020.138532

[30] Alloghani, Mohamed, et al. "Healthcare services innovations based on the state of the art technology trend industry 4.0." *2018 11th International Conference on Developments in eSystems Engineering (DeSE)*. IEEE. (2018): 64–70. https://doi.org/10.1109/DeSE.2018.00016

[31] Wamba, Samuel Fosso, and Maciel M. Queiroz. "Blockchain in the operations and supply chain management: Benefits, challenges and future research opportunities." *International Journal of Information Management* (2020): 102064. https://doi.org/10.1016/j.ijinfomgt.2019.102064

[32] Bhushan, Bharat, et al. "Blockchain for smart cities: A review of architectures, integration trends and future research directions." *Sustainable Cities and Society* 61 (2020): 102360. https://doi.org/10.1016/j.scs.2020.102360

[33] Verma, Surabhi, and Anders Gustafsson. "Investigating the emerging COVID-19 research trends in the field of business and management: A bibliometric analysis approach." *Journal of Business Research* 118 (2020): 253–261. https://doi.org/10.1016/j.jbusres.2020.06.057

[34] Zhu, Guiyang, Mabel C. Chou, and Christina W. Tsai. "Lessons learned from the COVID-19 pandemic exposing the shortcomings of current supply chain operations: A long-term prescriptive offering." *Sustainability* 12.14 (2020): 5858. https://doi.org/10.3390/su12145858

[35] McDonnell, Anthony, Chalkidou, Kalipso, Yadav, Prashant and Rosen, Dan. "Understanding the impact of COVID-19 on essential medicine supply chains." Center for Global Development, 17 June 2020. www.cgdev.org/blog/understanding-impact-covid-19-essential-medicine-supply-chains. Accessed on 28th November 2021

[36] Patrinley, James Randall, et al. "Lessons from operations management to combat the COVID-19 pandemic." *Journal of Medical Systems* 44.7 (2020): 1–2. https://doi.org/10.1007/s10916-020-01595-6

[37] Rizou, Myrto, et al. "Safety of foods, food supply chain and environment within the COVID-19 pandemic." *Trends in Food Science & Technology* 102 (2020): 293–299. https://doi.org/10.1016/j.tifs.2020.06.008

[38] Okeagu, Chikezie N., et al. "Principles of supply chain management in the time of crisis." *Best Practice & Research Clinical Anaesthesiology* 35.3 (2021): 369–376. https://doi.org/10.1016/j.bpa.2020.11.007

[39] Dwivedi, Sanjeev Kumar, Ruhul Amin, and Satyanarayana Vollala. "Blockchain based secured information sharing protocol in supply chain management system with key distribution mechanism." *Journal of Information Security and Applications* 54 (2020): 102554. https://doi.org/10.1016/j.jisa.2020.102554

[40] Heckmann, Iris, and Stefan Nickel. "Rethinking supply chain risk analysis – common flaws & main elements." *Supply Chain Forum: An International Journal* 18.2. Taylor & Francis (2017). https://doi.org/10.1080/16258312.2017.1348871

[41] Maitra, Sudip, et al. "Integration of internet of things and blockchain toward portability and low-energy consumption." *Transactions on Emerging Telecommunications Technologies* 32.6 (2021): 4103. https://doi.org/10.1002/ett.4103

[42] Litke, Antonios, Dimosthenis Anagnostopoulos, and Theodora Varvarigou. "Blockchains for supply chain management: Architectural elements and challenges towards a global scale deployment." *Logistics* 3.1 (2019): 5. https://doi.org/10.3390/logistics3010005

[43] Viegas, Cláudia Viviane, et al. "Reverse flows within the pharmaceutical supply chain: A classificatory review from the perspective of end-of-use and end-of-life medicines." *Journal of Cleaner Production* 238 (2019): 117719. https://doi.org/10.1016/j.jclepro.2019.117719

[44] Pagell, Mark. "Replication without repeating ourselves: Addressing the replication crisis in operations and supply chain management research." *Journal of Operations Management* 67.1 (2021): 105–115. https://doi.org/10.1002/joom.1120

[45] Andoni, Merlinda, et al. "Blockchain technology in the energy sector: A systematic review of challenges and opportunities." *Renewable and Sustainable Energy Reviews* 100 (2019): 143–174. https://doi.org/10.1016/j.rser.2018.10.014

[46] Treleaven, Philip, Richard Gendal Brown, and Danny Yang. "Blockchain technology in finance." *Computer* 50.9 (2017): 14–17. https://doi.org/10.1109/ICDMW51313.2020.00128

[47] Saberi, Sara, et al. "Blockchain technology and its relationships to sustainable supply chain management." *International Journal of Production Research* 57.7 (2019): 2117–2135. https://doi.org/10.1080/00207543.2018.1533261

[48] Min, Hokey. "Blockchain technology for enhancing supply chain resilience." *Business Horizons* 62.1 (2019): 35–45. https://doi.org/10.1016/j.bushor.2018.08.012

[49] Tijan, Edvard, et al. "Blockchain technology implementation in logistics." *Sustainability* 11.4 (2019): 1185. https://doi.org/10.3390/su11041185

[50] Efanov, Dmitry, and Pavel Roschin. "The all-pervasiveness of the blockchain technology." *Procedia Computer Science* 123 (2018): 116–121.

[51] Mohanta, Bhabendu Kumar, Soumyashree S. Panda, and Debasish Jena. "An overview of smart contract and use cases in blockchain technology." *2018 9th International Conference on Computing, Communication and Networking Technologies (ICCCNT)*. IEEE, 2018. https://doi.org/10.1109/ICCCNT.2018.8494045

[52] Pan, Xiongfeng, et al. "Blockchain technology and enterprise operational capabilities: An empirical test." *International Journal of Information Management* 52 (2020): 101946. https://doi.org/10.1016/j.ijinfomgt.2019.05.002

[53] Tseng, Jen-Hung, et al. "Governance on the drug supply chain via gcoin blockchain." *International Journal of Environmental Research and Public Health* 15.6 (2018): 1055. https://doi.org/10.3390/ijerph15061055

[54] Cumbler, Ethan, et al. "Contingency planning for health care worker masks in case of medical supply chain failure: Lessons learned in novel mask manufacturing from COVID-19 pandemic." *American Journal of Infection Control* 49.10 (2021): 1215–1220. https://doi.org/10.1016/j.ajic.2021.07.018

[55] Bocek, Thomas, et al. "Blockchains everywhere-a use-case of blockchains in the pharma supply-chain." *2017 IFIP/IEEE Symposium on Integrated Network and Service Management (IM)*. IEEE, 2017. https://doi.org/10.23919/INM.2017.7987376

[56] Radanović, Igor, and Robert Likić. "Opportunities for use of blockchain technology in medicine." *Applied Health Economics and Health Policy* 16.5 (2018): 583–590. https://doi.org/10.1007/s40258-018-0412-8

[57] Yoo, Minjae, and Yoojae Won. "A study on the transparent price tracing system in supply chain management based on blockchain." *Sustainability* 10.11 (2018): 4037. https://doi.org/10.3390/su10114037

[58] Etemadi, Niloofar, et al. "Supply chain disruption risk management with blockchain: A dynamic literature review." *Information* 12.2 (2021): 70. https://doi.org/10.3390/info12020070

[59] Ahmad, Raja Wasim, et al. "Blockchain-based forward supply chain and waste management for COVID-19 medical equipment and supplies." *IEEE Access* 9 (2021): 44905–44927. https://doi.org/10.1109/ACCESS.2021.3066503

[60] Kumar, Randhir, and Rakesh Tripathi. "Traceability of counterfeit medicine supply chain through Blockchain." *2019 11th International Conference on Communication Systems & Networks (COMSNETS)*. IEEE, 2019. https://doi.org/10.1109/COMSNETS.2019.8711418

[61] Dutta, Pankaj, et al. "Blockchain technology in supply chain operations: Applications, challenges and research opportunities." *Transportation Research Part E: Logistics and Transportation Review* 142 (2020): 102067. https://doi.org/10.1016/j.tre.2020.102067

[62] Badhotiya, Gaurav Kumar, et al. "Investigation and assessment of blockchain technology adoption in the pharmaceutical supply chain." *Materials Today: Proceedings* (2021). https://doi.org/10.1016/j.matpr.2021.01.673

[63] Arora, Monika, and Yogita Gigras. "Importance of supply chain management in healthcare of third world countries." *International Journal of Supply and Operations Management* 5.1 (2018): 101–106. https://doi.org/10.22034/2018.1.7

[64] Wan, Paul Kengfai, Lizhen Huang, and Halvor Holtskog. "Blockchain-enabled information sharing within a supply chain: A systematic literature review." *IEEE Access* 8 (2020): 49645–49656. https://doi.org/10.1109/ACCESS.2020.2980142

[65] Liu, Xinlai, et al. "Blockchain-based smart tracking and tracing platform for drug supply chain." *Computers & Industrial Engineering* 161 (2021): 107669. https://doi.org/10.1016/j.cie.2021.107669

[66] Chang, Shuchih Ernest, Yi-Chian Chen, and Ming-Fang Lu. "Supply chain re-engineering using blockchain technology: A case of smart contract based tracking process." *Technological Forecasting and Social Change* 144 (2019): 1–11. https://doi.org/10.1016/j.techfore.2019.03.015

[67] Niu, Baozhuang, Jian Dong, and Yaoqi Liu. "Incentive alignment for blockchain adoption in medicine supply chains." *Transportation Research Part E: Logistics and Transportation Review* 152 (2021): 102276. https://doi.org/10.1016/j.tre.2021.102276

[68] Queiroz, Maciel M., Renato Telles, and Silvia H. Bonilla. "Blockchain and supply chain management integration: A systematic review of the literature." *Supply Chain Management: An International Journal* (2019). https://doi.org/10.1108/SCM-03-2018-0143

[69] Jabbar, Sohail, et al. "Blockchain-enabled supply chain: Analysis, challenges, and future directions." *Multimedia Systems* (2020): 1–20. https://doi.org/10.1007/s00530-020-00687-0

[70] Chang, Shuchih E., and Yichian Chen. "When blockchain meets supply chain: A systematic literature review on current development and potential applications." *IEEE Access* 8 (2020): 62478–62494. https://doi.org/10.1109/ACCESS.2020.2983601

[71] Sunny, Justin, Naveen Undralla, and V. Madhusudanan Pillai. "Supply chain transparency through blockchain-based traceability: An overview with demonstration." *Computers & Industrial Engineering* (2020): 106895. https://doi.org/10.1016/j.cie.2020.106895

[72] Sharma, Toshender. "TOP 10 companies using blockchain for healthcare security." 22 June 2019. www.blockchain-council.org/blockchain/top-10-companies-using-blockchain-for-healthcare-security/. Accessed on 13 December 2021.

12 Big Data in Healthcare
Technological Implications and Challenges

Sushant Kumar Vishnoi[1], Naveen Virmani[1],
Divya Pant[1] and Ankit Garg[1]
[1] Institute of Management Studies, Ghaziabad, India

CONTENTS

12.1 EVOLUTION OF HEALTHCARE

The healthcare industry has revolutionised in aspects of services, trends and technology. Various developments have been witnessed in the healthcare industry when it comes to medication and care of patients. In the early times, hospital officials focused on meeting their budget, whereas over the last 10 years, there has been an alteration to concentrate on patient well-being in the hospitals. This section elaborates upon the traditional measures with respect to the modern procedures that are being taken up presently.

DOI: 10.1201/9781003217107-12

12.1.1 Traditional vs. Modern Techniques in the Healthcare Industry

12.1.1.1 Traditional Healthcare

Conventional practices in medical services incorporate several beliefs that have been recognised by indigenous individuals in various developing countries. Their practices frequently derive from the idea that an individual works as the basic component of nature and includes the utilisation of massage, herbs and, yoga practices for brain and body, which is accountable for the physical, mental and spiritual lifestyle.

Orthodox and recognised sorts of treatments are practiced under the conventional medical techniques, for instance, needle therapy, homeopathy and oriental practices. All these practices have been acknowledged since a long time, all around the world. Conventional medication may include:

- Acupuncture
- Ayurveda
- Homeopathy
- Naturopathy

But with the conventional practices, managing such vast data is difficult, and more than that, assessing that mass amount of data is even more difficult. Because of this reason, digitisation in healthcare was the need of the hour, where automated processes could intervene and help the traditional practices of managing this sector efficiently. Health systems required adapting new technologies in order to be capable of collecting, storing and examining the information of the data sets.

12.1.1.2 Modern Healthcare Techniques

Information technology in medical services has improved the quality of life by incorporating new advancements into medication. The immense growth of digitisation of the healthcare data and the advancement of value-based treatment has stimulated the healthcare sector to develop and use data analytics and construct tactical business evaluations. As healthcare is posed with ample number of challenges, such as volume, velocity, variety and veracity, a new system was important to manage and store all the information, for better and efficient workability of the healthcare sector [1].

Data innovation has offered significant commitments to the world, especially in healthcare industry. Big Data is a wonderful innovation that provides an overall holistic view of the patients, physicians and specialists and consumers. With the help of detailed profiles of the patient, Big Data aids in improving effectiveness of care personalisation and efficiency. Various geographic markets having immense potential for growth can be captivated with the help of Big Data. Physicians and patients both are benefitting from the advantages that the new innovations like tele-health services, use of electronic medical record (EMR) and continuous advancements of the mobile phones and tablets. Big Data manages the patient-physician relationship by taking care of their appointments, referrals, etc.

The healthcare sector has advanced from acquainting specialists with new tools to use inside private practices and medical clinics to bringing patients and specialists together even if they are miles away from each other, with the help of media communications. And Big Data has become very important for the healthcare sector as it converts the challenges into opportunities. As it focuses on three dimensions: the mass amount of data that is available, the rising costs in healthcare and an emphasis on consumerism, Big Data in healthcare has become very influential. The new model of Big Data in the healthcare industry emphasises quality, engagement and retention [2]. With an ever-increasing number of hospitals and clinics practicing medical innovations like cell phones at work, doctors are now able to approach any kind of data they need – from drugs data, research and studies and patient history – within seconds [3]. Moreover, because cell phones are easy to carry around, doctors are never away from the data they need. Applications that guide in distinguishing potential health risks and dangers and analyzing data like x-rays and computed tomography (CT) scans additionally add to the advantages that data innovation has brought to the healthcare industry.

With the advent of wearable technology, data will grow exponentially and the Internet of Things (IoT) is gaining popularity [4]. Patient monitoring with the help of wearable technology and IoT becomes constant, which helps in adding massive volumes of knowledge to big data sets. Furthermore, healthcare organisations will embrace Big Gata in more numbers, which will become more crucial for the success of this sector.

12.2 INTRODUCTION OF BIG DATA

Information is the greatest resource for the survival and growth of modern business, since Steve Jobs developed personal computers. Consistently, information is produced in such a quick way, that conventional database management techniques and other information storing frameworks will eventually store, recover and discover connections among information. Since consumerism gets incorporated into the product prototype and forms the core of final product features, business organisations are monitoring and accessing customer information on every possible touch point.

'Big Data' is the term used to define the datasets that are difficult to deal with, if one uses the traditional database management systems (DBMS). Big Data can also be defined when the size of these data sets goes beyond the working capabilities of the usual traditional software tools and storage systems where these tools have to encrypt the data, store it within the software, manage the stored data and then process it within an acceptable elapsed time [5]. Until 2019, yearly profits from the Big Data market from all over the world had reached 49 billion U.S. dollars, which gave a sure belief that this would increase more and more in the following years. The overall market of 2019 revealed that the largest share of Big Data revenue has been generated from Big Data service providers that include global names such as IBM, Splunk, Dell, Oracle and Accenture. Massive information volumes are persistently evolving, straightforwardly conflicting from few terabytes (TB) to a few petabytes (PB) of data in a self-sufficient informational directory. Thus, portions of the intricacies related to enormous information deal with capturing, storing, searching, sharing, examining and picturing. These days, firms are finding enormous volumes of data in order to reveal information and facts they didn't know before [6]. As indicated by Wikibon, Big Data analytics (BDA) will reach $49 billion with a compound annual growth rate

(CAGR) of 11%. Along these lines, every year, the market will pick up $7 billion in value. Because of this estimate, the BDA market should reach $103 billion by 2023. Hence, the role of Big Data analytics is practiced upon large data sets. Analytics practiced on massive data sets reveals and leverages business change [7].

This massive volume of data (Big Data) that gets generated every day is then studied with analytical tools and software to make it commercially viable or useful. Since time immemorial organisations have had access to these huge data sets which are stored into their complex computational architecture, but the success of modern business organisations dwells more around the process by which data is analysed and put into action. The Big Data that is created from sensor-empowered machines, cell phones, distributed or cloud computing, social networking sites or social media [8] contribute heavily to top-level policy formation and product design for gaining the satisfaction and loyalty customers. Big Data bestows organisations with the competence to transform the functioning of the government institutions and scholastic bodies into managing and empowering the market preparedness of their operations.

Big Data innovations have taken into account all the issues that have been identified with the help of hardware and dispersion. Organisations like Google, Yahoo!, Cornerstone, Microsoft, Kaggle, Facebook and Amazon are making huge investments into Big Data–related research. International Data Corporation (IDC) evaluated an estimation of the Big Data market to be about $ 6.8 billion in 2012, developing nearly 40% consistently to $17 billion by 2015. By 2020, Wikibon's Jeff Kelly predicts the Big Data market will top $50 billion. In sync with the functioning of modern businesses, BDA becomes imperative for strategic, tactical and operational decision making of organisations.

Examining complicated and bigger data sets can profit ventures or firms; in any case, this demonstrates a necessity for new information structures, scientific methodologies and analytical approaches. Hence, the later sections of this chapter will cover and clarify the Big Data concepts; the significance of the Big Data; and various tools that are being used to initiate Big Data storage, management and analysis in healthcare. Big Data is extensively being used in the healthcare industry, and the chapter will explore its implications and challenges in upcoming sections.

12.2.1 BIG DATA: CONCEPTUALISATION AND DEFINITIONS

Large information sets can either be classified as unstructured or structured. Organised data sets contain information in either databases or spreadsheets and are usually numeric in nature [9]. 'For improved perceptions and proper decision making, information assets of big Data like volume, velocity and variety need resourceful and advanced forms of data processing'. Unstructured information refers to the data that is complicated and doesn't fall into a preset model or format. It incorporates all the information and data that are gathered from online networking sources, which in the long run helps firms in understanding customer requirements [10]. Large information or data sets can be assembled from social stages and web-based interfaces and readily gathered from applications through polls, surveys or questionnaires. The existence of sensors in the advanced smart devices allows information to be gathered over a wide range of circumstances.

TABLE 12.1
Definition of Big Data

Author	Definition of Big Data
[13]	'Big data in healthcare comprises of collection of information from individual or groups pertaining to lifestyle, clinical, biological and environmental health and wellness quotient at different intervals of time.'
[14]	'Big healthcare data refers to the management of diverse datasets having dearth of unique features in addition to huge volumes, that not only expedite the processing of all relevant information but also enables the uprooting of concrete information about events and trends for decision making.'
[15]	'Big data in healthcare refers to the congregation of volumes of complex online data sets which otherwise are difficult to be analyzed with the traditional computational equipment's, database management systems and tools.'

Computer databases often store the Big Data and analyse it with the help of software that is especially created and designed to handle complicated and large data sets. This type of complex data is managed by various software as a service (SAAS) companies [11]. Relationships amidst varied data sets are studied and examined by data analysts – for instance, demographics or purchase history – to understand if there is any relation or not. Outsourcing or in-house examinations are conducted in order to focus on managing the large data sets into digestible structures, and this assessment of Big Data is generally used by firms to convert it into valuable information.

Since 2012, Big Data has created 8 million jobs in the United States and 6 million more over the globe. IT administration businesses earned significant shares of the Big Data benefits in 2019. The anticipated turnover is $77.5 billion. Likewise, the hardware purchases have yielded $23.7 billion, and business administrations produced benefits of roughly $20.7 billion. The insights uncover that Big Data benefits will thrive as high as $67.2 billion by 2020 [8, 12] as shown in Table 12.1.

12.2.2 SIGNIFICANCE OF BIG DATA

The importance of big data doesn't pivot around how much information a firm has, but on how that organisation is using the information. All organisations use information in their own particular manner; the more capably a firm uses data and information, the more enriched intelligence it will employ for operationalising the effective and efficient utilisation of its resources [15]. Business organisations are employing analysis tools for synthesising information from multichannel or omnichannel data sources to discover hidden trends and answers to enable the following:

2.2.1. Cost Savings: Techniques and instruments of Big Data like Hadoop and cloud-based analytics can help an organisation in achieving cost preferences, particularly when gigantic measures of information are to be warehoused. Big Data is helpful in recognising various productive methods for conducting business.

2.2.2. Time Reductions: The extreme quickness of Big Data instruments and analytics effectively perceives new origins of information, which helps firms in examining data and making quick assessments based on this.

2.2.3. Understand the ECONOMIC SITUATIONS: By assessing Big Data, one can accomplish improved comprehension of existing economic situations. For instance, by analyzing shoppers' purchasing habits, a firm can find the items that are sold the most and assembling items as per this measure. With the assistance of this evaluation, the firms can increase a competitive advantage.

2.2.4. Manage Online Anonymity: Big information approaches can likewise perform sentiment analysis. Henceforth, one can procure different audits about what is being seen about their firm. If one needs to manage and expand the online presence of their business, Big Data methods or tools can really be helpful.

2.2.5. Customer Acquisition, Retention and Satisfaction: The most important asset of any business is their consumer. No firm can claim their success without establishing a solid customer base. Nevertheless, even with a customer base, no business can afford to neglect the high competition it faces in the market [16]. With the use of Big Data, businesses tend to notice several consumer-related patterns and trends. Perceiving customer behaviour is important to understand customer loyalty.

2.2.6. Developing Marketing Insights: The integration and analysis of organisational data by using Big Data tools, techniques and capabilities helps generate customer insights. Hence, organisations sync these customer insights with product development and process improvement. This customisation and synergy between customer insights and requirements helps organisations match their customer expectations and simultaneously improve their satisfaction and loyalty quotients.

2.2.7. Innovations and New Product Development: Innovating and redeveloping the products is another importance of Big Data that companies practice.

12.2.3 CHALLENGES OF IMPLEMENTING BIG DATA IN HEALTHCARE

Even though there are enormous advantages of Big Data, there are a lot of challenges as well, which are difficult to handle and hence the potential of Big Data becomes limited because of those challenges. Few of these challenges are, however, functioned as attributes of Big Data, while a few of them behave in the form of present analysis methods and models and some, through the limitations of current data processing system [17]. The challenges of Big Data have engrossed on the dilemmas of understanding the impression of Big Data [18], the dynamics of what information and data must be created and accumulated uncertainties of privacy and security [12], implementation of intelligent automation [19–20] and moral consultations important to mining such information [6, 21]. [2] underlines that going for a practical approach is a challenge that firms are continuously learning. For example, one of the most challenging issues in regard to Big Data is the infrastructure's substantial expenses [22]. Hardware is exorbitant even with the accessibility of distributed computing advancements.

TABLE 12.2

Challenges of Big Data in Health Care

Challenge	Author	Description
Ethical Challenges	[25]	Healthcare: Discrimination in healthcare and insurance. Education: Using data for possible admissions discrimination.
Quality Challenges	[26]	Data Level: Unreliability, data copying, inconsistency General Level: Human data entry, missing values, social media Process Level: Collection and transmission of data.
Governance Challenges and Privacy Concerns	[27]	Administration and management issues of data in policy acceptance.
Management Challenges	[28]	Protection of patient identity. Privacy of the treatments that the patients undergo.
Volatility Challenges	[29]	Crashing of data due to the incapability of storing it.

Besides, to sort information so as to build significant data, human examination is frequently required. However, the computing technologies are essential, but human expertise is falling behind; this ends up being another enormous challenge. As reported by [23–24], the various challenges posed by Big Data can be categorised into three classes: information, procedure and the executive's challenges (Table 12.2).

12.2.4   BIG DATA IN HEALTHCARE: ENABLING TOOLS AND TECHNOLOGIES

The Internet transformation, cloud computing and the progression to self-service analytics have all together contributed to the altering dimensions of business intelligence [30]. To strive commendably in a digitally driven era, business/firm leaders must apprehend and address the acute modifications taking place in the field of analytics and how these alterations influence their whole strategy. The main motive of this section is to understand the various technologies of Big Data that aid in the successful implementation of analytics in organisations. This section looks at the probable profits of analytics, discovers the varying dimensions of analytics and offers a guide to some of the prospects that are available for using embedded technologies of Big Data in a business (Table 12.3).

12.2.4.1   Predictive Analytics

The extraction of knowledge or information through data to forecast the implications and behaviour repetitions through the analytics on big data is termed predictive analytics. All the future consequences and the possibility of any circumstance or incident that can take place can be established with the help of predictive analytics. It is a subset of data mining through which all the possible opportunities and their

TABLE 12.3

Enabling Technologies of Big Data

Parameter(s)	Information	Data	Big Data	Big Data Analytics
Tools	Surveys, personal interviews, questionnaires, case studies, etc.	Annual reports, experiments, published literature sources, etc.	Software like Hadoop, RapidMiner, Apache Storm, etc.	Tools like Cloudera Distribution Hadoop (CDH), Cassandra, Knime, Datawrapper, Lumify, High Performance Computer Cluster (HPCC), etc.
Era	Early 20th century	Late 1800s	Beginning of 2005	Beginning of 2013
Innovations	Digital education, communication, augmented reality, etc.	Safer supply chains, convenient travel, secure healthcare records, etc.	Blockchain, artificial intelligence (AI), Internet of things (IoT), automation, etc.	Big Data loan approval, predictive hospital staffing system, healthcare cost estimators, etc.

tendencies can be foreseen. Evaluation of huge data automatically is possible with the help of predictive analytics methods [31]. Many researchers and data scientists urge the design of an automated tool that can reason and further recognise the future situations and measures. To develop and assure proficiency and precision of the data extracted, the predictive analytics must be a constant.

There's an exponential potential and scope of predictive analytics in data mining [32]. The extraction of private, discrete or hidden information and data from varied data marts and warehouses is termed data mining. Knowledge discovery is one of the key methods that is used for the evaluation of arrays in the sources of data under the data mining process. Strategies like machine learning, statistics and pattern recognition are employed by data mining for knowledge discovery [33–34]. The extraction of data is done with the access of huge databases, which is the foremost step. This obtained data is managed through high-tech algorithms to disclose predictive knowledge and patterns.

12.2.4.2   Knowledge Discovery Tools

Knowledge discovery can be characterised as the non-insignificant practice of perceiving successful, unique, conceivably advantageous and ultimately sensible patterns or structures in information. It focuses on artificial intelligence (AI), measurable strategies, statistics and perception aptitudes to decide and introduce awareness in a manner that is clearly understood. Knowledge discovery considers crude and raw outcomes from data mining and carefully redesigns them into useful and reasonable data.

12.2.4.3   Data Virtualisation

Data virtualisation is the strategy for consolidating information from varied sources of data to encourage an individual, scientific and virtual understanding of data that can be recovered by front-end arrangements or solutions, for example, applications, dashboards and entries, without revealing the data's storage location. The whole strategy for data virtualisation involves abstracting, redesigning, partnering and dispersing information from various sources [35]. The premier objective of data virtualisation is to convey an individual point of approach to the information by collecting it from varied sources of data.

Data virtualisation includes abilities like:

- Abstraction of data related with the technical attributes of gathered information or data.
- Federation of informational originating from different, heterogeneous source frameworks (operational information or historical information or both).
- Flexibility of information delivery as information services are executed only when clients repurpose them.

Furthermore, data virtualisation also has the ability to disseminate skills for information safety, data quality and information management, for caching, optimisation and so on.

12.2.4.4 Data Integration

Organisations are employing a mix of both digital and physical sources for collecting data from individual customers and groups. As collected data pertains to both structured and unstructured data sources, data integration emerges as an important challenge.

The process by which organisations aggregate and transform this structured, semi-structured and unstructured data into analytical data structures is called data integration. Data integration begins with the ingestion action, and involves stages like, purging, ETL (extract, transfer and load) mapping and transformation [36]. Data reconciliation inevitably allows analytical methods to yield productive and significant business insights. There's no consistent strategy to integrate information. However, data integration explanations normally incorporates a pattern of confined basic components, including a network of information sources, a chief server and clients recovering information from the chief server.

Data integration methods tend to improve the value of a business' information over time. As information is integrated into a unified framework, quality issues get disclosed and vital upgrades are implemented, which eventually brings more precise information that is required for quality analysis.

12.2.5 Dimensions of Big Data

Big Data is significant on the grounds that it empowers firms to collect, store, control and employ or activate massive amounts of data at the right time for getting the right information for maximum impact. Likewise, Big Data managers must produce employable information (volume), diverse in nature (variety), at a manageable pace (velocity), while not losing the important attributes of raw data (veracity), for gaining

TABLE 12.4
Dimensions of Big Data

Dimension	Characteristics for Big Data	Author
Volume	Terabytes, Transactions, Tables, Records	[37]
Veracity	Authenticity, Availability, Accountability	[38]
Value	Statistical, Correlations, Hypothetical	[39]
Variety	Structured, Unstructured, Multifactor	[40]
Velocity	Batch, Real-time, Processes, Streams	[41]

customer loyalty and financial stability (value). These five attributes amalgamate to define big data capabilities (Table 12.4).

12.3 APPLICATIONS OF BIG DATA IN HEALTHCARE

In medical services, Big Data comprises heterogeneous, multi-dimensional, inadequate and uncertain perceptions (e.g. diagnosis, socioeconomics, treatment, prevention of ailment, disease, injury and physical and mental disabilities) derived from varied sources that use incongruent testing/sampling. A portion of this information is organised and they highlight genotype, phenotype, genomics information, International Classification of Diseases (ICD) codes and related health problems; however, the unstructured information also includes notices, clinical notes, medical prescriptions, clinical imaging, electronic health records (EHRs), human lifestyle and wellbeing information [42]. The major challenge for BA is to manage this heterogeneous information so as to create insights for improved healthcare.

12.3.1 GENERAL HEALTHCARE

Big Data in general healthcare or open medical services stresses on information related to physiological requirements of customers which is continuously collected by portable tools [43], like electrocardiogram, vitals, infection, wearable gadgets, everyday wellbeing record, sports and diet. Electrocardiogram is defined as the electrical chart recording the heartbeat movement of an individual in a timeframe, e.g. 60 seconds; this procedure includes putting anodes/electrodes on the skin. Vitals, short for indispensable signs, incorporate temperature, pulse rate, respiratory rate and blood pressure. These signs are the most significant four indications of the body's capacity. Wearable gadgets in context to the general healthcare refers to the wellbeing that is recorded by an equipment that offers insights regarding way of life and vitals of individuals, from which the doctors can aid treatment to their patients. Propelled gadgets, for example, cell phones with applications like HealthKit from Apple, Google Fit from Google and S Health structure Samsung, Android watches and Google Glasses have been created with sensors in the healthcare sector [44]. Since individuals have gotten progressively worried about their own wellbeing on an everyday basis, the outpatient diagnostic laboratory (ODL) performs a key job in recording an individual's day-by-day wellbeing and signs of any disease or illness [45]. Moreover, information related to sports and the diet of individuals contributes fundamentally to Big Data in general healthcare. In the Apple iTunes store alone, around 40,000 medical services applications can be accessed [46]. In 2017, more than 1.7 billion individuals downloaded applications related to healthcare. There is a notable case in which Google effectively anticipated the time and size of a flu by breaking down the web search tool results.

12.3.2 SERVICE DELIVERY SYSTEM

Big Data in the sector of healthcare offers one vital purpose – real-time cautioning and offering types of assistance when in a hurry. In emergency clinics, clinical decision support (CDS) examines clinical information on the spot, offering wellbeing experts with advice as they make prescriptive choices. Nevertheless, specialists want their patients to avoid medical clinics and hospitals to in order to get rid of expensive in-house medications and treatments. Analytics has been hailed as one of the chief business intelligence issues in 2020 and can possibly turn out to be another innovational technique [47]. Wearables help in gathering patients' health information persistently and send this information to the cloud.

Asthmapolis has begun to use inhalers with global positioning system (GPS)–empowered trackers help to recognise asthma patterns, both on an individual level and for huge sample sizes. This information is being utilised correlating with the data from the CDS so as to form and develop better treatment plans for asthmatics.

12.3.3 CLINICAL DIAGNOSIS AND RESEARCH

New Big Data techniques have the ability to turbocharge forces of perception in the healthcare sector. Just as the magnifying instrument improved vision, the refined scientific and computational methodologies can increase what can be 'seen' and comprehended from enormous amounts of datasets or information. Analysts can utilise approaches that are intended to uncover types of patient groups that may propose new scientific classifications as per an expansive scope of qualities, including results. It might be based on, natural, clinical, individual behaviour and reveals information that there are a lot more sorts of diabetes than previously though. The experimental arrangement is relatively helpful in choosing treatment procedures and anticipating results. This information can be helpful, even ahead of time in understanding the basic components of illness and reasons of diseases to approach for right treatment. In healthcare, there is a point of reference for finding compelling treatments (e.g. headache medicine like aspirin) before knowing why it delivered an advantage. AI can give inputs similar to that of a genuine specialist or master. However, the outcomes of these kinds of analyses should be assessed and deciphered by researchers with equivalent expertise in medication so that valuable information is produced.

Huge archives of potential information, populated by information from healthcare visits, gadgets, managerial cases and bio examples, are progressively accessible. The guarantee of enormous information resources lies not simply in their size, but in the manner in which they are utilised. For the clinical research undertaking to accomplish its latent capacity, it needs to find its general surroundings and encounter the intricacy inside it. Sufficiently, these repositories of information can be an essentially limitless source of information to fuel a learning medical services framework.

12.3.4 DISEASE TRANSMISSION AND PREVENTION

Big Data is frequently considered in regard to improving the healthcare sector, although it has a less valued but a significant task to carry out in hindering illness. Big Data can encourage activities for eliminating risks of common illnesses, for example, physical movement, diet, tobacco use and environmental pollution. It can be done by encouraging the disclosure of hazard factors for a disease at a large scale, both at a macro-level to associated subpopulations and at a micro-level to associated individuals, and by simultaneously improving the viability of convergence or intersections with the purpose of aiding individuals to accomplish more healthy practices in more healthy environments.

Big Data can both permit the establishment of new, customised illness risk factors correlated with individual's wellbeing and environment and also aid individuals to effectively change their lifestyle practices. With the expanding sicknesses in the United States, Big Data has improved people's wellbeing and has also managed to diminish medical costs and expenses. Policies identified in the federal healthcare arena are putting greater duty on medical services to avoid diseases, which include an extra budget for this 'goal-oriented Big Data–related prevention action'. One medical delivery in the current scenario is the inexpensive care association, wherein social healthcare suppliers get a fixed charge for each patient, regardless of the treatment that he or she undergoes, to give clinical care and consideration to a particular set of population. Under this framework, the monetary incentives are adjusted for social healthcare suppliers in order to keep away individuals from getting ill. This requires new inexpensive approaches to forestall illness by mediating on the determinants of health, with the objective of improving wellbeing while at the same time reducing costs.

12.4 CHALLENGES OF BIG DATA IN HEALTHCARE

Acquiring clean information: Every piece of information or data emerges from some source; however, for a few medical services suppliers, it doesn't constantly originate from sources having impeccable information. To get information that is clean, right, and organised that is fit for utilisation in different practices is a ceaseless challenge for organisations. Denied EHR usage, convoluted work processes and a deficient understanding of why Big Data is remarkable can add to data quality concerns during its lifecycle.

Cleaning the information: Healthcare providers are familiar with the importance of cleanliness in the hospitals and clinics and the operation theatre rooms; however, they may not know that it is imperative to clean their information as well. Unhealthy and dirty information can disturb a

Big Data analytics process, especially while conveying various information sources that have records of clinical or operational segments in varied arrangements.

However, most of the information cleaning techniques are achieved physically, but some of the IT experts propose mechanised cleaning software that with the help of some rules can contrast data, differentiate it, and rectify massive datasets. This software reduces the time and costs, protects accuracy and increases reliability in medical data warehouses.

Storage: The hospitals barely have an idea about where their information is being warehoused, but it's critical in regard to cost, security and execution for the IT department. While the size of the healthcare information increments exponentially, a few suppliers are unable to adapt to the expenses and impacts of on-premise data warehouses [48]. Nonetheless, different firms are content with 'on premise' information storage, which ensures administration over security and access, which is difficult to sustain is and is prone to making information across rare divisions.

Security of Data: Data security is one of the central needs for medical service providing firms, especially in the scenario of prominent encroachments, hackings and redemption cases. From phishing assaults to malware cases, medical services information is vulnerable to an array of challenges [49, 50]. Even the most safely held data warehouse could be obtained from the limitations of human staff individuals, who prefer ease over delayed programming updates and complex limitations on their access to information or software/application.

Stewardship: Healthcare information, primarily on the clinical edge, has an extended timeframe of realistic usability. To preserve information of the patients for any event in the preceding years, suppliers may have to use distinguished datasets for investigating research analysis, which makes steady stewardship a fundamental concern. Information may be reprocessed or reconsidered for reasons like quality estimation or performance benchmarking.

Picking up information about when the past information was framed, by whom, and for what reason is fundamental for specialists and information analysts. Mounting intensive, correct and the most recent metadata is a pivotal component of a successful information governance plan. An information analyst needs to protect all the segments that satisfy the guidelines, definitions and structures, and are likewise sorted out appropriately from origination to obliteration and can be of help in carrying out these tasks.

Querying: Powerful metadata and flexible stewardship techniques make it less difficult for organisations to query their information and procure the appropriate responses that they are foreseeing. The capacity to query information is the initial step for detailing and analytics; however, medical services affiliations should conquer the difficulties before they can take part in significant analysis of their Big Data resources.

12.5 BIG DATA ANALYTICS IN HEALTHCARE: PROMISES AND FUTURE PROSPECTS

Presently, huge volumes of data are generated by applications based on biomedical devices, healthcare tools and associated biometric sensors. Therefore, organisations must carefully plan for the implications of this existing healthcare data. This data holds great prominence as organisations are deriving business insights aiding further technological, medical, procedural and clinical improvements. Based on these data-centered developments, a new world of personalised medicine and patient-specific medical or clinical specialty is possible. The reigning future prospects and promises that Big Data technologies will enrich the healthcare industry are as follows:

- The volume of data collected from digitalisation of health, medical records (EHR and EMR) and clinical records are reshaping the future of disease diagnostic and prognostic systems. The business organisations are extending their contribution towards this cause of facilitating examination and audit of medical services and simultaneously enabling smooth transition of clinical change management are better placed to this ride this digital wave.
- CDS frameworks provide a platform for improved diagnostic policies and recognising and reducing the probability of malicious practices related to Big Data. However, practically, most of them face difficulties on government issues like handling of private data, sharing of data and its security. The information collected from medical organisations and researchers provides improved results and diagnostic solutions to ailments. This has additionally helped in building a superior and better customised medical care structure. The importance of Big Data has been realised by healthcare associations, and they have executed Big Data investigations in medical services and clinical practices. Better computing powers are being used to draw out relevant information from Big Data, which has drastically decreased time frames. Clinical preliminaries and investigation of drug store and insurance claims are indicators to analyse the medical Big Data.
- BDA is using the distance between structured and unstructured data sources. The shift to a coordinated data climate is a notable obstacle to survive. The guideline of Big Data vigorously depends on the possibility of the more data one has, the more experiences one can acquire from this data and can make expectations for future occasions. Expansion and growth of Big Data is legitimately projected by different by healthcare organisations and various research organisations. Nonetheless, a limited ability to focus has seen a range of examination presently being used that altogether affects the navigation and execution of medical services industry.
- The high volume of clinical data gathered across heterogeneous stages has put a test on data researchers for cautious incorporation and execution. It is consequently proposed that transformation in medical care is additionally expected to assemble bioinformatics, wellbeing informatics and examination to advance customised and more successful therapies. Moreover, new methodologies and advances ought to be created to comprehend the nature

(organised, semi-organised, unstructured), intricacy (aspects and traits) and volume of the data to determine its significance. The best resource of Big Data lies in its boundless conceivable outcomes. The emergence and growth of Big Data have considerably impacted the progressions of the medical industry, which includes medical data management and drug development for several ailments.

12.6 REFERENCES

[1] Ellaway, R. H., Pusic, M. V., Galbraith, R. M., & Cameron, T. (2014). Developing the role of big data and analytics in health professional education. *Medical Teacher*, 36(3), 216–222.

[2] Sukumar, S. R., Natarajan, R., & Ferrell., R. K. (2015). Quality of big data in health care. *International Journal of Health Care Quality Assurance*, 1–14.

[3] Dimitrov, D. V. (2016). Medical internet of things and big data in healthcare. *Healthcare Informatics Research*, 22(3), 156–163.

[4] Liu, C., Yang, C., Zhang, X., & Chen, J. (2015). External integrity verification for outsourced big data in cloud and IoT: A big picture. *Future Generation Computer Systems*, 49, 58–67.

[5] Mehta, N., & Pandit, A. (2018). Concurrence of big data analytics and healthcare: A systematic review. *International Journal of Medical Informatics*, 114, 57–65.

[6] Andrew, E. B., Davenport, T. H., Patil, D. J., & Barton, D. (2012). Big data: The management revolution. *Harvard Business Review*, 90(10), 60–68.

[7] Davenport, T. H. (2014). How strategists use "big data" to support internal business decisions, discovery and production. *Strategy & Leadership*, 45–50.

[8] Bagga, T. (2012). A study on perception of various social networking sites with special reference to Delhi/NCR. *ZENITH International Journal of Business Economics & Management Research*, 2(10), 64–79.

[9] Mannering, F., Bhat, C. R., Shankar, V., & Abdel-Aty, M. (2020). Big data, traditional data and the tradeoffs between prediction and causality in highway-safety analysis. *Analytic Methods in Accident Research*, 25, 1–9.

[10] Vishnoi, S. K., & Bagga, T. (2020). *Marketing Intelligence: Antecedents and Consequences. 3rd International Conference on Innovative Computing and Communication* (pp. 1–9). New Delhi: Elsevier.

[11] Demirkan, H., & Delen, D. (2013). Leveraging the capabilities of service-oriented decision support systems: Putting analytics and big data in cloud. *Decision Support Systems*, 55(1), 412–421.

[12] Lazer, D., Pentland, A., Adamic, L., & Roy, D. (2009, February 6). Computational social science. *Social Science*, 721–722.

[13] Auffray, C., Balling, R., & Zanetti, G. (2016). Making sense of big data in healthcare. *Genome Medicine*, 1–13.

[14] Dinov, I. (2018). *Data Science and Predictive Analytics*. Spain: Springer International Publishing.

[15] Mishra, D., Luo, Z., Jiang, S., Papadopoulos, T., & Dubey, R. (2017). A bibliographic study on big data: Concepts, trends and challenges. *Business Process Management Journal*, 555–573.

[16] Singh, A., Vishnoi, S. K., & Bagga, T. (2018). A study on customer preferences towards travel and tourism sector and their services. *International Journal of Research in Advent Technology*, 6(12), 3847–3854.

[17] Jin, X., Cheng, X., & Wang, Y. (2015). Significance and challenges of big data research. *Big Data Research*, 59–64.

[18] Hargittai, E. (2015). Is bigger always better? Potential biases of big data derived from social network sites. *The ANNALS of the American Academy of Political and Social Science*, 63–76.

[19] Vishnoi, S. K., Bagga, T., Sharma, A., & Wani, S. N. (2018). Artificial Intelligence enabled marketing solutions: A review. *Indian Journal of Economics & Business*, 167–177.

[20] Vishnoi, S. K., Tripathi, A., & Bagga, T. (2019). Intelligent automation, planning & implementation: A review of constraints. *International Journal on Emerging Technologies*, 174–178.

[21] Tole, A. (2013). Big data challenges. *Databse Systems Journal*, 31–40.

[22] Wang, Y., & Wiebe, V. J. (2014). Big data analytics on the characteristic equilibrium of collective opinions in social networks. *Internation Journal of Cognitive Informatics and Natual Intelligence*, 29–44.

[23] Akerkar, R. (2013). *Big Data Computing*. Norway: Taylor & Francis Group.

[24] Zicari, R. (2013). Big data: Challenges and opportunities. In R. Akerkar (ed.), *Big Data Computing* (pp. 103–128). Norway: Taylor & Francis Group.

[25] Martin, K. (2015). Ethical issues in the big data industry. *MIS Quarterly Executive*, 67–85.

[26] Dssouli, R. (2018). *Big Data Quality: A Survey. Big Data Congress* (pp. 4066–4081). San Francisco: IEEE.

[27] Giest, S. (2018). Big data application in governance and policy. *Politics and Governance*, 1–4.

[28] George, G. (2014). Big data & management. *The Academy of Management Journal*, 321–326.

[29] Gu, M., Rubel, O., & Wu, K. (2013). A big data approach to analyzing market volatility. *SSRN*, 1–32.

[30] Tripathi, A., Bagga, T., & Aggarwal, R. K. (2020). Strategic impact of business intelligence: A review of literature. *Prabandhan: Indian Journal of Management*, 35–48.

[31] Power, D. J. (2014). Using 'big data' for analytics and decision support. *Journal of Decision Systems*, 23(2), 222–228.

[32] Zaman, M., & Mirza, S. (2016). A review of data mining literature. *IJCSIS*, 437–442.

[33] Lee, C. H., & Yoon, H.-J. (2017). Medical big data: Promise and challenges. *Kidney Research and Clinical Practice*, 36(1), 32–45.

[34] Sun, J., & Reddy, C. K. (2013). Big data analytics for healthcare. In *Proceedings of the 19th ACM SIGKDD International Conference on Knowledge Discovery and Data Mining,* Association for Computing Machinery, New York, NY: United States. (pp. 1525–1534).

[35] He, P., Wang, P., & Tang, J. G. (2015). City-wide smart healthcare appointment systems based on cloud data virtualization paas. *International Journal of Multimedia and Ubiquitous Engineering*, 10(2), 371–382.

[36] Sensmeier, J. (2003). Advancing the state of data integration in healthcare. *Journal of Healthcare Information Management: JHIM*, 17(4), 58–61.

[37] Lycett, M. (2013). Datafication': Making sense of (big) data in a complex world. *European Journal of Information Systems*, 381–386.

[38] Gandomi, A., & Haider, M. (2015). Beyond the hype: Big data concepts, methods, and analytics. *International Journal of Information Management*, 35(2), 137–144.

[39] Watson, H. (2014). Big data concepts, technologies & applications. *Communications of the Association for Information Systems*, 1247–1268.

[40] Ivan, M., & Trifu, M. (2014). Big data: Present & future. *Database Systems Journal*, 32–41.

[41] Uddin, M. F., & Gupta, N. (2014). Seven V's of big data understanding big data to extract value. In *Proceedings of the 2014 Zone 1 Conference of the American Society for Engineering Education* (pp. 1–5). IEEE: United States.

[42] Raghupathi, W., & Raghupathi, V. (2014). Big data in healthcare: Promise & potential. *Health Information Science and Systems*, 1–10.

[43] Yan, V., Qin, X., & Fan, J. (2015). A review of big data research in medicine and healthcare. In Y. Zhu & S. Guo (eds.), *Collaborative Computing* (pp. 3–16). Wuhan: Springer.

[44] Safavi, S., & Shukur, Z. (2014). Conceptual privacy framework for health information on wearable device. *PLOS*, 1–16.

[45] Backonja, K., Irving, R., & Webster, P. (2012). Mood and cognition by nutraceutical interventions. In R. Watson & V. Preedy (eds.), *Bioactive Nutraceuticals* (pp. 122–148). Elsevier: Netherlands.

[46] Marston, H., & Hall, A. (2018). Gamification: Application for health promotion and health information technology engagement. In *Handbook of Research on Holistic Perspectives in Gamification for Clinical Practice*, IGI GLOBAL, (pp. 78–104).

[47] Lai, P., Mai, C., & Lim, P. (2019). Healthcare big data analytics: Re-engineering healthcare delivery through innovation. *IeJSME*, 10–13.

[48] Wamba, S. F., Akter, S., Edwards, A., Chopin, G., & Gnanzou., D. (2015). How 'big data' can make big impact: Findings from a systematic review and a longitudinal case study. *International Journal of Production Economics*, 165, 234–246.

[49] Sivarajah, U., Kamal, M. M., Irani, Z., & Weerakkody, V. (2017). Critical analysis of big data challenges and analytical methods. *Journal of Business Research*, 70, 263–286.

[50] Crawford, K., & Boyd, D. (2012). Critical questions for big data. *Information, Communication & Society*, 662–679.

13 An Efficient System for Predictive Analysis on Brain Cancer Using Machine Learning and Deep Learning Techniques

Akshita S. Chanchlani[1], Vilas M. Thakare[1], Vijay M. Wadhai[2], Dhanashri H. Gawali[1] and Minakshee Patil[3]

[1] Sant Gadge Baba Amravati University, Amravati, India
[2] D.Y. Patil College of Engineering, Pune, India
[3] Sinhgad Academy of Engineering, Pune, India

CONTENTS

DOI: 10.1201/9781003217107-13

13.1 INTRODUCTION

In brain tumour diagnosis, doctors integrate their medical domain knowledge with brain magnetic resonance imaging (MRI) scans to obtain the characteristics of the brain tumour and decide on further treatment options. However, in brain MRI scans, a large number of MRI scans are taken for every patient (more than 500 image scans). Given this, the system must be able to work on real-time data to generate qualitative input images. The most important task for any brain MRI image analysis is pre-processing (noise removal), efficient segmentation (edge detection), feature extraction (pixel extraction) and masking (morphological operations) using various classification and segmentation algorithms.

In conventional practices, radiologists, clinical practitioners and neurosurgeons perform disease detection and analysis of brain cancer MRIs manually and that becomes a time-consuming process. The segmentation of brain tumours in magnetic resonance high-resolution images is a challenging and difficult task because of the variety of their possible shapes, locations and image intensities. This may lead to inaccurate results. Accurate automatic brain image segmentation in magnetic resonance (MR) images is a prerequisite for the quantitative assessment of the brain. Therefore, there is a need for computer-aided brain tumour detection and segmentation from brain MR images to overcome the problems involved in the manual segmentation. Various techniques of image processing when combined with algorithms of advanced machine learning for performing accurate segmentation, classification and prediction of brain cancer will increase the performance and reduce the time required by radiologists. A proposed system is implemented and developed from brain cancer MRI data. Automated brain cancer diagnosis from MRI scans is one of the medical image analysis methodologies. The automated diagnosis involves two steps: (1) image classification and (2) image segmentation.

Image classification is performed by learning (training) on MRI high-resolution image scans and its structure using machine learning algorithms. Image segmentation is used for extraction of abnormal tumour portions, which is essential for volumetric analysis on the region of interest.

This chapter presents the study of imaging technologies for detection, classification, segmentation, analysis and prediction of existing brain cancer techniques. In addition, it describes the development of a system for classification of brain cancer disease based on MRI images using machine learning and deep learning techniques for improving accuracy and efficiency. This research work will enable all stakeholders like doctors, radiologists and neurosurgeons to detect and predict brain cancer precisely, efficiently and accurately with speedy performance.

13.2 LITERATURE SURVEY

The human brain is a vital part of the human body and has a complex structure [1]. Brain cancer is a very serious type of malignancy that occurs when there is an uncontrolled growth of cancer cells in the brain [2]. With the increase in globalisation of medical issues and growth of medical data, there is a necessity for a robust and fast method of retrieving the medical data across different hospitals for the same patient from multiple locations in order to facilitate early diagnosis and care.

Brain cancer is caused by a malignant brain tumour. Not all brain tumours are malignant (cancerous). Some types of brain tumour are benign (non-cancerous). Tumour grade is the description of a tumour based on how abnormal the tumour cells and the tumour tissue look under a microscope [3]:

Grade I: The tissue is benign. The cells look nearly like normal brain cells, and they grow slowly.

Grade II: The tissue is malignant. The cells look less like normal cells than do the cells in a Grade I tumour.

Grade III: The malignant tissue has cells that look very different from normal cells. The abnormal cells are actively growing (anaplastic).

Grade IV: The malignant tissue has cells that look most abnormal and tend to grow quickly.

Using various computer-aided algorithms and deep learning technology, it is a challenging task of classifying, detecting and predicting of brain cancer/tumour MRI scans. Because of the humongous growth of the medical data, there is a necessity to move the data from one place to another in order to facilitate early patient diagnosis and care. With the increase in globalisation of medical issues and medical tourism, there is a need for a robust and fast method of retrieving the medical data across different hospitals for the same patient from multiple locations. The patient should not be forced to carry the bundles of scan reports across the world to discuss his medical problem. Cloud technology makes access to the medical data easier. The main advantage of using the cloud is that the quality of medical care is improved as well as patient safety and the cost for the treatment is reduced. As represented in Figure 13.1, machine learning methods basically try to discover a model (e.g. rules or parameters) by using a set of input data points and some way to guide the algorithm in order to learn from this input. The computer learns to perform a task by studying a training set of examples. Machine leaning [4] employs two categories: supervised (we have examples of expected output) and unsupervised (some assumption is made in order to build the model). In supervised learning, the training set

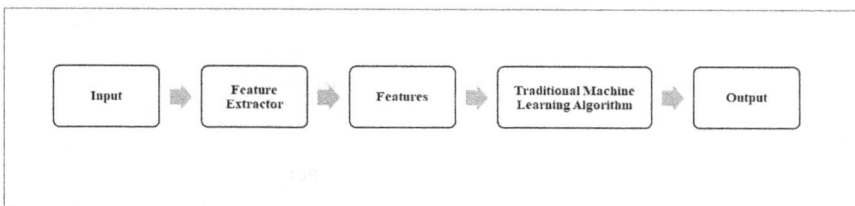

FIGURE 13.1 Machine learning flow.

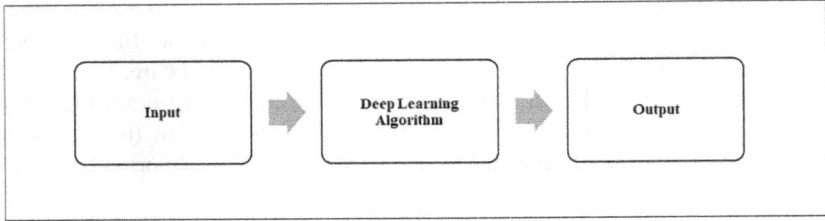

FIGURE 13.2   Deep learning flow.

contains data and the correct output of the task with that data. Supervised learning includes various classification and regression algorithms. With unsupervised learning, the training set contains data but no solutions; the computer must find the solutions on its own. Unsupervised learning includes clustering and dimension reduction algorithms.

It is important to have a good representation of the input data, i.e. a good set of features that produces a feature space in which an algorithm can use its bias in order to learn. Artificial intelligence (AI) involves machines that can perform tasks that are characteristic of human intelligence.

As represented in Figure 13.2, deep learning [5] allows computational models that are composed of multiple processing layers to learn representations of data with multiple levels of abstraction. Deep learning is a subfield of machine learning concerned with algorithms inspired by the structure and function of the brain called artificial neural networks.

Figure 13.1 and Figure 13.2 represent the learning flow of feature extraction in the case of machine learning and deep learning. Feature engineering and feature extraction are important but time-consuming parts of the machine learning workflow. The difference is that in traditional machine learning the features have to be hand-crafted, whereas in deep learning the features are learned. In brain tumour diagnosis, doctors integrate their medical domain knowledge and brain MRI scans or they analyse histopathology [6] biopsy images to obtain the characteristics of brain tumour for cancer confirmation and to decide on further treatment options. However, to detect brain cancer, initially a large number of MRI scans are taken for every patient (approximately 500 image scans). Those images are manually observed by radiologists for detection of a tumour and then those images are segmented. In case of histopathology brain images, pathology diagnosis has been performed by a human pathologist observing the stained specimen on the slide glass using a microscope [7]. The segmentation [8] of brain tumour in MRI is a challenging and difficult task because of the variety of their possible shapes, locations and image intensities. This may lead to inaccurate results. There is no such automated technique used by doctors in the clinical floor for accurate brain MR image segmentation. Accurate automatic brain image segmentation [9] in MRIs [10] is a prerequisite for the quantitative assessment of the brain. There are various challenges in recent years in terms of the classification, detection of findings and recommendations for further actions.

Image classification [11] is one of the most active research and application areas of neural networks [12]. A classification problem occurs when an object needs to be assigned into a predefined group or class based on a number of observed attributes related to that object. Image classification plays an important role in computer vision. Image classification [13] is a process including image pre-processing, image segmentation [14], key feature extraction and matching identification. One key ingredient of deep learning in image classification is the use of convolution architectures [15].

Previous projects have worked on the following areas individually:

- Pre-processing of brain MRI images
- Segmentation of brain MRI images
- Data mining techniques for medical image analysis and diagnosis

Also, some of the challenges faced in recent years are:

- Large number of brain atlas in multiple dimensions and deep learning [16] requires massive training datasets, as the accuracy of a deep learning classifier is largely dependent on the quality and size of the dataset; however, the unavailability of a dataset is one the biggest barriers in the success of deep learning in medical imaging.
- Variations in image acquisition, image intensities, image scale and orientation may lead to errors in annotations. As annotation requires extensive time from medical experts, it especially requires multiple expert opinion to overcome human error.
- Different readers have different perspectives on the same image.

As mentioned earlier, there are many challenges in predictive analysis of brain cancer. Therefore, there is a need for computer-aided brain tumour detection and segmentation from brain MR images to overcome the problems involved in the manual segmentation. Various techniques of image processing, when combined with algorithms of machine learning and deep learning, can be used to perform segmentation, classification and prediction of brain cancer. Automated brain cancer diagnosis from MRI scans is one of the medical image analysis methodologies.

The automated diagnosis involves two steps: (1) image classification and (2) image segmentation. In image classification [17] MRI scans are categorised in normal and abnormal input images into different tumour groups based on some similarity measures using deep learning technology [18]. This is done by learning (training) on MRI image scans and its structure using deep learning algorithms. This system also classifies the images based on normal or abnormal. The second step, image segmentation, is used for extraction of abnormal tumour portion, which is essential for volumetric analysis. The system essentially performs accurate brain MR image segmentation and classification.

Some brain cancer datasets are available that are open-access databases of medical images for cancer research like MICCAI Brats (Multimodal Brain Tumour Segmentation[15] Challenge dataset), figshare.com, TCGA (The Cancer Genome Atlas Program), The Cancer Imaging Archive (TCIA), etc.

13.2.1 MEDICAL IMAGE MODALITIES

Medical imaging techniques help doctors, medical practitioners and researchers view inside the human body and analyse internal activities without incisions. Cancer diagnosis, grade estimation, treatment response assessment, patient prognosis and surgery planning are the main steps and challenges in cancer treatment.

There are various medical imaging techniques [19] or image modalities like computed tomography (CT), MRI, biopsy, etc., that are used by hospitals across the world for different treatments. CT and MRI are used for brain tumour analysis and are able to capture different cross-sections of the body without surgery.

In a CT scan, an x-ray beam circulates around specific part of the body and a series of images are captured from various angles. The computer uses this information to create a series of two-dimensional (2D) cross-sectional image of the organ and combines them to make a three-dimensional (3D) image, which provides a better view of the organs. Positron emission tomography (PET) is a variant of CT where a contrast agent is injected into the body in order to highlight abnormal regions. CT scans are recommended by doctors in many conditions such as hemorrhages, blood clots or cancer. However, CT scans use x-rays which emit ionising radiation and have the potential to affect living tissues, thereby increasing the risk of cancer.

MRI [20] is a radiation-free and therefore a safer imaging technique than CT and provides finer details of the brain, spinal cord and vascular anatomy due to its good contrast. Axial, sagittal and coronal are the basic planes of MRI to visualise the brain's anatomy (Figure 13.3). Biopsies are the gold standard for all cancer diagnosis and grade estimation. In a biopsy, the colour, shape and size of the cell nuclei of tumour sample are observed.

The most commonly used MRI sequences for brain analysis are Tl-weighted, T2-weighted and FLAIR. A Tl-weighted scan provides grey and white matter contrast. T2-weighted is sensitive to water content and therefore well suited to diseases where the water accumulates inside brain tissues. T1- and T2-weighted images are also used to differentiate cerebrospinal fluid (CSF). The CSF is colourless and found

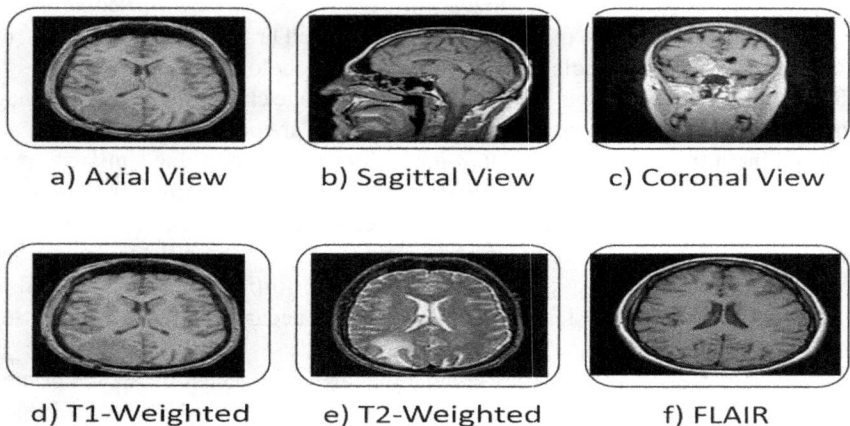

a) Axial View   b) Sagittal View   c) Coronal View

d) T1-Weighted   e) T2-Weighted   f) FLAIR

FIGURE 13.3 Basic planes of MRI. a) Axial View; b) Sagittal View; c) Coronol View; d) T1-Weighted; e) T2-Weighted; and f) Flair.

in the brain and spinal cord. It looks dark in T1-weighted imaging and bright on T2-weighted imaging. The third sequence is fluid attenuated inversion recovery (FLAIR), which is similar to T2-weighted image except for its acquisition protocol. FLAIR is used in pathology to distinguish between CSF and brain abnormalities. FLAIR can locate an edema region from CSF by suppressing free water signals, and hence periventricular hyperintense lesions are clearly visible in the images.

Many tools and techniques are used for classification and detection of brain cancer MRI. Also, the images in the dataset come from different models and types of cameras, which can affect the visual appearance of the image. This chapter focuses only on MRI brain cancer images for classification and segmentation.

13.3 METHODOLOGY

Figure 13.4 presents the methodology of the proposed system.

13.3.1 COLLECTION OF DATA SET AND PRE-PROCESSING ON IMAGE DATA OF BRAIN CANCER

- Medical image processing is a most important and challenging field. Image pre-processing of the brain MRI and its analysis is an act of examining images for identifying objects and analysing their significance.

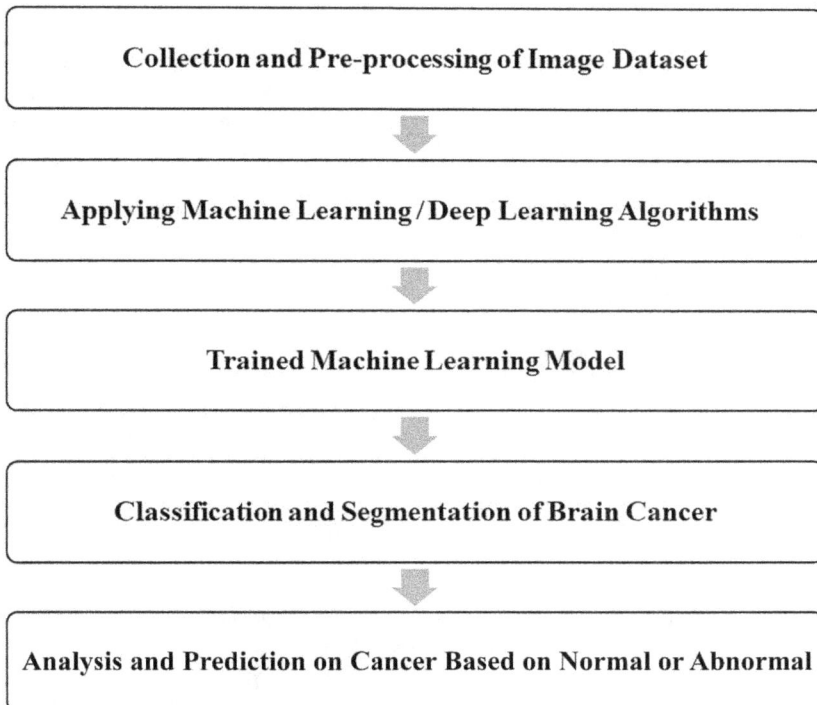

Collection and Pre-processing of Image Dataset

Applying Machine Learning / Deep Learning Algorithms

Trained Machine Learning Model

Classification and Segmentation of Brain Cancer

Analysis and Prediction on Cancer Based on Normal or Abnormal

FIGURE 13.4   Proposed methodology.

- Removal of unwanted noise and image enhancement are the two main objectives of pre-processing. The image characteristics can be enhanced by using image pre-processing techniques. The image enhancement depends upon different factors like computational time, computational cost, quality of the uncorrupted image and the techniques used for noise elimination. The goal of medical imaging is to extract meaningful and accurate information from these images with the least error possible.
- Table 13.1 presents some of the pre-processing techniques [21].
- Image pre-processing includes the collection, analysis, enhancement and display of images captured via MRI. Image processing converts an image into digital form and perform some operations like pre-processing, noise removal, image enhancing and feature extraction, etc., in order to get an enhanced image and to extract some useful information from it. The brain MRI scan image dataset is collected and pre-processed by applying image processing techniques.

TABLE 13.1
Image Pre-Processing Techniques

Pre-Processing Method	Advantages	Disadvantages
Adaptive Histogram Equalization (AHE)	1. Suitable for enhancing the edges in each region of an image. 2. Removes associated dark black edge pixels and labels.	1. Over-amplifies noise in relatively homogeneous regions of an image. 2. Unable to retain the brightness with respect to the input image.
Median Filter	1. It maintains the sharpness of the picture boundaries. 2. Effective in non-linear smoothing.	1. It can't distinguish fine details from the noise
Adaptive Median Filter	1. It can handle impulse noises with larger probabilities. 2. It preserves the details, and smoothen the non-impulse noises. 3. It reduces distortion, like excessive thinning or thickening of object boundaries.	1. It distinguishes fine details from the existing noise in the images to a limited extent.
Weiner Filter	1. It de-blurs and removes the additive noise from the image simultaneously. 2. It is used to measure the contrast between original image and low-pass filter image. 3. It minimises the mean squared estimation (MSE) error.	1. This filter assumes that the process dynamics are linear. 2. It can handle additive and unimodal noise only.
Gaussian Filter	1. Fast processing, 2. More effective while smoothening is applied on the images.	1. It might not preserve image brightness. 2. Not particularly effective at removing salt and pepper noise.

13.3.2   Classification and Segmentation of Brain MRI Images

- Machine learning techniques employed include support vector machine (SVM), K-nearest neighbour (KNN), linear discriminant, tree, ensemble and logistic regression. The best prediction accuracy based on classification is achieved by using deep learning features extracted by a pre-trained convolutional neural network (CNN) and was trained by a linear discriminant.
- There are various classification and segmentation algorithms [6, 9, 12–15], as represented in Table 13.2.
- Using deep learning algorithms and frameworks in the proposed system classifies brain MRI scans based on normal and abnormal. Further brain cancer MRI is evaluated using the machine learning model.
- For automatic extraction of the region of interest, various segmentation algorithms are applied.
- CNN is used for classification, as it has been found to provide higher accuracy than other machine learning algorithms.

TABLE 13.2
Various Classification and Segmentation Techniques

Algorithm	Working
Watershed	This algorithm is used in combination with active contour or edge detection, methods or with some colour space model or distance measure or with a conditioned random field for its simplicity, less computational overhead and accuracy validation.
Patch-Based	This method basically works on the similarity between images or sub-images, represented by a weighted graph or a sparse matrix computed from intensity-based distances between patches or group of pixels or pixel-level groups defined. This method is used for labelling.
Concatenated, Connected Random Forest with Multiscale Patch-Driven Active Contour Model	Detection of complete tumour, tumour core, pr enhancing tumour Accuracy: 90%, 80% and 73%, respectively
Ensembles of Classifications/ Decision Tree/ Random Forest	Tumour cells frequently lurk outside the 2-centimetre radius and its type is found by analysing the cell type characteristics, which means that each tumour cells in the image content will show some different visual texture, shape, etc. Decision trees help to make such an array of factors predictable for detection with ease by using if-then-else analysis at every threshold, calculated by the decision tree or ensemble method–based algorithms
Support Vector Machine	Non-linear, non-separable data, non-parameterised classification method which is extensively used in the medical field due the large number of advantages over regression methods, but the advantage is debatable as compared to neural networks, since this method provides information straight and distinct (which is a typical characteristic of brain tumour feature sets).

(Continued)

TABLE 13.2 (CONTINUED)

Algorithm	Working
K-Means	This method has a large number of citations, which shows its extensive use for unsupervised methods of images segmentation which uses the intensities in terms of colour which may be grey or some other texture-based feature to group the pixels of tumour and non-tumour parts. K-means provides approximately 76% accuracy.
Fuzzy Clustering	The boundary of tumour tissue is highly irregular and non-crisp. Region-based methods are extensively used for medical image segmentation. to locate the boundary of the tumour. However, fuzzy clustering which may use single or multiple criteria, helps in getting better results in terms of accuracy with some computational cost. It can be used in combination with other methods like K-means.
Artificial Networks (CNN)/Neural Network	This machine algorithm has used in both ways in terms of supervised and in unsupervised to find the tumour part. The accuracy, however, in both methods depends on the right kind of feature.
	This requires the selection and right combination of input, hidden and output layers. Having it automated has the advantage of speeding it up, and the faster we can be, the more efficient we can be and treat more patients in an efficient manner. This is possible by taking advantage of the I-H-O model of artificial networks, which accepts 'n' number of inputs (I), hidden layer (H), and gives 'n' number of (O) outputs, which means it can scale for inputs, processing power and outputs for detecting tumours with a large set of input features.

13.3.3 Analysis and Prediction

Once the region of interest is extracted with the segmentation technique, it is analysed with pre-trained data. Based on the extracted region of interest, prediction on normal or abnormal tumour is evaluated using machine learning and deep learning algorithms.

13.4 EXPERIMENTAL RESULTS, DISCUSSION, AND THEORETICAL IMPLICATIONS

As mentioned in Figure 13.4, the proposed methodology is implemented using Python packages and libraries. This section will elaborate on the performance parameters and analysis of various techniques applied to brain MRI for cancer detection.

13.4.1 Collection of Data Set and Pre-Processing on Image Data of Brain Cancer

For this proposed system brain cancer MRI data are collected and used for further processing. Image pre-processing converts an image into digital form and performs some operations like pre-processing, noise removal, image enhancing and feature extraction, etc., in order to get an enhanced image and to extract some useful information from it. A brain MRI scan image dataset is collected and is pre-processed by applying various image processing techniques. Identification of brain tumours in MR images involves in removing noise followed by enhancing the images using image segmentation.

13.4.2 SEGMENTATION AND CLASSIFICATION OF BRAIN MRI IMAGES

The following section describes various segmentation and classification techniques implemented for the proposed system.

13.4.2.1 Image Segmentation Using Various Techniques

For extracting the region of interest, image segmentation is required. There are different types of image segmentation techniques [14] like thresholding, clustering, edge-based segmentation, region-based segmentation, artificial neural network–based segmentation, etc. The following are some of the image segmentation techniques implemented using Python libraries.

13.4.2.1.1 Image Thresholding

It is one of the techniques for image segmentation to binarize the image based on pixel intensities as it partitions the image into two groups of pixels. As shown in Figure 13.5 and Figure 13.6 the methods of image thresholding have been implemented. The

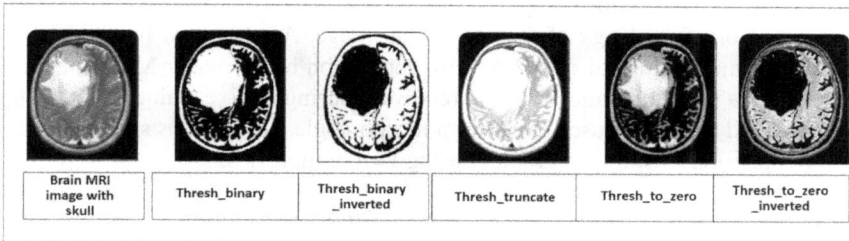

FIGURE 13.5   Simple thresholding techniques.

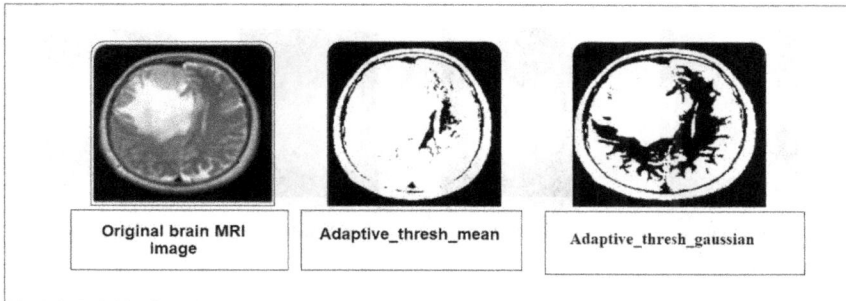

FIGURE 13.6   Adaptive thresholding technique.

techniques are simple thresholding and adaptive thresholding are applied specifically on brain cancer MRI image.

Figure 13.5 represents simple thresholding is applied to brain cancer MRI. All the styles of simple thresholding techniques have been implemented on the brain cancer MRI image. The first technique is binary. This means that if pixel intensity is greater than the set threshold, the value set to 255, or else set to 0 (black). Binary inverted is the second technique which is exactly opposite of the binary technique. The third technique is Trunc, and in this if the pixel intensity value is greater than threshold, it is truncated to the threshold. The pixel values are set to be the same as the threshold. All other values remain the same. The threshold to zero technique indicates the pixel intensity is set to 0 for all the pixels with less than the threshold value.

Adaptive thresholding is the method where the threshold value is calculated for smaller regions and therefore, there will be different threshold values for different regions. This leads to different threshold values for different regions with respect to the change in lighting. There are two types of adaptive thresholding: mean and gaussian. In the first type, the threshold value is the mean of the neighbourhood area, and in the second technique, the threshold value is the weighted sum of neighbourhood values where weights are a gaussian window. Figure 13.6 represents adaptive thresholding on a brain cancer MRI image, and it depicts the output of adaptive mean and adaptive gaussian.

13.4.2.1.2 Segmentation Using Morphological Operation

Morphological image processing is a collection of non-linear operations related to the shape or morphology of features in an image. As shown in Figure 13.7 and Figure 13.8, morphological operations are applied on brain cancer MRI images for segmentation. These operations rely on relative ordering of pixel values. A structural element called a kernel is used to perform morphological operations such as erosion, dilation, opening, closing and gradient using Python libraries.

13.4.2.1.3 Region-Based and Edge Detection Segmentation

The region-based technique is also known as 'similarity-based segmentation' and is used to find a region directly. It partitions an image into uniform sub-regions based

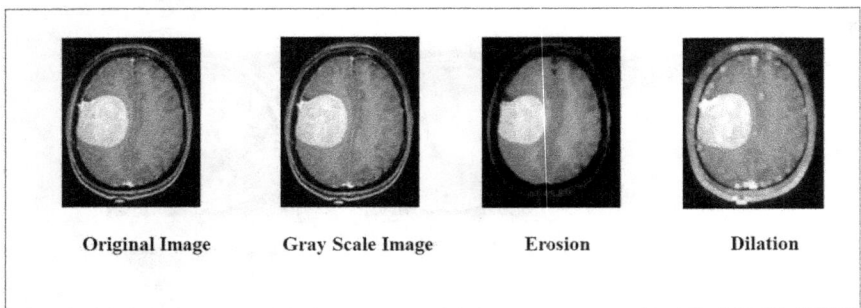

| Original Image | Gray Scale Image | Erosion | Dilation |

FIGURE 13.7 Morphological transformation operations.

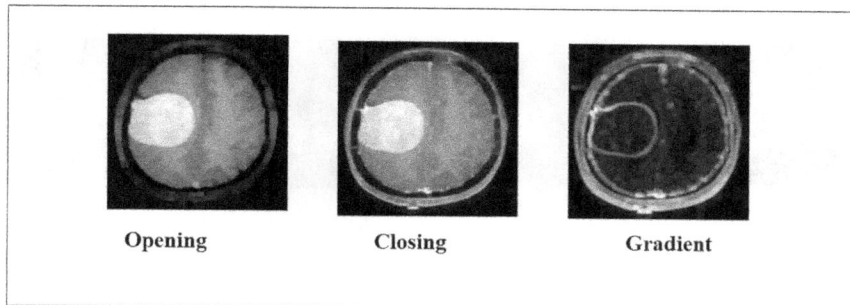

FIGURE 13.8 Morphological transformation operations.

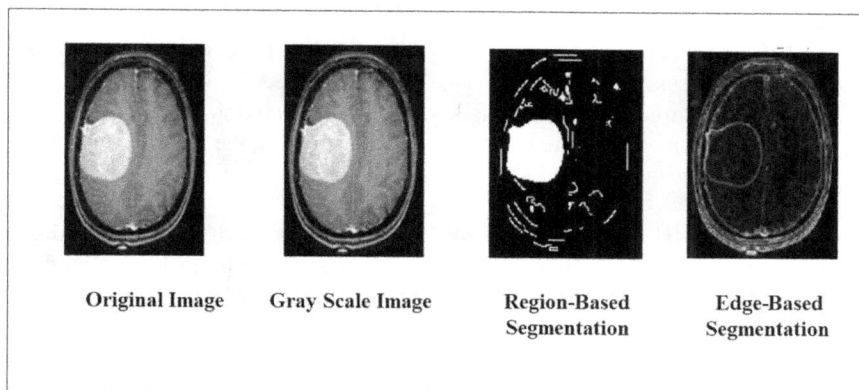

FIGURE 13.9 Region- and edge-based segmentation.

on some properties such as texture, colour, intensity, etc. Edge detection is mainly used for object detection and image segmentation. The edge detection technique is based on the discontinuities in image values between different regions and highlights intensity changes. Figure 13.9 represents the output generated by implementing region-based and edge-based segmentation using machine learning libraries.

13.4.2.2 Image Classification

Image classification of brain cancer MRI using a CNN enables analysis and prediction. The proposed system uses various machine learning algorithms and libraries by classifying brain cancer MRI as normal or abnormal. This involves the following steps:

Step 1: Collection of image dataset and converted into grey scale images.
Step 2: Pre-processing of image dataset by resizing.

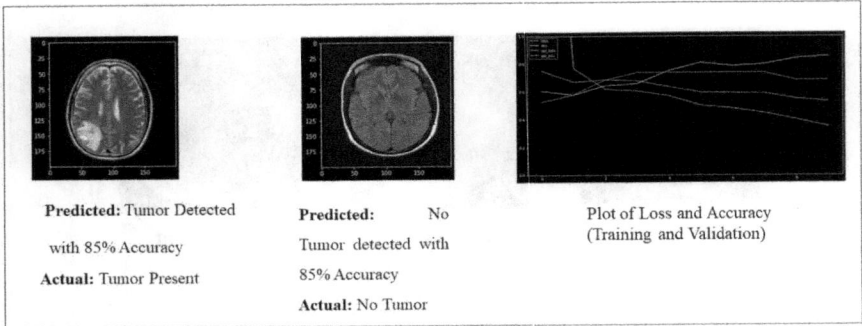

Predicted: Tumor Detected	**Predicted:** No	Plot of Loss and Accuracy
with 85% Accuracy	Tumor detected with	(Training and Validation)
Actual: Tumor Present	85% Accuracy	
	Actual: No Tumor	

FIGURE 13.10   Classification and prediction result.

Step 3: Using machine learning sklearn library, data is divided into training
  and test datasets.
Step 4: Model implementation using keras sequential model.
Step 5: Prediction on test data is performed by evaluating the machine learning
  model, as shown in Figure 13.10.

Normally a model trained on a classification problem with a validation dataset
may produce the following listing: 'Training accuracy', 'Training loss', 'Validation
accuracy' and 'validation loss'. This can be represented by graph or plots, as in
Figure 13.10.

13.4.2.3   Theoretical Implications
With the proposed system, the following implications can be made:

- Development of an intelligent system for brain cancer detection, classification and prediction will help the radiologists to detect and classify the
  cancer in a shorter span of time. This will also help the patients for planning
  treatment at an early stage.
- The proposed system is able to find region of interest by applying various
  segmentation algorithms.
- It will improve the accuracy of already existing algorithms that will help the
  neurosurgeons for better treatment planning with brain cancer MRI.
- This system will reduce the time to diagnosis that will save the time of
  patients and radiologists.
- As per our communication with some of the medical professionals, bringing
  this exclusive product to the public would be a big relief for patients. Sec-
  ondly, introducing this product in the semi-urban cities would increase the
  valuation of this patent and the product at least by 25% to 30%.

13.5   CONCLUSION

The development of a system for brain cancer detection, classification and prediction that can help the radiologists to detect and classify cancer in a shorter span of time is needed. This will also help the patients for early treatment planning. The proposed system is able to find a region of interest by applying various segmentation algorithms and is able to classify the brain cancer MRI as normal or abnormal using various machine learning algorithms. This system can improve the diagnosis accuracy in comparison with the accuracy of already existing algorithms. This will help the neurosurgeons provide better treatments.

Hence, there is a huge requirement for a system that can do predictive analysis on brain cancer detection and analysis with advanced image technologies using machine learning and deep learning considering the present demand, circumstances and requirements of the public and medical practitioners.

13.6   LIMITATIONS OF THE STUDY AND SCOPE FOR FURTHER RESEARCH

- Since human brain structure varies in adults and children, the present system is based on an adult image dataset. In the future, a system can be developed which can detect, classify and perform prediction on pediatric brain cancer.
- In the future, a system can be implemented which can provide a recommendation system to list out the possible treatments for the patient.
- Further, the system can be expanded to analyse tumours of other parts of the human body.

13.7   REFERENCES

[1] Luxit Kapoor et al., "A Survey on Brain Tumor Detection Using Image Processing Techniques," 7th International Conference on Cloud Computing, Data Science & Engineering, IEEE, 2017.

[2] Pariwat Ongsulee, "Artificial Intelligence, Machine Learning and Deep Learning," 15th International Conference on ICT and Knowledge Engineering, IEEE, 2017.

[3] Gopal S. Tandel et al., "A Review on a Deep Learning Perspective in Brain Cancer Classification," *Cancers Rev.*, 2019. doi:10.3390/cancers11010111.

[4] P. Louridas and C. Ebert, "Machine Learning," *IEEE Softw.*, vol. 33, no. 5, pp. 110–115, 2016.

[5] J. Schmidhuber, "Deep Learning in Neural Networks: An Overview," *Neural Netw.*, vol. 61, pp. 85–117, 2015.

[6] P. Sobana Sumi and R. Delhibabu, "Glioblastoma Multiforme Classification by Deep Learning Techniques on Histopathology Images," *Int. J. Innov. Technol. Explor. Eng.*, vol. 8, no. 12, pp. 4741–4748, 2019.

[7] D. Komura and S. Ishikawa, "Machine Learning Methods for Histopathological Image Analysis," *Comput. Struct. Biotechnol. J.*, vol. 16, pp. 34–42, 2018.

[8] I. Despotović, B. Goossens, and W. Philips, "MRI Segmentation of the Human Brain: Challenges, Methods, and Applications," *Comput. Math. Methods Med.*, vol. 2015, 2015.

[9] S. Kumar, A. Negi, and J. N. Singh, "Semanitc Segmentation Using Deep Learning for Brain Tumor MRI Via Fully Convolution Neural Network," in *Intelligent Systems, Smart Innovation, Systems and Technologies*, Singapore: Springer, 2017.

[10] A. Ari and D. Hanbay, "Deep Learning Based Brain Tumor Classification and Detection System," *Turkish J. Electr. Eng. Comput. Sci.*, vol. 26, no. 5, pp. 2275–2286, 2018.

[11] Tianmei Guo, Jiwen Dong, Henjian Li, and Yunxing Gao, "Simple Convolution Neural Network on Image Classification, Institute of Electrical and Electronics Engineers," IEEE 2nd International Conference on Big Data Analysis (ICBDA 2017): March 10–12, Beijing, China, pp. 721–724, 2017.

[12] E. Cengil, A. Çinar, and E. Özbay, "Image Classification with Caffe Deep Learning Framework," 2nd International Conference on Computational Science, Engineering. UBMK 2017, pp. 440–444, 2017.

[13] A. Sawant, M. Bhandari, R. Yadav, R. Yele, and S. Bendale, "Brain Cancer Detection from Mri: A Machine Learning Approach (Tensorflow)," *Int. Res. J. Eng. Technol.*, vol. 9001, p. 2089, 2018.

[14] A. Işin, C. Direkoğlu, and M. Şah, "Review of MRI-based Brain Tumor Image Segmentation Using Deep Learning Methods," *Procedia Comput. Sci.*, vol. 102, no. August, pp. 317–324, 2016.

[15] A. Krizhevsky, I. Sutskever, and G. E. Hinton, "ImageNet Classification with Deep Convolutional Neural Networks," *Commun. ACM*, vol. 60, no. 6, pp. 84–90, 2017.

[16] R. Miotto, F. Wang, S. Wang, X. Jiang, and J. T. Dudley, "Deep Learning for Healthcare: Review, Opportunities and Challenges," *Brief. Bioinform.*, vol. 19, no. 6, pp. 1236–1246, 2017.

[17] P. Moeskops, M. A. Viergever, A. M. Mendrik, L. S. De Vries, M. J. N. L. Benders, and I. Isgum, "Automatic Segmentation of MR Brain Images with a Convolutional Neural Network," *IEEE Trans. Med. Imaging*, vol. 35, no. 5, pp. 1252–1261, 2016.

[18] P. Ongsulee, "Artificial Intelligence, Machine Learning and Deep Learning," *Int. Conf. ICT Knowl. Eng.*, pp. 1–6, 2018.

[19] G. S. Tandel et al., "A Review on a Deep Learning Perspective in Brain Cancer Classification," *Cancers (Basel).*, vol. 11, no. 1, 2019.

[20] E. Cengil, A. Çinar, and Z. Güler, "A GPU-Based Convolutional Neural Network Approach for Image Classification," *IDAP 2017 – Int. Artif. Intell. Data Process. Symp.*, pp. 1–6, 2017.

[21] L. Kapoor and S. Thakur, "A Survey on Brain Tumor Detection Using Image Processing Techniques," *IEEE*, pp. 117–151, 2017.

14 A Review Study on Different Machine Learning Algorithms Used for COVID Outbreak Prediction

Saumya Satija[1], Mohd Tajuddin[2] and Meena Agrawal[3]

[1] Indira Gandhi Delhi Technical University for Women (IGDTUW), India

[2] Jeddah Regional Lab, Mahjar, Jeddah, Saudi Arabia

[3] Maulana Azad National Institute of Technology, Bhopal, Madhya Pradesh, India

14.1   INTRODUCTION

In December 2019 the novel coronavirus started spreading from the city of Wuhan and soon engulfed the entire world, leading to declaration of a world health emergency in January 2020 by the World Health Organization (WHO). Since then the virus has affected the lived of people all over.

The novel coronavirus (SARS-CoV-2) causes severe acute respiratory congestion and is an airborne disease which easily spreads from the infected person. People across the world have presented different numbers and theories related to its spread. The initial symptoms include dry cough, fever, shortness of breath, fatigue, loss of taste and sense of smell, diarrhoea and congestion. Still symptoms vary from person to person and the body's immune response. Some people have no symptoms but still are carriers of the virus and have the potential to spread and infect others.

DOI: 10.1201/9781003217107-14

The high transmission ability of this virus led to the declaration of a global pandemic in March 2020. According to Bioassay the COVID-19 pandemic is not only the most serious global health crisis since the 1920 but is one of the costliest pandemics in recent history. Initially the only option that countries were relying on to break the chain of transmission was lockdown. Countries were forced to close their businesses, borders, economic activities, schools and colleges and put their population in self-quarantine.

As of May 2021, the total confirmed cases recorded of COVID-19 is more than 150 million and more than 3 million people have lost their lives. To tackle this outbreak researchers are using different computer-aided, artificial intelligence (AI), machine learning (ML) and deep learning techniques, big data analytics and blockchain technologies to predict and prepare themselves in overcoming and effective management of covid outbreak.

Due to less accessibility to data, the traditional data analysis techniques were of no use.

ML algorithms play an important role in epidemic analysis, forecasting and prediction. ML techniques have been widely used and helped in providing better assistance of healthcare and administrative professional to better manage and tackle disease outbreak. ML is a subset of AI and has different applications in various domains. ML is broadly categorised into three categories, namely supervised learning, unsupervised learning and reinforcement learning.

ML techniques help in identification of the disease patterns and help in tracking the spread and devising strategies to stop the spread of the disease. Additionally, ML techniques are used in drug discovery and even in carrying out vaccine trials. With the use of ML algorithms the detection, diagnosis and prediction of the virus can be better analysed which helps in devising an effective preparedness strategy.

Even though scientists are working and developing the vaccines and medicines for tackling COVID, still people are worried about their existence and when their lives will become normal.

This chapter largely focuses on reviewing and doing a comparative analysis of the different ML techniques and algorithms used for predicting the spread of COVID.

14.2 LITERATURE REVIEW

In recent years, ML has been attracting many researchers and is successfully being applied for data analysis in various domains like medical engineering, financial sector, business sector, educational domains and other related sectors [1].

The method of learning is simply learning from experience or observations from previous instances. The basic aim of ML is to make systems learn automatically identify patterns, analyse data and make correct decisions with no or less human intervention.

Historical data is used to train the model, and the trained model is used to test new data which is used for making prediction. The trained ML model performance is appraised using some portion of available historical data (which is not present during training). This is known as the validation process. In this process, the ML model is assessed for its performance measure, such as accuracy. Accuracy describes the ML model performance over unseen data in terms of the ratio of the number of correctly predicted instances to the total number of instances to be predicted. Figure 14.1 depicts the ML process.

ML is broadly categorised into categories which are:

1. Supervised learning
2. Unsupervised learning
3. Reinforcement learning
4. Semi-supervised learning

In supervised learning, learning takes place with help of labelled datasets i.e. the class-level information is available in the training datasets. Whereas unsupervised learning means learning or training is done without labelled datasets, or in other words learning algorithms learn dynamically with the help of a partitioning or clustering algorithm. Most of the clustering algorithms available in the literature are K-means, fuzzy C-means, hierarchical clustering methods and so on. Reinforcement learning is a combination of supervised and unsupervised learning methods [3]. Semi-supervised algorithms are between the category of supervised and unsupervised learning. The algorithm uses both unlabelled and labelled datasets for training purposes; generally a small amount of labelled data and a large amount of unlabelled data is used. The advantage of this learning technique is that it improves the accuracy of learning [2].

In the last few decades ML has been used in solving complex and sophisticated real-world problems. ML algorithm learning is typically based on a trial and error method, quite the opposite of traditional algorithms, which follow include the traditional instruction set of if-else. One of the most important areas in which ML is being

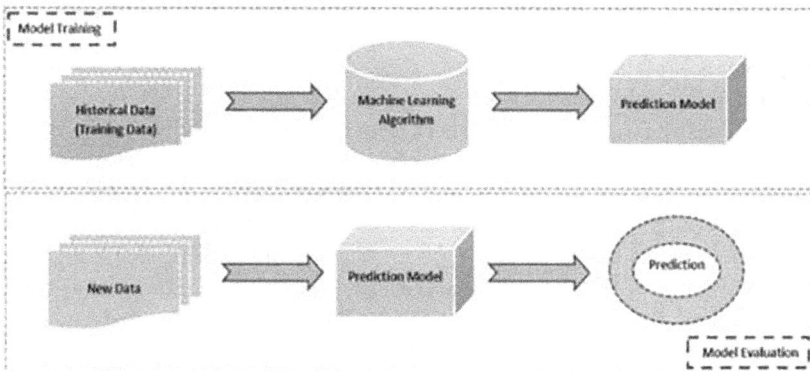

FIGURE 14.1   The machine learning process (Painuli, D et al. [2]).

used today is forecasting. Various standard ML algorithms have been used to predict the future course of actions needed in countless application areas including weather forecasting, disease forecasting, stock market forecasting and disease prognosis.

In healthcare, the correct diagnosis at the correct time is the key to successful treatment. If the treatment has a high error rate, it may cause several mortalities. Therefore, healthcare practitioners have started using artificial intelligence applications in medical diagnosis. The task is complicated because the practitioners have to choose the correct tool as it is a matter of life or death.

ML has revolutionised the field of healthcare. ML techniques are used to interpret and analyses large datasets to predict and identify the symptoms of disease and classify samples into different classes and treatment groups. ML helps hospitals to maintain administrative data and to process and find new findings about their patients [2].

ML techniques were previously used to detect and treat cancer, pneumonia, diabetes, Parkinson disease, arthritis, neuromuscular disorders and many more diseases; they give more than 90% accurate results in prediction and forecasting [4–5].

ML is also used to analyse the ailments based on medical imagining techniques such as x-ray scans, which can be used to detect whether a patient has been infected with COVID-19 or not [6–7].

Moreover, social distancing can be monitored with the help of ML, which can help in tracking effective distancing from one another and keeping ourselves safe from COVID-19.

Figure 14.2 shows the basic machine learning flowchart.

14.3   RELATED WORK

Singh V et al. [8] used a prediction model to forecast the confirmed cases of the COVID-19 using the support vector machine (SVM) method. The data collected was used to explore the impact on identification, deceased and recovered case estimates. The prediction helped in to plan resources, determine government policy and provide survivors with immunity passports and use the same plasma for treatment of infected persons.

Sengupta, S et al. [9] used time series forecasting techniques including ML models like linear regression, support vector regression, polynomial regression and deep learning forecasting model like long short-term memory (LSTM) to study the plausible hike in cases to help public welfare professionals plan the preventive measures to be taken, keeping the economic equilibrium of the country in their minds.

Tiwari S et al. [10] used a time series forecasting method to predict the outbreak trends in India based on the pattern of the outbreak in China, considering that the population density of both countries is very high. The prediction model was built from the publicly available dataset of COVID-19. The aim of the study was to prepare the government and citizens of India to take control measures to reduce the impact of COVID-19.

Yadav, R.S. [3] used different regression analysis models on the datasets extracted from Kaggle. Six regression analysis based models had been utilised on the COVID-2019 dataset, and Root Mean Square Error (RMSE) of these six regression analysis

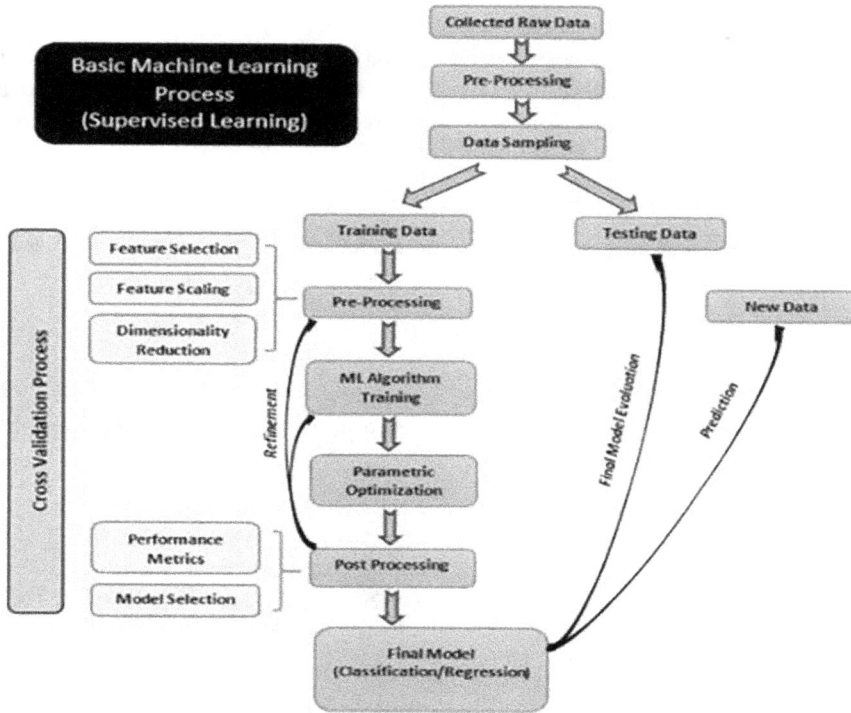

FIGURE 14.2 Machine learning (ML) process flowchart (Painuli, D et al. [2]).

models was calculated and concluded that the sixth-degree polynomial regression model is very good models for forecasting the next six days for COVID-2019 data analysis in India which would help Indian doctors and the government in preparing their plans in the next seven days. Based on further regression analysis study, this model can be tuned for forecasting long-term intervals.

Žmuk, B. et al. [11] used linear regression, gaussian processes, SMOreg and neural network multilayer perceptron to predict the number of cases and fatalities of COVID-19 disease for 10 days in the future. The accuracy of the forecasts was measured using Mean Absolute Percentage Error (MAPE) and RMSE error metrics. The results of the analysis had shown that algorithms can be successfully used for prediction of COVID-19 spread in the world. The results of the investigation indicated that the gaussian processes and multilayer perceptron neural network were the most precise algorithms for the prediction of new and total cases of COVID-19 disease on a global scale and on an individual country level.

F. Rustam et al. [12] used ML models to estimate the number of forthcoming patients affected by COVID-19. In particular, they used four regular forecasting models which were linear regression (LR), least absolute shrinkage and selection operator (LASSO), support vector machine (SVM) and exponential smoothing

(ES) to forecast the threatening impacts of COVID-19. Three types of predictions were made by each of the models which were newly infected cases, the number of deaths and the number of recoveries in the next 10 days. The results showed that the ES performed best amongst all the used ML techniques followed by LR and LASSO which performed fine in forecasting the new confirmed cases, death rate and recovery rate, while SVM performed worst in all the prediction scenarios.

Table 14.1 shows a comparative analysis of the different ML techniques used, their advantages and disadvantages, and datasets used in predicting and forecasting COVID-19 outbreak.

TABLE 14.1

Comparative Analysis of Different ML Technique Used and Advantages and Disadvantages

S. No.	Authors	ML Technique Used	Advantages of ML Techniques	Disadvantages of ML Techniques	Dataset
1	Kafieh R et al. [13]	Multilayer perceptron, random forest and LSTM	High accuracy LSTM reduces errors in prediction	Sensitive to data quality	Johns Hopkins CSSE Data repository updated on regular basis [14]
2	Sumayh S et al. [15]	Logistic regression, random forest (RF) and extreme gradient boosting (XGB).	Efficient prediction ability High accuracy	Sensitive to outliers and imbalanced data High computational costs	287 COVID-19 samples of patients from the King Fahad University Hospital, Saudi Arabia.
3	Yeung AY et al. [16]	Random forest and adaptive boosting (AdaBoost) regression.	Easy to use with less tweaking parameters Better accuracy	Prone to outliers and sensitive to noisy data and highly depended upon data quality High computational costs	Oxford COVID-19 Government Response Tracker data set
4	Painuli, D et al. [2]	ARIMA	Good prediction performance	Depends upon data accuracy and quality of data	COVID-19 tracker by govt. of India [17]

5	Yuan Tian et al [18]	Hidden Markov chain model (HMM), hierarchical Bayes model and LSTM using RMSE.	High realistic prediction ability	Depends upon data consistency and quality of data	Johns Hopkins CSSE Data repository updated on regular basis [14]
6	O. Istaiteh et al [19]	ARIMA, ANN, LSTM and CNN models	High prediction ability LSTM reduces errors in prediction	Limited to data availability Long-term predictability yet to be tested	Johns Hopkins CSSE Data repository updated on regular basis [14]
7	Serkan Ballı [20]	SVM, MLP	SVM works well structured, unstructured and semi-structured data. MLP has higher accuracy	Limited to data availability Long-term predictability yet to be tested	Data of COVID-19 between cases 20/01/2020 and 18/09/2020 for USA and Germany and the global was obtained from World Health Organization
8	Saba, T et al. [21]	Random forest, KNN, SVM, decision trees	Works well with categorical and continuous data Reduces overfitting	Limited to data availability	Johns Hopkins CSSE Data repository updated on regular basis [14]
9	Punn, N et al. [22]	LSTM, SVM	High prediction ability	High computational costs	Johns Hopkins CSSE Johns Hopkins CSSE Data repository updated on regular basis [14]
10	Watson, G et al [23]	Bayesian time series model and random forest algorithm	High accuracy Reliable predictions and uncertainty estimates	Limited to data availability Long-term predictability yet to be tested	COVID 19 Tracking Project [24]

14.4 CONCLUSIONS

A comprehensive analysis has been carried out on previous research focusing on the usage of different ML algorithms used to predict the COVID outbreak. The ML algorithms have shown their efficiency in the area of therapeutic and epidemiological data analysis and in the estimation of pandemic outgrowth. These predictions helped the governments and citizens to equip the medical infrastructure of their country and devise strict measures to reduce the impact of this deadly disease and even designing manufacturing and devising vacation programs for citizens to combat the disease.

14.5 LIMITATIONS AND CHALLENGES

COVID-19 has spread throughout the globe, posing a threat to human existence. As a result, a number of studies have been carried out in order to find an intelligent medical diagnosis system that employs AI techniques and control the virus's consequences. However, there are number of obstacles that limit scholarly works. Because of the complexity of this epidemic, it is incredibly difficult to understand how the virus spreads and how people become infected.

The lack of a substantial dataset on coronavirus in the academic literature creates a hindrance for AI researchers since it makes it difficult to understand viral patterns and features.

14.6 FUTURE WORKS

The present work can be improved further by merging new factors and ML algorithms with existing ones. Also the comparative analysis of different ML techniques for their long-term predictability can be evaluated.

14.7 REFERENCES

[1] Machine learning research towards combating COVID-19: Virus detection, spread prevention, and medical assistance Osama Shahid-Mohammad Nasajpour-Seyedamin Pouriyeh-Reza Parizi-Meng Han-Maria Valero-Fangyu Li-Mohammed Aledhari- Quan Sheng. *Journal of Biomedical Informatics*, 2021;117:103751.
[2] Forecast and prediction of COVID-19 using machine learning Deepak Painuli-Divya Mishra-Suyash Bhardwaj-Mayank Aggarwal. *Data Science for COVID-19,* 2021:381–397. https://doi.org/10.1016/B978-0-12-824536-1.00027-7
[3] Data analysis of COVID-2019 epidemic using machine learning methods: a case study of India Ramjeet Yadav. *International Journal of Information Technology*, 2020. https://doi.org/10.1007/s41870-020-00484-y
[4] Quinlan R. *C4.5: Programs for Machine Learning*. Morgan Kaufmann Publishers; San Mateo, CA, 2014.
[5] Turaiki I, Alshahrani M, Almutairi T. Building predictive models for MERS-CoV infections using data mining techniques. *Journal of Infection and Public Health,* 2016;9:744–748.
[6] Sreeja S, Bhavya L, Swamynath S, Dhanuja R. Chest x-ray pneumonia prediction using machine learning algorithms. *International Journal for Research in Applied Science and Engineering Technology*, 2019;7(4):3227–3230.

[7] Kose U, Guraksin GE, Deperlioglu O. Diabetes determination via vortex optimization algorithm based support vector machines. *2015 Medical Technologies National Conference*, pp. 1–4. IEEE: United States.

[8] Prediction of COVID-19 corona virus pandemic based on time series data using support vector machine Vijander Singh-Ramesh Poonia-Sandeep Kumar-Pranav Dass-Pankaj Agarwal-Vaibhav Bhatnagar-Linesh Raja. *Journal of Discrete Mathematical Sciences and Cryptography*, 2020. doi: 10.1080/09720529.2020.1784535

[9] Sengupta, S., Mugde, S., & Sharma, G. (2020). Covid-19 pandemic data analysis and forecasting using machine learning algorithms. medRxiv.

[10] Tiwari S, Kumar S, Guleria K. Outbreak trends of CoronaVirus (COVID-19) in India: A prediction. *Disaster Medicine and Public Health Preparedness*, 2020;14:1–9. doi: 10.1017/dmp.2020.115.

[11] Žmuk B, Jošić H. Predicting COVID-19 spread using machine learning algorithms. *Contemporary Economic and Business Issues*, 2021; 233.

[12] F. Rustam et al. COVID-19 future forecasting using supervised machine learning models. *IEEE Access*, 2020;8:101489–101499. doi: 10.1109/ACCESS.2020.2997311.

[13] COVID-19 in Iran: Forecasting pandemic using deep learning Rahele Kafieh-Roya Arian-Narges Saeedizadeh-Zahra Amini-Nasim Serej-Shervin Minaee-Sunil Yadav- Atefeh Vaezi-Nima Rezaei-Shaghayegh Javanmard. *Computational and Mathematical Methods in Medicine*, 2021, Article ID 6927985, 16 pages. https://doi.org/10.1155/2021/6927985

[14] https://github.com/CSSEGISandData/COVID-19

[15] Machine learning-based model to predict the disease severity and outcome in COVID19 Patients, Sumayh Aljameel-Irfan Khan-Nida Aslam-Malak Aljabri-Eman Alsulmi. *Scientific Programming*, 2021, Article ID 5587188, 10 pages. https://doi.org/10.1155/2021/5587188

[16] Machine Learning – Based prediction of growth in confirmed COVID-19 infection cases in 114 countries using metrics of non pharmaceutical interventions and cultural dimensions: Model development and validation Arnold Yeung-Francois Roewer-Despres-Laura Rosella-Frank Rudzicz. *Journal of Medical Internet Research*, 2021. doi: 10.2196/26628

[17] www.covid19india.org/

[18] Yuan Tian, Ishika Luthra, Xi Zhang. Forecasting COVID-19 cases using machine learning models. *medRxiv*, 2020;7(2):20145474. https://doi.org/10.1101/2020.07.02.20145474

[19] Istaiteh O, Owais T, Al-Madi N, Abu-Soud S. Machine learning approaches for COVID-19 forecasting. *2020 International Conference on Intelligent Data Science Technologies and Applications (IDSTA)*, pp. 50–57. doi:10.1109/IDSTA50958.2020.9264101.

[20] Serkan Ballı, Data analysis of Covid-19 pandemic and short-term cumulative case forecasting using machine learning time series methods. *Chaos, Solitons and Fractals*, 2021;142:110512. ISSN 0960–0779. https://doi.org/10.1016/j.chaos.2020.110512

[21] Saba T, Abunadi I, Shahzad MN, Khan AR. Machine learning techniques to detect and forecast the daily total COVID-19 infected and deaths cases under different lockdown types. *Microscopy Research and Technique*, 2021;84(7):1462–1474.

[22] Punn NS, Sonbhadra SK, Agarwal S. COVID-19 epidemic analysis using machine learning and deep learning algorithms. *MedRxiv*, 2020: 1–10.

[23] Watson GL, Xiong D, Zhang L, Zoller JA, Shamshoian J, Sundin P, Ramirez CM. Pandemic velocity: Forecasting COVID-19 in the US with a machine learning & Bayesian time series compartmental model. *PLoS Computational Biology*, 2021;17(3):e1008837.

[24] https://github.com/COVID19Tracking/covid-public-api

15 Designing a Rough-PSO–Based COVID-19 Prediction Model

Shampa Sengupta[1], Sourik Pyne[1]
and Sangya Chattopadhyay[1]
[1] MCKV Institute of Engineering, India

CONTENTS

15.1 INTRODUCTION

In December 2019, a pneumonia outbreak was reported in the Wuhan City of China. The outbreak was traced to a novel strain of coronavirus on 31 December 2019, which was given the interim name 2019-nCoV by the World Health Organization (WHO), later renamed SARS-CoV-2 by the International Committee on Taxonomy of Viruses. The Wuhan strain has been identified as a new strain of beta coronavirus from group 2B having approximately 70% genetic similarity to the SARS-CoV. The virus has a 96% similarity to a bat coronavirus and hence is widely suspected to be originated from bats as well. CoVs are a large family of viruses from the Coronaviridae family, including Middle East Respiratory Syndrome (MERS)-CoV, Severe Acute Respiratory Syndrome (SARS)-CoV and the new virus named SARS-CoV-2 [1–2]. Since it was first reported, the disease has spread exponentially across the world. However, currently there is no approved human vaccine that can prevent the disease with 100% accuracy. It has been observed that the spread of COVID-19 has been fastest when people are in close proximity. Travel restrictions were thus imposed in countries to control the spread of the virus, and frequent hand washing/sanitising is recommended to prevent potential virus infections. The most common infection symptoms are cough and mild fever and may appear in COVID-positive patients. However, other symptoms including chest discomfort, sputum development and sore throat may also occur.

As we know pros and cons are available for everything is happening, likewise due to the starting of this deadly coronavirus, the science and technology sector becomes richer with their new discoveries of different digital technologies. Various applications are already built for the healthcare system to handle diseases to save people. Various emerging technologies include artificial intelligence (AI) [3], big data analytics [4], Internet of Things (IoT) [5] and blockchain technology [6], which uses different machine learning (ML) [7] and deep learning (DL) [8–9] approaches to develop the intelligent healthcare system. We can see that AI is gradually doing all the work of human experts in medical practice too. Researchers have already developed a few methods for the prediction of the diseases and are continuously doing work on the real CoV datasets to predict the disease. Developing prediction systems that can accurately predict and diagnose still remains a challenge. ML techniques are the key technologies to identify epidemiological risks in advance for the improvement in the prevention, prediction and detection of future worldwide health problems.

The objective of this work is to design a novel intelligent prediction model to predict the severity of the COVID-19 disease by selecting the most important and optimised feature set by using the rough set theory [10] (RST) and particle swarm optimisation (PSO) algorithm [11]. There are two modules of the proposed work. The first module selects the important features through rough-PSO based (named SPSO) method from the original disease feature set, and the second module deals with the prediction on the severity of the disease is done through generating classification rules for different level of severity by the classifiers from the reduced data. Finally, classification accuracy is measured for the prediction of the disease. Other performance evaluation metrics related to classification are also being measured to prove the efficiency of the method.

The chapter is structured as follows: Section 2 discusses the basic background theory of rough set theory and particle swarm optimisation algorithm. Section 3 discusses the recent AI based works for the prediction of COVID-19 disease, and Section 4 discusses the designing of the proposed prediction model. Section 5 shows the experimental results and comparisons with some existing methods. Section 6 discusses the salient features of the proposed method with the conclusion of the work.

15.2   OVERVIEW OF SOFT COMPUTING TECHNIQUES USED

For the designing of the proposed COVID-19 prediction model (SPSO), soft computing tools such as RST [11–24] and PSO algorithm [11, 25–29] have been used. Soft computing tools are very much useful for handling the inconsistent, ambiguous and uncertain data. A brief description of the Rough Set Theory [19–24] and Particle Swarm Optimisation algorithm [11, 26–29] are provided next.

15.2.1 ROUGH SET THEORY

Rough Set Theory [19–24] is a very popular soft computing tool to handle the different uncertainties in the data. The technique is popular as it does not need any extra parameter except the data itself to find out the insight of different aspects of the data. The concept of reduct [19–21], core [21], lower approximation [21] upper approximation [21], positive region [21–22], boundary region [21] and attribute significance [21–24] of RST are very important to design any RST-based intelligent model. Many papers discussed these concepts with the derived formulas with examples [24]. Here in our chapter, the concept of positive region overlapping of RST is being used [25] to find out the important feature subset from the dataset. It actually finds out the overlapping region formed by the original feature set and the targeted feature subset. A positive region overlapping value determines the number of common objects identified in the positive region both by the original feature set and the targeted feature subset. The good positive region overlapping value indicates that the selected feature subset is interesting and important one. The detail concept of positive region overlapping is discussed in Section 4.

15.2.2 PARTICLE SWARM OPTIMISATION ALGORITHM

In 1995, Kennedy and Eberhart proposed an interesting and popular swarm-based evolutionary algorithm known as particle swarm optimisation algorithm. In PSO, a population called swarm is formed by the randomly initialised particles in the search space. The whole swarm is moved in the search space by updating the position of all the individual particles to find out the best targeted solution based on the previous experiences of its own and its neighbouring particles. In an n-dimensional search space, a particle can be represented as $P(i) = (p(j,1), p(j,2), \ldots, p(j,n))$ where the coordinate $p(j,k)$ of the particle $P(i)$ is associated with the velocity (i.e. rate of change of position) $v(j,k)$ where $k = 1, 2, \ldots, n$. Here in this PSO [11, 26] the concept of velocity and neighbourhood topology is very important. Each particle actually associated with a velocity vector and which updates in every generation to generate new particle. Each current particle $P(i)$ maintains a record of its previous best position known as *cpbest* and can be represented as *PBi*. Based on the swarm, by considering all the particles position, a global best position known as *gpbest* is also recorded and can be represented as *G*. The neighbourhood topology defines how *cpbest* and *gpbest* are connected to each particle. Basically PSO [26] is a three-step method where in the first phase, all particles' ability/quality is evaluated to check how these particles are able to solve the problem or be the target solution based on the fitness function. Then in the second phase, a comparison is made to choose the best particles, and finally in the evolution phase, a set of new particles is generated based on the some of the best particles already found. The steps are repeated until the convergence criteria is met to get the best particle as the final optimal solution.

15.3   RECENT WORK ON THE PREDICTION OF COVID-19

Researchers are continuously working on the COVID-19 data to provide some insights to help medical science manage the pandemic efficiently by saving lives. Various IT-based solutions have already been developed to assist the medical practitioners. Still, the development of a total IT-based healthcare solution for handling the disease data in this moment is challenging.

A paper [1] proposed a prediction model to determine the positivity or the negativity of the disease through smartphone or smart devices, as many times it is seen that setting up of the infrastructure is very time consuming and costly for many people. Smartphone sensors were used to detect COVID-positive patients using a set of AI algorithms. They studied [1] the general characteristics of COVID-19 symptoms i.e. fever, cough, computed tomography (CT) scan features and difficulty in breathing. The usefulness of the powerful and extraordinary smartphone sensors is mentioned in this research work for COVID-19 prediction. For example, the microphone sensor can be used to detect the abnormality in breath and cough, camera sensors can be used too for different purposes, fingerprint sensors can be used to get the temperature measurement, etc. Another work of the camera sensor is to analyse the pre-processed CT scan images for the detection of the virus. Different features from different images make a large database that help to identify the affected patient. When it comes to get the temperature, the study shows that the patient has to put his or her index finger in front of the flash and the camera will take the sample images, and using the algorithm, it will convert into heart rate and consequently to the temperature. X-ray images that are pre-processed can be analysed by the camera sensor and compared with the previously obtained data from the COVID-positive patient to get the result.

The paper [2] presented an improved prediction process where one of the most widely used algorithms is the random forest algorithm applied on the dataset from Kaggle. This database comprises datasets from various sources, including the WHO and John Hopkins University. The data analysis contains the basic symptoms of COVID-19 disease. Data pre-processing includes columns with relations between each and every feature with a unique value. They used the boosted random forest algorithm that includes two parts: 'Boosting Algorithm' and 'Random Forest Algorithm' which includes decision tree. This algorithm divides the data set into smaller subset for more efficiency. This algorithm reduces the depth and increases the estimation to get a high variance in model and provides accurate precision. The paper [12] discusses the role of artificial intelligence to detect the disease. A deep learning–based approach [8–9] such as convolutional neural network (CNN) [12] is used for the prediction of coronavirus. CNN [12] is a deep learning algorithm which is mostly used for imagery analysis. They focused on the use of CNN and other deep learning methods in various way to predict COVID-19 disease. According to their study the computer models are trained to perform the classification task directly from the picture, sound and text. However, their x-ray diagnosis comes into two parts. They preferred the X-ray over CT scan as it is a quick process, safer, less harmful and budget friendly. Their proposed methodology comprises several phases to detect the COVID-19 virus. They depend on the x-ray images (CNN is an image-based method) for the dataset and applied the deep learning algorithm to get the final result. The dataset comes from two kinds of people: one is a healthy person and the other is a COVID-positive patient. To overcome the limitation of x-ray images, they used data augmentation to increase the number of images with various sample iterations. They evaluated some evaluation metrics to get the accurate prediction. The paper [13] proposed that unlike the previous research papers, they worked on the prediction as well as the severity of the cases. The dataset distinguished by age and the respected symptoms. Their proposed method works with an AI approach called predictive analysis (PA) which extracts the insights and rules from the historical dataset collected from the hospitals for a better result. The attributes hold the features of each patient considered in this analysis, which represents the base characteristics. These data help to identify the feature related to acute respiratory distress syndrome (ARDS). The feature selection method is used to minimise the feature set and maximise the prediction power for ARDS. This study reveals two types of feature selection methods. One is the filter method, based on the entropy that measures how much information is encapsulated in the feature to predict the final result of the ARDS sample. Valuable information goes upwards with higher entropy. Information gain is a measure to rank the features. This helps to prioritise the features acquired. However, the wrapper method chooses the best-ranked features and adds them to an empty set until it stops improving the framework performance. The proposed experiment shows a range of accuracies (50–80%), with different classifiers according to the study [13]. The paper [14] did a deep analysis of the COVID pandemic with the techniques such as neural language processing and regression analysis to get more accurate prediction and reduce the mortality rate. Their ML approach works on the segmentation area of the images and assign the precise image samples. The authors also gave an idea that poly-protein preparation is an important part of the viral replication. The forecasting technique for artificial intelligence [7] is an efficient way to predict the infection. A deep learning model is used for the two numerical methods: SIER and ARIMA [14]. Long-term memory model and simulation neural organisation models were the best match for them according to the author of this paper, although the estimation of these models was not within the range of 15%. The outcome of this experiment is a detailed and significant data sheet of the COVID cases with confirmed, recovery and deaths with a statistical overview of increment and decrement rate. The paper [15] discusses that to gain a worldwide knowledge of how COVID-19 is affecting the population, the severity and which part of the area needs be recognised as critical, and Tuli et al. have proposed to a method based on machine learning that continuously updates the spread prediction information on the cloud server. The decision of taking the dataset from Our World in Data by Hannah Ritchie for this research work is an excellent decision as the dataset is updated by WHO eventually. This reduces the risk of getting inaccurate data. The authors of this research work proposed the way to enhance the ML working performance. They deployed a cloud data centre with the features of fail-safe computation and quick data analysis. The hospitals and other health care centres will update their information of recovery, positive cases, deaths, etc., on this cloud server by which the machine learning algorithm will analyse the data to predict the spread of the disease on the population. They have used a susceptible-infected-recovered model and gaussian distribution model for better estimation and graph representation. Their research also says to get the best fitted distribution model, they came up with the five best distribution models by daily disease data analysis. However, their experiment gives a fairly accurate result, though there are some biases in the data. The paper [16] presents a study containing a methodology or technique to perform prediction for upcoming COVID cases for updating public awareness. Most of the work is for evaluating the efficiency of the enforced policy and to control the spread of the disease. Kavadi et al. designed a partial derivative regression and non-linear machine learning (PDR-NML) model for predicting upcoming cases in a timely fashion. The data are collected from the Indian database for an updated and accurate database. The Exposed Affected Cured Dead model is used to create the mathematical formula for the research work. The progressive partial derivative regression model evaluates the parameter i.e. number of exposed people, affected people, cured people and dead people. On the other hand, the global pandemic predictions in big data datasets are created utilising the non-linear global pandemic machine learning model. The test cases and results are based on the input and output of the NGP-MP prediction model. Faster foresight refers to faster prevention of the coronavirus spread. The paper [17] is based on the CT images for predicting the severity of the disease in the host's body. According to this paper, the method is approved by the Institutional Review Board of Shanghai Public Health Clinical Center, Fudan University. They mentioned the criteria of only patients who are coronavirus positive, and a CT scan of the patient must show pneumonia. The pneumonia was calculated for all patients. For image resources the patient would have to pass through 64 CT scans. The V-Net or a CNN [1] quantified the infected area from the CT scan images. The neural network model was trained by the old images of infected region and compared it with new set of CT scan images. The statistical analysis is also done. The result shows the severe patient has a history of exposure in an outbreak area than a non-severe patient. Logistic regression was applied to get the best feature. Authors stated the use of nomogram model to measure the severity of the disease. The sensitivity, specificity and accuracy were 86.1%, 80.0% and 84.7% for this experiment. The paper [18] proposed a method based on the CT images to predict COVID-19, but in a more elaborate way. In this paper, deep learning algorithm [18] is used to detect COVID in order to control the spread of the disease, provide appropriate quarantine and treatment and lower the chances of getting false negativity. The datasets are collected from two type of people, i.e. normal pneumonia patient and actual COVID-positive patient for better comparison. Their proposed trained neural network model works in two parts which is helpful to increase the efficiency of the framework. The first part is for conversion of image into a one-dimensional vector, and other part is for classification. They used pixel spacing to get more features from the images which is very helpful for the prediction.

15.4   DEVELOPMENT OF THE PREDICTION MODEL

In the proposed work, an intelligent prediction system has been developed to predict the COVID-19 severity level by selecting important features from the disease data using the RST [19–25] and PSO algorithm [26–28]. Only a few research papers are available on the prediction of COVID-19 by using intelligent soft computing techniques [30] and optimisation techniques [31]. The proposed work is divided into two parts where in the first part, important disease features are selected through the devised algorithm based on the RST [21–24] and PSO algorithm [26–29] (SPSO). In the later phase, state-of-the-art learning algorithms are applied to find out the rule set to determine the classification accuracy of the learning algorithms on the reduced dataset to predict the severity level of the disease. In the work, one variant of the original PSO method named the discrete PSO method [29] is used where the fitness function is designed using rough set theory [21–24]. The proposed rough-PSO based intelligent algorithm finds out the important feature subset P from the whole disease data (decision system DS). The method starts with generating a swarm of particles of size S randomly [29]. A heuristic is used to define the fitness function for evaluation of each particle. The concept of positive region overlapping value [25] of RST [21–24] is used to design the fitness function of the PSO algorithm [29]. Suppose for a decision system DS, the positive region of DS with feature set P and target feature subset P_1 are $POS_p(D)$ and $POS_{P1}(D)$, then overlapping positive Region $OP_P(D) = POS_p(D) \cap POS_{P1}(D)$ indicates the magnitude of the correctly classified common objects by both P and P_1. Here, importance is given to maximise the fitness value for getting the target feature subset with a lesser number of features in the feature subset P_1 as well. In our method, equation (15.1) describes the fitness function $fitness(p)$ for a particle p to find out the optimised target feature subset R of the system DS.

$$fitness(p) = \left(\left(\frac{OP_P(D)}{|U|} \right) / P_1 \right) \qquad (15.1)$$

To find out the optimised target feature subset, we have used one variant of traditional PSO algorithm [28]. Let a decision system $DS = \{U, A, D\}$, where U is the set of objects, $A = \{C_1, C_2, \ldots C_n\}$ is the set of conditional attributes and $D = \{d_1, d_2 \ldots dq\}$ is the decision attribute with q class labels. Fitness function is already defined in equation (15.1). Convergence criteria can be anything like no of iterations, no average fitness value change between successive iterations, etc. For our SPSO method, the convergence criteria is the same average fitness value for the whole swarm for two successive generations. After convergence of the algorithm, the optimised feature subset is generated from the final population for DS. The proposed algorithm named as SPSO is given here:

Algorithm: SPSO (DS, F)
Inputs: $DS = (U, A, D)$, swarm_size, convergence criteria
Outputs: Best Feature subset F of DS
Begin
Set No_of_runs = 100.
For each No_of_runs {
Create initial swarm of size swarm_size

Initialise velocity array of each particle.
Repeat {
For every particle in the swarm {
Calculate fitness value using Eq. (1).
cpbest = current best position of the particle.
gpbest = global best position among all particles.
Update the velocity of the particle using cpbest and gpbest.
Formation of new particle by replacing old particles
} //end-for
}Until convergence criteria is reached.
Insert gpbest into F.
} //end-for
Return (F)
End

15.5   RESULTS AND DISCUSSION

A benchmark 'COVID-19 Symptoms Checker' dataset is collected from Kaggle [32] and used in the experiment. The SPSO method is developed using Python programming language. The dataset contains 3, 16, 800 instances with 21 attributes, and after pre-processing the same we consider 50,000 instances by the stratified sampling method with 13 numeric conditional attributes such as Fever, Tiredness, Difficulty in breathing, Dry cough, sore throat, Pains, Nasal Congestion, Runny Nose, Diarrhoea, Age, None_Experience, Gender and Contact and one decision attribute with four different severity class labels such as Severity_Mild, Severity_Moderate, Severity_ Severe and Severity_none.

First of all, the proposed method SPSO is applied on the considered dataset to generate the optimised feature subset from 13 conditional features. Then the classification algorithms are run on the reduced dataset with selected feature subset to evaluate the efficiency of SPSO algorithm. Here k-fold cross validation method [33] is used to measure the classification accuracy of SPSO method where the value of k has been considered to be 10.

Now SPSO is compared with the standard feature selection methods such as CFS [34], CON [35], from the weka tool [36] and one implemented static rough-GA based method [25] in terms of selecting the number of features and the execution efficiency. For checking the classification capability of the generated feature set the standard classifiers such as Naïve Bayes (NB) [33], partial decision tree algorithm (PART) [33], random forest [33], bagging [33], tree-based classifier (j48) [33] and multi-layer perceptron (MLP) [33] are considered.

For running the static version of the rough-GA based method [25], the following parameters were used:

For fitness function evaluation $k = 2$, $z = 0.05$ and $w = 0.55$ have been fixed and GA parameters are as population size $(M) = 200$, crossover probability $= 0.9$ and mutation rate $= 0.001$, termination criteria: same average fitness value for 2 successive generations.

To run the SPSO method, certain parameter values have been fixed experimentally for SPSO. The SPSO parameter values are as follows:

Swarm Size: 200, termination criteria: average fitness value for 2 successive generations remains same, The constant updating factors a, b, c to determine the strength of the contribution of the individual best, personal best and global best values fixed experimentally as: $a = 0.14$, $b = 0.16$ and $c = 0.18$ respectively.

The proposed method of SPSO was run on 'COVID-19 Symptoms Checker' [32] data, and the following eight important features were selected: fever, tiredness, difficulty in breathing, dry cough, sore throat, nasal congestion, runny nose and age to predict the severity label of the disease. Classification accuracy of all the severity classes are computed, and after that the average prediction results is given with the selected features.

Table 15.1 represents the 'COVID-19 Symptoms Checker' dataset with original feature number and the selected feature subset after applying the proposed SPSO method and the standard existing feature selection methods leading to corresponding classification accuracies by the different classifiers. Not only the classification accuracy but other statistical methods measures like Precision [33], Recall [33], F-Measure [33] and Fall_out [33] are also evaluated and tabulated in Table 15.2 to prove the efficiency of the method.

From the results, it is seen that SPSO performed very well compared to other popular feature selection methods as shown in Table 15.1 and Table 15.2. Though the CFS method [34] gives good results by selecting a lesser number of features, accuracy wise it gives poorer results than SPSO. For finding out the best feature subset, the SPSO method converges faster than rough-GA method [25]. Thus it is claimed that SPSO method is an efficient method to select the important features without losing too much information.

To make the method a standardised one, the proposed method was run on some other benchmark datasets collected from the UCI repository [37]. Table 15.3 provides the results of the experiment on the other datasets as well. It is again seen that the performance of SPSO is quite well on the other datasets in terms of feature selection and classification.

TABLE 15.1
Severity Prediction Results Obtained for the COVID-19 Dataset

Dataset (#original Features)	Methods (#features)	Classifiers (%)					
		NB	Bagging	PART	Random Forest	J48	MLP
COVID-19	Whole Data (13)	76.30	75.65	75.48	75.44	75.82	75.12
Symptoms	CFS (7)	77.90	76.10	76.07	76.21	77.28	76.14
Checker (13)	CON (6)	76.68	76.17	76.73	76.86	76.32	76.09
	Rough-GA (7)	77.70	76.94	76.08	77.76	77.25	77.34
	SPSO (8)	78.76	77.43	76.32	78.31	77.68	77.67

TABLE 15.2
Detail Statistical Results Obtained for the COVID-19 Dataset

Dataset (#Selected Feature)	Classification Methods	Precision	Recall	F-Measure	Fall_out
			Classifier Parameters		
COVID-19	NB	0.780	0.785	0.789	0.179
Symptoms	Bagging	0.776	0.771	0.771	0.210
Checker (8)	PART	0.762	0.762	0.763	0.237
	Random Forest	0.786	0.786	0.785	0.215
	J48	0.772	0.772	0.773	0.227
	MLP	0.778	0.779	0.778	0.212

TABLE 15.3
Prediction Results for Other Datasets

Dataset (#original Features)	Feature Selection Methods (#features)	NB	Bagging	PART	Random Forest	J48	MLP
				Classifier Accuracy (%)			
Breast Cancer (9)	CFS (4)	95.71	94.85	94.34	94.42	94.56	94.13
	CON (5)	95.99	94.70	94.50	94.70	93.56	94.56
	Rough-GA (5)	95.93	94.82	93.46	94.01	93.75	94.27
	SPSO (3)	95.75	94.89	95.98	95.34	93.88	95.42
	CFS (9)	98.76	98.06	98.10	98.64	98.07	98.62
Dermatology (33)	CON (9)	98.52	98.25	98.21	98.73	98.86	98.67
	Rough-GA (11)	98.72	98.45	98.50	98.48	98.76	98.46
	SPSO (8)	99.86	98.87	98.78	98.90	98.91	99.32
Mushroom (21)	CFS (4)	97.52	96.01	97.01	97.19	97.01	97.01
	CON (5)	98.52	98.85	98.67	99.01	99.05	98.16
	Rough-GA (5)	97.04	98.03	98.12	98.22	98.10	98.10
	SPSO (3)	99.87	99.85	98.82	99.60	99.01	98.36

Tables 15.3 and 15.4 describe the accuracy results and the detail statistical parameter values of the considered classifiers based on the SPSO method.

15.6 CONCLUSION AND FUTURE WORK

Development of an intelligent healthcare system is the need of the hour in this pandemic period where medical professionals and IT professionals are working together to build these kinds of expert systems to monitor the health condition of people to save them from this deadly virus. The proposed method uses meta-heuristic approach to build a solution. A rough set theory–based PSO algorithm has been devised to

TABLE 15.4

Detail Statistical Results for the Other Dataset

Dataset with Selected Number of Features Generated by the Proposed Method	Classification Methods	Classifier Parameters			
		Recall	Fall_out	Precision	F-Measure
Dermatology (8)	NB	0.99	0.01	0.98	0.98
	PART	0.99	0.01	0.98	0.99
	Bagging	0.98	0.02	0.98	0.98
	J48	0.99	0.01	0.98	0.97
	MLP	0.99	0.01	0.99	0.97
	Random Forest	0.98	0.02	0.98	0.99
Mushroom (3)	NB	0.99	0.01	0.98	0.98
	PART	0.99	0.01	0.99	0.99
	Bagging	0.99	0.01	0.98	0.98
	J48	0.97	0.03	0.97	0.97
	MLP	0.99	0.01	0.96	0.96
	Random Forest	0.99	0.01	0.99	0.99
Breast Cancer (3)	NB	0.96	0.04	0.95	0.96
	PART	0.95	0.05	0.96	0.95
	Bagging	0.95	0.05	0.96	0.95
	J48	0.94	0.06	0.94	0.94
	MLP	0.95	0.05	0.95	0.94
	Random Forest	0.95	0.05	0.95	0.94

build the system with greater prediction accuracy. The method is simple and efficient in terms of selecting features by achieving better classification accuracy. As a future work, a big data approach including Hadoop clusters and a map reduce approach will be used to solve the problem with more data in a shorter time.

15.7 REFERENCES

[1] Halgurd S. Maghdid, Kayhan Zrar Ghafoor, Ali Safaa Sadiq, Kevin Curran, Danda B. Rawat, & Khaled Rabie (2020) A Novel AI-enabled Framework to Diagnose Coronavirus COVID-19 Using Smartphone Embedded Sensors: Design Study. 2020 IEEE 21st International Conference on Information Reuse and Integration for Data Science (IRI), pp. 180–187. IEEE.

[2] Celestine Iwendi, Ali Kashif Bashir, Atharva Peshkar, R. Sujatha, Jyotir Moy Chatterjee, Swetha Pasupuleti, Rishita Mishra, Sofia Pillai, & Ohyun Jo (2020) COVID-19 Patient Health Prediction Using Boosted Random Forest Algorithm. *Frontiers in Public Health*, 8. Available at: www.frontiersin.org/articles/10.3389/fpubh.2020.00357/full.

[3] K.H. Yu, A.L. Beam, & I.S. Kohane (2018) Artificial Intelligence in Healthcare. *Nat. Biomed. Eng.*, 2(10), pp. 719–731.

[4] I.E. Agbehadji, O.A. Bankole, B. Alfred, & C.M. Richard (2020) Review of Big Data Analytics, Artificial Intelligence and Nature-Inspired Computing Models Towards Accurate Detection of COVID-19 Pandemic Cases and Contact Tracing. *Int. J. Environ. Res. Public Health*, 17(15), pp. 1–16.

[5] S. Swati, & M. Chandana (2020) Application of Cognitive Internet of Medical Things for COVID-19 Pandemic. *Diabetes Metab Syndr: Clin. Res. Rev.*, 14(5), pp. 911–915.

[6] C. Antonio, A. Ruggeri, M. Fazio, A. Galletta, M. Villari, & A. Romano (2020) Blockchain-Based Healthcare Workflow for Telemedical Laboratory in Federated Hospital IoT Clouds. *Sensors*, 20(9), pp. 2590–2600.

[7] S. Abhimanyu, P. Vineet, & M. Oge (2020) Artificial Intelligence and COVID-19: A Multidisciplinary Approach. *Integr. Med. Res.*, 9(3), pp. 111–125.

[8] Z. Abdelhafid, H. Fouzi, D. Abdelkader, & S. Ying (2020) Deep Learning Methods for Forecasting COVID-19 Time-Series Data: A Comparative Study. *Chaos Solit. Fractals*, 140, pp. 1–13.

[9] O. Gozes, M. Frid-Adar, H. Greenspan, P.D. Browning, H. Zhang, W. Ji, E. Siegel, (2020) Rapid AI Development Cycle for the Coronavirus (COVID-19) Pandemic: Initial Results for Automated Detection & Patient Monitoring Using Deep Learning CT Image Analysis. *Arvix*, pp. 1–120.

[10] Z. Pawlak (1982) Rough Sets. *Int. J. Comput. Inf. Sci.*, 1(5), pp. 341–356.

[11] Trelea, I.C. (2003). The Particle Swarm Optimization Algorithm: Convergence Analysis and Parameter Selection. *Inf. Process. Lett.*, 85, pp. 317–325.

[12] Moutaz Alazab, Albara Awajan, Abdelwadood Mesleh, Ajith Abraham, Vansh Jatana, & Salah Alhyari (2020) COVID-19 Prediction and Detection Using Deep Learning. *Int. J. Comput. Inf. Syst. Ind. Manag. Appl.*, 12(2150–7988), pp. 168–181 [Online]. Available at: www.mirlabs.net/ijcisim/index.html.

[13] Xiangao Jiang, Megan Coffee, Anasse Bari, Junzhang Wang, Xinyue Jiang, Jianping Huang, Jichan Shi, Jianyi Dai, Jing Cai, Tianxiao Zhang, Zhengxing Wu, Guiqing He, & Yitong Huang (2020) Towards an Artificial Intelligence Framework for Data Driven Prediction of Coronavirus Clinical Severity (2020). *Comput. Mater. Contin.*, 63(01), pp. 537–551.

[14] Swarn Avinash Kumar, Harsh Kumar, Vishal Dutt, & Pooja Dixit (2020) Deep Analysis of COVID-19 Pandemic using Machine Learning Techniques. *Global Journal on Innovation, Opportunities and Challenges in AAI and Machine Learning*, 4(2).

[15] Shreshth Tuli, Shikhar Tuli, Rakesh Tuli, & Sukhpal Singh Gill (2020) Predicting the Growth and Trend of COVID-19 Pandemic Using Machine Learning and Cloud Computing. *IOT*, 11, pp. 100222 [Online]. Available at: https://doi.org/10.1016/j.iot.2020.100222.

[16] Durga Prasad Kavadi, Rizwan Patan, Manikandan Ramachandran, & Amir H. Gandomi (2020) Partial Derivative Nonlinear Global Pandemic Machine Learning Prediction of COVID 19. *Chaos Solit. Fractals*, 139, pp. 110056 [Online]. Available at: https://doi.org/10.1016/j.chaos.2020.110056.

[17] Weiya Shi, Xueqing Peng, Tiefu Liu, Zenghui Cheng, Hongzhou Lu, Shuyi Yang, Jiulong Zhang, Mei Wang, Yaozong Gao, Yuxin Shi, Zhiyong Zhang, & Fei Shan (2021) A Deep Learning-Based Quantitative Computed Tomography Model for Predicting the Severity of COVID-19: A Retrospective Study of 196 Patients. *Ann Transl Med.*, 9(3), p. 216 [Online]. Available at: http://dx.doi.org/10.21037/atm-20-2464.

[18] Shuai Wang, Bo Kang, Jinlu Ma, Xianjun Zeng, Mingming Xiao, Jia Guo, Mengjiao Cai, Jingyi Yang, Yaodong Li, Xiangfei Meng, & Bo Xu (2021) A Deep Learning Algorithm Using CT Images to Screen for Corona Virus Disease (COVID-19). *Imaging Informatics And Artificial Intelligence*, pp. 1–9 [Online]. Available at: https://doi.org/10.1007/s00330-021-07715-1.

[19] T.R. Li, D. Ruan, W. Geert, J. Song, & Y. Xu (2007) A Rough Set Based Characteristicrelation Approach for Dynamic Attribute Generalization in Data Mining. *Knowl.-Based Syst.*, 20(5), pp. 485–494.

[20] J.Y. Liang, F. Wang, C.Y. Dang, & Y.H. Qian (2012) An Efficient Rough Feature Selection Algorithm with a Multi-Granulation View. *Int. J. Approx. Reason.*, 53, pp. 912–926.

[21] K. Thangavel, & A. Pethalakshmi (2009) Dimensionality Reduction Based on Rough Set Theory: A Review. *J. Appl. Soft Comput.*, 9(1), pp. 1–12.

[22] R.W. Swiniarski (2011) Rough Sets Methods in Feature Reduction and Classification. *Int. J. Appl. Math. Comput. Sci.*, 11(3), pp. 565–582.

[23] Z. Pawlak, & A. Skowron (2007) Rudiments of Rough Sets. *Inf. Sci.*, 177(1), pp. 3–27.

[24] G.Y. Wang, Z. Zheng, & Y. Zhang (2002) RIDAS-A Rough Set Based Intelligent Data Analysis System, Beiing. *Proc. 1st Int. Conf. Mach. Learn. Cyber.*, 2, pp. 646–649.

[25] A. Das, S. Sengupta, & S. Bhattacharyya (2018) A Group Incremental Feature Selection for Classification Using Rough Set Theory Based Genetic Algorithm. *Appl. Soft Comput.*, 65. Doi:10.1016/j.asoc.2018.01.040.

[26] A.A. Freitas (2002) *Data Mining and Knowledge Discovery with Evolutionary Algorithms*. Springer-Verlag.

[27] J. Kennedy, & R.C. Eberhart (1997) A Discrete Binary Version of the Particle Swarm Algorithm. *Proc. 1997 IEEE Conf. Syst. Man Cyber.*, pp. 4104–4109.

[28] F. Van den Bergh (2002) An Analysis of Particle Swarm Optimizers. PhD thesis. Department of Computer Science, University of Pretoria.

[29] Elon S. Correa, Alex A. Freitas, & Colin G. Johnson (2006) A New Discrete Particle Swarm Algorithm Applied to Attribute Selection in a Bioinformatics Data Set. *Proc. GECCO'06*, pp. 35–42.

[30] An_Overview_of_Soft_Computing. Available at: www.researchgate.net/publication/309452475.

[31] M. Dorigo, M. Birattari, C. Blum, M. Clerc, T. Stützle, & A. Winfield (2008) *Ant Colony Optimization and Swarm Intelligence*. Springer.

[32] www.kaggle.com/iamhungundji/covid19-symptoms-checker.

[33] E. Alpaydin (2010) *Introduction to Machine Learning*, 2nd edition, PHI.

[34] M.A. Hall (1998) Correlation-Based Feature Selection for Machine Learning. PhD thesis. Department of Computer Science, University of Waikato, Hamilton, New Zealand.

[35] M. Dash, H. Liu, & H. Motoda (2000) Consistency Based Feature Selection. Proceedings of Fourth Pacific-Asia Conference on Knowledge Discovery and Data Mining (PAKDD), pp. 98–109.

[36] WEKA. Machine Learning Software. Available at: www.cs.waikato.ac.nz/%E2%88%BCml/.

[37] P. Murphy, W. Aha (1996) UCI Repository of Machine Learning Databases. Available at: www.ics.uci.edu/mlearn/MLRepository.html.

16 Transitions in Machine Learning Approaches for Healthcare-Sector Applications

Juli Kumari[1], Deepak Kumar[2] and Ela Kumar[1]
[1] Indira Gandhi Delhi Technical University for Women, India
[2] Amity Institute of Geoinformatics & Remote Sensing, India

CONTENTS

16.1 INTRODUCTION

From the evolution of human life, good health is more precious than anything. Various researchers have been interested in developing new ideas, processes, classifications and architecture for advancements in healthcare. Healthcare is an advancement in human health conditions through proper handling, management and analysis of physical impairment, mental illness, injury and disease [1]. In the present scenario, healthcare is facing three major challenges at the global level such as shortage of medical professionals, inappropriate management and high medical cost. According to the annual report of the World Health Organization (WHO), global necessity and the actual amount of health personnel were 60.4 million and 43 million, respectively, in 2013 [2]. These figures will increase to 81.8 million and 67.3 million, respectively, by 2030. Therefore, the scarcity of healthcare workers is a more serious and unsolved issue. So, computer-aided diagnosis and treatment is a huge emerging field of research in medical science. Researchers are continuously trying to improve the accuracy of perception and diagnosis of disease [3] using more potential machine learning techniques. Deep learning is a sub-field of machine learning and it uses multiple-step learning techniques. It is widely applied on a larger dataset and filtered

DOI: 10.1201/9781003217107-16

through several multiple layers. Due to multiple layer filtering approaches, it produces more and more accurate outcomes than traditional machine learning, while handling the larger dataset with structure.

Among these areas, healthcare is the largest growing field, which has attracted more researchers, academicians and health professionals to contribute to the improvement of the healthcare facility. Healthcare facilities comprise services like hospitals, medical tools and clinical trials, telemedicine, medical tourism, health insurance, medical equipment, etc. It provides an enormous opportunity to improve health facilities by adopting more advanced technology. Hence, the advent of more advanced technology facilitates large-scale data and provides a massive transformation in healthcare, in the context of providing easy access to the best diagnostic tools, latest cutting-edge treatments and a variety of simple invasive procedures resulting in less pain and faster healing. Healthcare also plays a most important role in different prospects like drug discovery, personalised medicine, robotic surgery, disease monitoring, etc.

This technique has a vast capacity to build a system for diagnosis, treatment and improved accuracy of the clinical test [4]. A machine learning technique is usually used to build a system model, providing earlier data prediction, removing an anomalies in data, classification of data, etc. In healthcare, this technique is mainly used for disease diagnosis, disease prediction and automatic surgery and produces more accurate results of the clinical test. Various machine learning techniques i.e. supervised, unsupervised, semi-supervised, reinforcement and deep learning algorithms methods are more popular for this purpose [5–6].

The purpose of this chapter is to study the implementation of the machine learning technique in different diseases and the accuracy of this technique. Here we also focus on exploring its future aspect.

1. **Supervised learning** uses any previous experience to produce the outcomes. There are two types of datasets used: trained and test sets. The test set is a dataset that is used to predict, and the training dataset is a resultant variable that needs to predict. All algorithms follow a set of rules from training datasets and apply them to the test datasets for prediction and classification [7].

2. **Unsupervised learning** is another type of technique, which is used to classify the datasets. These algorithms classify datasets based on similarity among input data. It is referred as density estimation [8] and is mainly used to make clusters and classification of data.

3. **Semi-supervised learning** is a sub-class of supervised learning techniques. The method is used to produce results among larger numbers of unlabelled datasets with smaller numbers of labelled datasets [9]. It is a combination of unsupervised learning (unlabelled data) and supervised learning (labelled data) methods.

4. **Reinforcement learning** is supported by behavioural psychology. This system is trained to do a particular job and learns by itself on its prior knowledge while doing a similar kind of job [10].

5. **Evolutionary learning** is used to study biological evolution. The method deals with the adaptation process of a biological organism with its survival

rate and the evolution of its offspring [11]. It uses the concept of fitness to ensure the correctness of the solution. It can also use the model in the computer system.

6. **Deep learning** uses the combined result of all back-propagation classical parameters to optimise the output of the task [12]. It is based on deep graph generation through different process layers and made up many linear and non-linear transformations.

16.2 LITERATURE SURVEY

The supervised learning-based model is applied to data for classification, regression and prediction of the labelled dataset. An unsupervised learning-based model is used on unlabelled datasets for clustering, dimensionality reduction of a dataset, detection, etc. Also, the machine learning approaches are applied in several fields and is responsible for revolutionising changes in the healthcare sector. It is mostly used for early-stage disease prediction, detection and monitoring the patient condition based on clinical datasets. Machine learning techniques are also applied to medical image–related datasets for automatic object feature detection. Among the different machine learning models, the deep neural network–based technique has attracted more attention for handling the image datasets and larger datasets. Machine learning approaches are extensively applied to handle healthcare problems. Here, we have tabulated the various machine learning approaches, which are applied to several disease predictions and diagnoses with their accuracy (Table 16.1).

16.3 META-ANALYSIS

The literature of survey reports that the machine learning technique is widely used to solve the data complexity problem. It has several techniques to classify analyse and predict the data. Due to this potential, the machine learning technique has played a significant role in the healthcare sector. Currently, machine learning approaches are used in disease prediction, disease diagnosis, medical discovery, biomedical data analysis and robotic surgery. It has solved several problems in medical science and is widely implemented for early disease prediction. This technique has increased the human life rate, saved the doctors time and increased the accuracy of clinical data results.

Previously, there was a huge challenge for medical personnel to manage, handle and analyse the larger amount of patient data for precise handling and earlier predictions of medical data, since there were no tools and technologies available. So, it was a huge waste of time and money. In the same era, healthcare professionals used risk calculators to find the disease possibility. This calculator was based on the basic patient information like life routines, physical condition, demographics, etc., for calculating the possibility of developing a certain disease. This calculation used the mathematical equation-based method.

The development of new tools and techniques such as machine learning techniques has made it quite easy to handle wide-scale data and also helpful for data

TABLE 16.1
Summary of Various Machine Learning Algorithms and Their Accuracy

Sl. No.	Machine Learning Methods	Author(s)	Year	Type of Disease	Accuracy
1.	Joint Localisation, Active Shape Models	Yinghe Huo [13]	2017	Rheumatoid Arthritis	96%
2.	Manual, Colour and K-Means Image Segmentation	A. B. Suma [14]	2016	Rheumatoid Arthritis	93%
3.	Joint Localisation, Contour Delineation, ASM-Driven Snakes	Georg Langs [15]	2009	Rheumatoid Arthritis	92%
4.	ANN, PCA	Smita Jhajharia [16]	2016	Cancer	96%
5.	FROC, ANN	Juan Wang [17]	2017	Lung Disease	96.24%
6.	Feedforward and Back-propagation Neural Network	Shubhangi Khobragade [18]	2017	Lung Disease	86%
7.	Naïve Bayes J48	Iyer [19]	2015	Diabetes Disease	79.56%, 76.95%
8.	CART, Adaboost, Logiboost, Grading	Sen and Dash [20]	2014	Diabetes Disease	78.64%, 77.86%, 77.47%, 66.40%
9.	Hough, Supervised Learning	R. Catherine Silvia [21]	2013	Diabetes Disease	74%
10.	C4.5, ID3, CART	Sathyadevi [22]	2011	Hepatitis Disease	71.4%, 64.8% 83.2%
11.	Statistical Parametric Mapping, Stochastic Searches	Ruben Armananzas [23]	2017	Alzheimer Disease	97.14%
12.	Discriminative Sparse Learning, Relational Regularisation	Baiying Lei [24]	2017	Alzheimer Disease	94.68%
13.	Sparse Representation techniques	Tong Tong [25]	2016	Alzheimer Disease	92%
14.	DWT,SVM	Priyanka Thakare [26]	2016	Alzheimer Disease	94%
15.	Nonlinear Registration, Shape-Constrained Regression-Forest Algorithm	Jun Zhang [27]	2016	Alzheimer Disease	83.7%
16.	SVM Naive Bayes	Vijayarani and Dhayanand [28]	2015	Liver Disease	79.66%, 61.28%

17.	Random Forest, SVM, Bayesian Network, Naive Bayes	Gulia et al [29]	2014	Liver Disease	71.86%, 71.35%, 69.12%, 96.52%
18.	K Star, FT Tree	Rajeswari and Reena [30]	2010	Liver Disease	96.52%, 83.47%, 97.10%
19.	Decision Tree, ANN, RS	Tarmizi et al.[31]	2013	Dengue Disease	99.95%, 99.98% 100%
20.	SVM	Fathima and Manimeglai [32]	2012	Dengue Disease	90.42%
21.	MFNNN	Ibrahim [33]	2005	Dengue Disease	90%
22.	Boosted Logistic Regression	Kamal Nayan Reddy Challa [34]	2016	Parkinson Disease	97.15%
23.	Gaussian Radial Basis Function Kernel-Based SVM	Sachin Shetty Y. S. Rao [35]	2016	Parkinson Disease	83.33%

statistics, real-time data analysis and more accurate data analytics for disease data, clinical test results, blood pressure, family details and lab trial data, etc., to healthcare professionals. In the medicine industry, it has increased the rates of drug discovery, reduced the time in drug discovery and reduced the cost of medicine and drug failure in the clinical trial due to better predictive methods. Earlier, a pharmaceutical company faced various problems during drug development due to a lack of technologies for the prediction of the potential drug molecule and also for prediction of its effect on target and non-target subjects. Thus, drugs are more likely to fail in a clinical trial. This scenario makes drug discovery a very costly and time-consuming process.

Various studies have been performed on several diseases such as hepatitis, lung diseases, rheumatoid arthritis, cancer, diabetic retinopathy, heart diseases, dengue disease, Alzheimer's disease, liver disease and Parkinson disease using machine learning techniques for diagnosis and prediction [36–39]. This technique has many different methods for the analysis of clinical data and bio-medical image data.

16.4 CONCLUSION

In healthcare, control of disease is the main serious issue along with improvements in treatment. Several air-borne diseases are spreading very rapidly, so this requires more advanced technology which quickly controls such types of problems. It is most important to use more accurate tools for disease diagnosis and analysis of disease and also more reliable treatment. In this respect, it is also necessary to recognise the actual treatment through clinical analysis and evaluation. The effective disease diagnosis along with reliable cost management requires an automated assistant system based on computer-based systems, as the healthcare sector creates a larger amount of data during the clinical test, report handling of patients, regular monitoring of the patient condition, patients cure, medication and regular follow-up, etc. It is a complex task to handle all these issues manually. Quality of treatment affects the inappropriate management of data. Machine learning techniques have played a vital role in this by self-trained or decision methods and classifying diseases based on different characteristics. It processes data more quickly and accurately than other techniques. Therefore, it is very popular in the diagnosis of several diseases, i.e. cancer, lung cancer, brain tumour, arthritis detection, dengue, heart disease, diabetes and liver etc.

16.4.1 FUTURE SCOPE

Machine learning is a sub-area of artificial intelligence, and the current scenario requires more efforts towards its advancement in the healthcare sector. It is used in the area of disease diagnosis/identification, disease prediction, drug discovery and biomedical image analysis. Different machine learning techniques haves been used for the improvement of the treatment and diagnosis accuracy. This study will help in the development of biomedical image analysis, disease diagnosis and prediction model with more accuracy from previously used tabulated technique (see Table 16.1) for this purpose, and a Python programming language will be used. The Python programming language has various supporting libraries for data analysis and graph plotting and also has different machine learning technique, i.e. support vector machine, decision tree, naïve Bayes, neural network and random forest algorithms for building models. This work will serve in biomedical image analysis, generation of the clinical test result sand early prediction of diseases accurately. It will contribute to improve healthcare treatment techniques and control human health problems.

16.5 REFERENCES

[1] K.T. Chui, W. Alhalabi, S.S.H. Pang, P.O. de Pablos, R.W. Liu, and M. Zhao, 2017, "Disease diagnosis in smart healthcare: Innovation, technologies and applications," *Sustain*, Volume: 9, Issue: 12, pp. 1–23.

[2] R. Scheffler et al., 2016, "Health workforce requirements for universal health coverage and the sustainable development goals", *Hum. Resour. Heal. Obs. Ser.*, Issue: 17, pp. 1–40.

[3] A.J. Dinu, R. Ganesan, F. Joseph, and V. Balaji, 2017, "A study on deep machine learning algorithms for diagnosis of diseases", *International Journal of Applied Engineering Research*, Volume: 12, Issue: 17, pp. 6338–6346.

[4] D. Yu, and L. Deng, 2011, "Deep learning and its applications to signal and Information Processing", *IEEE Signal Processing Magazine*, Volume: 28, Issue: 1, pp. 145–154.

[5] J. Shi, and J. Malik, 2000, "Normalized cuts and image segmentation", *IEEE Transactions on Pattern Analysis and Machine Intelligence*, Volume: 22, Issue: 8, pp. 888–905.

[6] A. Kumar, J. Kim, W. Cai, and D. Feng, 2013, "Content-based medical image retrieval: a Survey of applications to multidimensional and multimodality data", *The Journal of Digital Imaging*, Volume: 26, Issue: 6, pp. 1025–1039.

[7] S.B. Kotsiantis, 2007, "Supervised machine learning: A review of classification techniques", *Informatica*, Volume: 31, pp. 249–268.

[8] S. Geman, E. Bienenstock, and R. Doursat, 2008, "Neural networks and the bias/variance dilemma", *Neural Network*, Volume: 4, pp. 1–58.

[9] D.F. Nettleton, A. Orriols-Puig, A. Fornells, 2010, "A study of the effect of different types of noise on the precision of supervised learning techniques", *Artificial Intelligence Review*, Volume: 33, pp. 275–306.

[10] Z. Akata, F. Perronnin, Z. Harchaoui, C. Schmid, 2014, "Good practice in large-scale learning for image classification", *IEEE Transactions on Pattern Analysis and Machine Intelligence*, Volume: 36, pp. 507–520.

[11] D.D. Lewis, and J. Catlett, 1994, "Heterogeneous uncertainty sampling for supervised learning", Proceedings of the Eleventh International Conference on Machine Learning, New Brunswick, NJ, USA, 10–13 July 1994; Morgan Kaufmann Publishers: San Francisco, CA, USA.

[12] A. Under, A. Murat, R.B. Chinnam, 2011, "MR 2 PSO: A maximum relevance minimum redundancy feature selection method based on swarm intelligence for support vector machine classification", *Information Sciences*, Volume: 181, pp. 4625–4641.

[13] Yinghe Huo, Koen L. Vincken, Floris P. Lafeber, and Max A. Viergever, 2016, "Automatic quantification of radiographic finger joint space width of patients with early rheumatoid arthritis", *IEEE Journals & Magazines*, Volume: 63, Issue: 10, pp. 2177–2186.

[14] A.B. Suma, U. Snekhalatha, and T. Rajalakshmi, 2016, "Automated thermal image segmentation of knee rheumatoid arthritis", IEEE International Conference on Communication and Signal Processing (ICCSP).

[15] Georg Langs, Philipp Peloschek, Horst Bischof, and Franz Kainberger, 2009, "Automatic quantification of joint space narrowing and erosions in rheumatoid arthritis", *IEEE Transactions on Medical Imaging*, Volume: 28, Issue: 1.

[16] Smita Jhajharia, Harish Kumar Varshney, Seema Verma, and Rajesh Kumar, 2016, "A neural network based breast cancer prognosis model with PCA processed features", IEEE, International Conference on Advances in Computing, Communications and Informatics (ICACCI).

[17] J. Wang, H. Ding, F.A. Bidgoli, B. Zhou, C. Iribarren, S. Molloi, and P. Baldi, 2017, "Detecting cardiovascular disease from mammograms with deep learning", *IEEE Transactions on Medical Imaging*, Volume: 36, Issue: 5, pp. 1172–1181.

[18] Shubhangi Khobragade, Aditya Tiwari, C.Y. Patil, and Vikram Narke, 2017, "Automatic detection of major lung diseases using Chest Radiographs and classification by feed-forward artificial neural network", IEEE, International Conference on Power Electronics, Intelligent Control and Energy Systems (ICPEICES).

[19] A. Iyer, S. Jayalalitha, and R. Sumbaly, 2015, "Diagnosis of diabetes using classification mining techniques", *International Journal of Data Mining & Knowledge Management Process (IJDKP)*, Volume: 5, pp. 1–14.

[20] S.K. Sen, and S. Dash, 2014, "Application of meta-learning algorithms for the prediction of diabetes disease", *International Journal of Advanced Research in Computer Science and Management Studies*, Volume: 2, pp. 396–401.

[21] R. Catherine Silvia, and R. Vijayalakshmi, 2013, "Detection of non-proliferative diabetic retinopathy in fundus images of the human retina", International Conference on Information Communication and Embedded Systems (ICICES).

[22] G. Sathyadevi, 2011, "Application of CART algorithm in hepatitis disease diagnosis", IEEE International Conference on Recent Trends in Information Technology (ICRTIT), MIT, Anna University, Chennai, 3–5 June 2011, 1283–1287.

[23] Rubén Armañanzas, Martina Iglesias, Dinora A. Morales, and Lidia Alonso-Nanclares, 2017, "Voxel-based diagnosis of Alzheimer's disease using classifier ensembles", *IEEE Journal of Biomedical and Health Informatics*, Volume: 21, Issue: 3, pp. 778–784.

[24] Baiying Lei, Peng Yang, Tianfu Wang, Siping Chen, and Dong Ni, 2017, "Relational-regularized discriminative sparse learning for Alzheimer's disease diagnosis", *IEEE Transactions on Cybernetics*, Volume: 47, Issue: 4, pp. 1102–1113.

[25] Tong Tong, Qinquan Gao, Ricardo Guerrero, Christian Ledig, Liang Chen, and Daniel Rueckert, 2017, "A novel grading biomarker for the prediction of conversion from mild cognitive impairment to Alzheimer's disease", *IEEE Transactions on Biomedical Engineering*, Volume: 64, Issue: 1, pp. 155–165.

[26] P. Thakare, and V. R. Pawar, 2016, "Alzheimer disease detection and tracking of Alzheimer patient", *2016 International Conference on Inventive Computation Technologies (ICICT), IEEE*, Volume: 1, pp. 1–4.

[27] Jun Zhang, Yue Gao, Yaozong Gao, Brent C. Munsell, and Dinggang Shen, 2016, "Detecting anatomical landmarks for fast Alzheimer's disease diagnosis", *IEEE Transactions on Medical Imaging*, Volume: 35, Issue: 12, pp. 2524–2533.

[28] S. Vijayarani, and S. Dhayanand, 2015, "Liver disease prediction using SVM and naïve bayes algorithms", *International Journal of Science Engineering and Technology Research (IJSETR)*, Volume: 4, pp. 816–820.

[29] A. Gulia, R. Vohra, and P. Rani, 2014, "Liver patient classification using intelligent techniques", *(IJCSIT) International Journal of Computer Science and Information Technologies*, Volume: 5, pp. 5110–5115.

[30] P. Rajeswari, and G.S. Reena, 2010, "Analysis of liver disorder using data mining algorithm", *Global Journal of Computer Science and Technology*, Volume: 10, pp. 48–52.

[31] N.D.A. Tarmizi, F. Jamaluddin, A. Abu Bakar, Z.A. Othman, S. Zainudin, and A.R. Hamdan, 2013, "Malaysia dengue outbreak detection using data mining models", *Journal of Next Generation Information Technology (JNIT)*, Volume: 4, pp. 96–107.

[32] A.S. Fathima, and D. Manimeglai, 2012, "Predictive analysis for the arbovirus- dengue using SVM classification", *International Journal of Engineering and Technology*, Volume: 2, pp. 521–527.

[33] F. Ibrahim, M.N. Taib, W.A.B.W. Abas, C.C. Guan, and S. Sulaiman, 2005, "A novel dengue fever (DF) and dengue haemorrhagic fever (DHF) analysis using artificial neural network (ANN)", *Computer Methods and Programs in Biomedicine*, Volume: 79, pp. 273–281.

[34] Kamal Nayan Reddy Challa, Venkata Sasank Pagolu, Ganapati Panda, and Babita Majhi, 2016, "An improved approach for prediction of Parkinson's disease using machine learning techniques", Signal Processing, Communication, Power and Embedded System (SCOPES), 2016 International Conference, IEEE.

[35] S. Shetty, and Y. S. Rao, 2016, "SVM based machine learning approach to identify Parkinson's disease using gait analysis", *Inventive Computation Technologies (ICICT), International Conference*, pp. 1–5.

[36] Meherwar Fatima1, and Maruf Pasha2, 2017, "Survey of machine learning algorithms for disease diagnostic", *Journal of Intelligent Learning Systems and Applications*, Volume: 9, pp. 1–16.

[37] L. Zheng, and A.K. Chan, 2001, "An artificial intelligent algorithm for tumour detection in screening mammogram", *IEEE Transactions on Medical Imaging*, Volume: 20, Issue: 7, pp. 559–567.

[38] F.M. Ba-Alwi and H.M. Hintaya, 2013, "Comparative study for analysis the prognostic in hepatitis data: Data mining approach", *International Journal of Scientific & Engineering Research*, Volume: 4, pp. 680–685.

[39] Indrajit Mandal, and N. Sairam, 2012, "New machine-learning algorithms for prediction of Parkinson's disease", *International Journal of Systems Science*, pp. 1–20.

Index

For Product Safety Concerns and Information please contact our EU
representative GPSR@taylorandfrancis.com
Taylor & Francis Verlag GmbH, Kaufingerstraße 24, 80331 München, Germany

* 9 7 8 1 0 3 2 1 0 8 0 1 8 *